T0296689

Men's Health

Jeannette M. Potts

Editor

Men's Health

A Head to Toe Guide for Clinicians

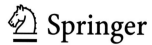 Springer

Editor
Jeannette M. Potts
Vista Urology & Pelvic Pain Partners
San Jose, CA, USA

ISBN 978-1-4939-3236-8   ISBN 978-1-4939-3237-5   (eBook)
DOI 10.1007/978-1-4939-3237-5

Library of Congress Control Number: 2015957062

Springer New York Heidelberg Dordrecht London

© Springer Science+Business Media New York 2016
This work is subject to copyright. All rights are reserved by the Publisher, whether the whole or part of the material is concerned, specifically the rights of translation, reprinting, reuse of illustrations, recitation, broadcasting, reproduction on microfilms or in any other physical way, and transmission or information storage and retrieval, electronic adaptation, computer software, or by similar or dissimilar methodology now known or hereafter developed.
The use of general descriptive names, registered names, trademarks, service marks, etc. in this publication does not imply, even in the absence of a specific statement, that such names are exempt from the relevant protective laws and regulations and therefore free for general use.
The publisher, the authors and the editors are safe to assume that the advice and information in this book are believed to be true and accurate at the date of publication. Neither the publisher nor the authors or the editors give a warranty, express or implied, with respect to the material contained herein or for any errors or omissions that may have been made.

Printed on acid-free paper

Springer Science+Business Media LLC New York is part of Springer Science+Business Media (www.springer.com)

To my patients.

Contents

Contributors

Loutfi S. Aboussouan Cleveland Clinic, Respiratory Institute, Cleveland, OH, USA

Dan E. Azagury Department of Surgery, Stanford University School of Medicine, Stanford, CA, USA

Michael L. Eisenberg Department of Urology, Stanford University School of Medicine, Stanford, CA, USA

Kathleen Fagan Department of Environmental Health Sciences, Case Western Reserve University, School of Medicine, Cleveland, OH, USA

Irving Franco Heart and Vascular Institute, Cleveland Clinic, Cleveland, OH, USA

Harcharan Gill Department of Urology, Stanford University Hospital, Stanford, CA, USA

David P. Guo Department of Urology, Stanford University School of Medicine, Stanford, CA, USA

Lyen C. Huang Department of Surgery, Stanford University School of Medicine, Stanford, CA, USA

Shilpi Khetarpal Department of Dermatology, Cleveland Clinic Foundation, Cleveland, OH, USA

Cindy Kin Department of Surgery, Stanford University School for Medicine, Stanford, CA, USA

Rony Lahoud Department of Cardiology, Cleveland Clinic Foundation, Cleveland, OH, USA

Christopher K. Payne Emeritus Professor of Urology, Stanford University, Stanford, CA, USA

Vista Urology & Pelvic Pain Partners, San Jose, CA, USA

Jeannette M. Potts Vista Urology & Pelvic Pain Partners, San Jose, CA, USA

Gary K. Roberts Oral Medicine and Maxillofacial Surgery, Department of Surgery, Stanford University Medical Center and Lucille Packard Children's Hospital, Palo Alto, CA, USA

Rosemary Sokas Department of Human Science, Georgetown University School of Nursing and Health Studies, Washington, DC, USA

Kenneth J. Tomecki Department of Dermatology, Cleveland Clinic Foundation, Dermatology and Plastic Surgery Institute, Cleveland, OH, USA

Dean A. Tripp Department of Psychology, Anesthesiology & Urology, Queen's University, Kingston, ON, Canada

Alok Vij Department of Dermatology, Cleveland Clinic Foundation, Dermatology and Plastic Surgery Institute, Cleveland, OH, USA

Sarah C. Vij Department of Urology, Cleveland Clinic, Cleveland, OH, USA

Hayley Yurgan Department of Psychology, Queen's University, Kingston, ON, Canada

His Occupation: Safety and Fulfillment

Kathleen Fagan and Rosemary Sokas

Work and health are inextricably linked. While toxic exposures, ranging from coal dust to unfair supervisors, shorten life and degrade its quality, work itself is essential for human flourishing. The International Labour Organization uses the term "decent work" for paid employment that provides a living wage, additional benefits (such as retirement, health insurance, family leave, etc.), safe working conditions, and the opportunity for development and respect [1]. Work plays a central but complicated role in the life of every adult. On the one hand, we shape our world, participating in the act of creation through growing food, framing houses, cleaning offices, repairing engines, exploring energy sources, treating cancer, selling insurance, plowing streets, teaching algebra, or any of the thousands of activities that combine to shape modern society. Especially for men, work may take on an outsized portion of their identity, although both men and women experience negative health outcomes from lack of work as well as from overwork.

1.1 Absence of Work

The big picture, of course, is that the absence of work can kill. Perhaps the most compelling evidence for the deadly impact of work loss comes from information gathered in the wake of the collapse of the former Soviet Union, when mortality rates for middle-aged men in Russia and the newly independent states of Eastern Europe skyrocketed and life expectancy precipitously declined [2]. Sweden, a

K. Fagan, M.D., M.P.H. (✉)
Department of Environmental Health Sciences, Case Western Reserve University School of Medicine, 10900 Euclid Avenue, Cleveland, OH 44106, USA
e-mail: occmeddoc@sbcglobal.net

R. Sokas, M.D., M.O.H.
Department of Human Science, Georgetown University School of Nursing and Health Studies, St. Mary's Hall Room 258, 3700 Reservoir Rd, NW, Washington, DC 20057, USA
e-mail: sokas@georgetown.edu

© Springer Science+Business Media New York 2016
J.M. Potts (ed.), *Men's Health*, DOI 10.1007/978-1-4939-3237-5_1

country with an exceptionally strong safety net and linked health records, experienced a prolonged recession in the early 1990s that provided a virtual laboratory to explore the adverse effects of unemployment, including long-term unemployment [3, 4]. Male mortality associated with unemployment (compared to those never unemployed and adjusted for prior health status) peaked after 5 years of unemployment with a hazard ratio (HR) of 1.6. While female mortality also increased significantly among the unemployed, it peaked at an all-cause HR of 1.13. Among men, increased deaths from alcohol-related causes peaked at an HR of 2.87 after approximately 3 years of continuous unemployment, accompanied by a peak stroke HR of 1.55 and cancer HR of 1.18. Mortality from suicide, transportation, and other external causes in this Swedish cohort continued to increase and drove the overall increase seen after 5 years of continuous unemployment. A meta-analysis of suicide following unemployment found a relative risk of 2.50 (CI 1.83–3.17) within 5 years and 1.70 (CI 1.22–2.18) after 5 years and remained significantly elevated among those unemployed for up to 16 years of follow-up [5].

In the United States, periods of unemployment predict nonfatal myocardial infarctions. Using data collected by the National Institute on Aging's Health and Retirement Study, Dupre et al. reviewed prospective cohorts who were interviewed every 2 years from 1992 to 2010. Among 13,451 participants who reported ever having worked, 1061 reported having experienced acute myocardial infarctions during follow-up surveys. The risk was significantly higher among those who had been previously unemployed at any time (HR 1.35, CI 1.10–1.6). Not only was any period of unemployment a risk factor but also myocardial infarction risk increased with multiple job loss. Risk was highest during the first year of unemployment [6].

1.2   Workplace Fatalities

Work itself can kill. In 2012, fatal traumatic injuries occurring at work claimed the lives of 4628 people in the United States; 92 % of those killed were men [7]. Mortality rates for miners, agricultural workers, transportation workers, and construction workers are higher than for other occupations, and most of these workers are men. As the tragic case described in Box 1.1 illustrates, small business owners and the self-employed are at higher risk than the workforce as a whole. Extremely high mortality rates among those who log, fish, build structural steel or residential buildings, or fly airplanes in the bush for a living mostly affect men. Transportation incidents claim the most lives, followed by falls to a lower level, assaults (intentional or by livestock), contact with objects and equipment, exposure to hazardous environments, and fires and explosions.

Boring work can kill in the long run. Amick et al. demonstrated that working in low-control jobs for a working lifetime was associated with increased mortality (odds ratio 1.43, CI 1.13–1.81) [8], while others have found that workers in passive jobs (low control and low demands) are less likely to engage in leisure time physical activity [9]. The Whitehall II studies, providing longitudinal data about a cohort of British civil servants, has explored a number of work characteristics for their impact

Box Case 1.1

It was a family business. The 40-year-old business owner had been painting and performing maintenance on towers, such as radio and cell towers, for over 20 years. The new job involved painting a 1500-ft radio tower, replacing the beacon light on top of the tower, and installing rest platforms at various locations on the tower. On the day of the incident, the business owner was riding the hoist rope to the top of the tower to replace the beacon light. His 16-year-old stepson and a 19-year-old employee were riding the same hoist rope 1200 ft up the tower to continue painting. The owner's wife was operating the hoist rope system, when the rope began to slip. She was unable to gain control of the rope, and her husband, son, and the young employee fell to their death. She was later transported to the hospital for treatment of shock and severe rope burns on her hands.

The National Institute for Occupational Safety and Health (NIOSH) conducted an investigation of the incident but was unable to determine exactly why the hoist system failed. They did find that the hoist rope system was not rated for lifting people. Additionally, the total weight being lifted that day was likely over the amount for which the system was rated. Multiple safe work practice recommendations were made, and it was noted that child labor laws were violated. The Fair Labor Standards Act prohibits workers under the age of 18 from performing hazardous work, such as those leading to the tragic deaths of these three men.

To read the complete report, follow this link: http://www.cdc.gov/niosh/face/In-house/full200007.html#recommendations (NIOSH FACE Report 2000-07).

on cardiac and other outcomes. Controlling for other risk factors, workers followed for an average of 11 years who routinely work 3–4 h overtime daily were 67 % more likely to die from a fatal MI or CHD (HR 1.67, CI 1.02–2.76) [10]. In a series of studies, workers who self-reported more unfair supervisory treatment at baseline were also more likely to sustain fatal cardiovascular events at follow-up, had a greater risk of developing metabolic syndrome, had increased inflammatory markers, and had poorer cognitive function [11–13].

1.3 Injuries in the Workplace

Injuries result from safety hazards, all of which can be identified and reduced. The Bureau of Labor Statistics [14] reports that, in 2013, US workers suffered over three million nonfatal work-related injuries and illnesses. The cost and scope of nonfatal work-related illness and injury are difficult to ascertain because diseases often go unrecognized as work related and injuries may go unreported if the individual has other forms of insurance and wants to avoid stigmatization [15]. Some of the highest rates, particularly for the more serious injuries, are in male-dominated industries, such as construction and agriculture, and occupations, such as laborers, truck drivers, and warehouse workers.

The industrial revolution and assembly-line work, and later the computer and cubicle workplace transformation, gave rise to an ongoing epidemic of injuries variously known as "cumulative trauma disorders," "repetitive motion injuries," or more recently "musculoskeletal disorders" (MSDs). MSDs, such as sprains and strains, tendinitis, and carpal tunnel syndrome, are more commonly associated with upper extremity injuries; however, lower extremity and back injuries may also fall into this category. In 2013, MSDs accounted for 33 % of all occupational injuries [16]. Again, male-dominated jobs, such as truck driving, construction, farming, movement of materials, and warehousing, have some of the highest MSD rates. Early studies of computer users and, subsequently, numerous studies in a wide variety of industries have strongly linked the following physical job exposures to MSDs: repetition, high force, awkward postures, vibration, cold temperatures, and tool use [17]. A combination of these factors can increase the risk of developing MSDs severalfold. Early recognition of MSD symptoms by workers and early diagnosis and treatment by clinicians can significantly improve outcomes, both in terms of severity and resolution. Prevention of work-related MSDs is accomplished through ergonomics, which is the science of fitting the workplace to the worker, through the design of tasks, processes, tools, and equipment to control and eliminate the above-mentioned physical exposures [18, 19].

1.4   Work Exposures and Disease

Illnesses result from a variety of health hazards, which may be chemical, biologic, physical, biomechanical, or psychosocial. Toxic exposures may cause systemic illness or may target specific end organs or both. Some illnesses are associated with specific job tasks. For example, metal-fume fever, a flu-like illness associated with welding on galvanized steel, is recognized as an occupational disease based on the exposure history. A discussion regarding the exposure history is found later in this chapter.

The two most common routes of exposure in the workplace are the skin and the lungs, although ingestion may occur through handling of contaminated food, nail biting, smoking at work, and other activities that result in gut absorption. The route of absorption is often the target organ, e.g., nickel exposure and contact dermatitis, chlorine gas and reactive airway disease. But this is not always the case. Inhaled lead fumes may affect the kidneys and nervous and GI systems; dermal absorption of organophosphate pesticides may lead to systemic symptoms. Pneumoconioses or dust diseases of the lung, such as asbestosis, silicosis, and coal workers' pneumoconiosis (black lung), are familiar to most clinicians and not difficult to diagnose when the history of exposure has been elicited and characteristic chest X-ray findings are seen. However, because the history is not always obtained, cases can be misdiagnosed as idiopathic pulmonary fibrosis or other entities. Thus, underreporting of occupational diseases is surprisingly common. Occupational asthma, the most common occupational respiratory disease, is often not recognized either by clinicians or by the worker experiencing the symptoms, again because the appropriate exposure history is often not asked.

Asthma in the United States has been on the rise for over three decades [20], and exposures at work are estimated to cause 15–17 % of adult-onset asthma [21, 22]. An even larger percentage of workers with underlying asthma will have exacerbations of their asthma at work [23]. Lack of recognition and management of work-related asthma can lead to worsening symptoms, increased use of medications, more emergency department visits and hospitalizations, and fatal asthma attacks. The Centers for Disease Control and Prevention (CDC) estimates asthma healthcare costs at $56 billion a year. Almost 1/3 of adults with asthma miss work because of asthma attacks [20]. Preventing and managing work-related asthma depends on workplace controls to minimize or eliminate exposure, worker training on exposure health effects and symptoms, medical surveillance and early diagnosis, and removal from further exposure [24, 25]. Clinicians, employers, and workers all play a part in prevention.

Physical hazards include noise, heat, cold, hypo- or hyperbaric atmospheres, and ionizing and nonionizing radiation. Noise-induced hearing loss is a clear example of a prevalent and potentially disabling work-related condition that should be preventable [26]. Clinicians can identify noise exposure on and off the job as a hazard, offer advice on noise reduction, and request to review any workplace audiometry testing (or provide it for self-employed individuals). Heat stress and heatstroke impact young, healthy populations of workers, athletes, and others, in addition to frail elderly. Clinicians can help educate workers and identify predisposing conditions that require additional acclimatization or accommodation. The case described in Box 1.2 offers a clear example of a missed opportunity for identifying an at-risk individual whose need for appropriate worksite interventions would have been life sustaining.

> **Box Case 1.2**
> A 43-year-old previously unemployed cement worker began his first day at a new job with a cement contractor in midsummer of 2010. He worked for 5 hours installing forms for poured concrete walls. He took a lunch break in an air-conditioned truck and then returned to work. Shortly thereafter, he complained of light-headedness and fell backward, striking his head on the concrete. He initially refused medical treatment and was given some water and then moved to an air-conditioned trailer. He asked to be driven home; however, en route he lost consciousness and was taken to the local emergency department (ED). On arrival, he was in cardiopulmonary arrest with a core body temperature of 108 °F. He was resuscitated twice in the ED before his transfer to the intensive care unit. He died the next day of multi-organ system failure due to heat stroke.

(continued)

Box Case 1.2 (continued)
The deceased worker was obese with a BMI of 39.9. Cirrhosis of the liver was found on autopsy, but he had no other underlying medical conditions and toxicology was negative for alcohol or other drugs. On the day he collapsed, the outdoor temperature was 82 °F with 76 % humidity, which results in a heat index of 88 °F [43]. He had been unemployed for a significant amount of time before hiring onto this job. The Occupational Safety and Health Administration (OSHA) opened an investigation into this worker's death. Although the employer had provided water and an air-conditioned break area, OSHA identified several deficiencies in the employer's safety practices that lead to this worker's death. These deficiencies included lack of worker training, inadequate work/rest cycles, and most importantly, no period of acclimatization for new workers.

Psychosocial hazards in the workplace include long hours, shift work, violence, harassment, and discrimination. Recently, we have witnessed dramatic examples of the psychological effects of that most devastating work hazard—war—in military personnel returning from Iraq and Afghanistan. Anxiety, depression, post-traumatic stress disorder, and suicide rates in this population have reached historic highs [27]. Studies funded by the National Institutes of Health (NIH) and US Army identified the following risk factors for suicide in army personnel: being male, being white, recent demotion, and previous suicidal thoughts or actions [28, 29]. These mental health sequelae reach beyond the soldiers to their families, relatives, and friends. Workplace violence is encountered in a wide variety of occupations ranging from law enforcement to driving taxicabs to providing healthcare and social services. Workplace homicides are the fourth leading cause of fatal occupational injuries [30]. More subtle but pervasive is stress in the workplace from job insecurity, increased workload demands, and changing employment practices, such as greater use of temporary workers. The National Institute for Occupational Safety and Health (NIOSH) supports research on work organization and other factors that influence job stress with the goal of identifying ways to redesign jobs to create safer, healthier workplaces [31].

1.5   Reproductive Health and the Workplace

Reproductive health is a leading public health concern. More than two million couples in the United States suffer from infertility; 10–20 % of pregnancies end in spontaneous abortion; and 3 % of children are born with major birth defects [33]. Box 1.3 describes a case of reversible male infertility from exposure to lead, a hazard that has not yet been eliminated in the workplace. Table 1.1 (adapted from references 34–36) lists chemical and physical occupational exposures known to adversely affect the male reproductive system. These exposures may cause harmful effects to

Box Case 1.3

A 41-year-old law enforcement officer ("Mr. B.") presented to his family physician with a 3-month history of nonspecific symptoms of headache, dizziness, irritability, and trouble sleeping. During the visit, he raised an additional concern: he and his wife had been unsuccessfully attempting to conceive a child. No cause for the infertility had been diagnosed, and he had successfully fathered a child 14 years previously. Among other tests, the physician ordered a semen analysis which revealed a low sperm count.

Taking a work history, the physician learned that Mr. B. had been working full time as a firearms instructor for 2 years, first on an outdoor range but in the last 6 months at an indoor range. In addition to instruction, his duties involved cleaning and maintaining the range, including sweeping up the dust. Although Mr. B. used a respirator when sweeping, he noted that the ventilation system was not always operational. The astute physician drew a blood lead level, which was markedly elevated at 88 µg/dl. Mr. B. was initially removed from work and treated with a short course of chelation. Subsequently, Mr. B. was able to adjust his job duties to classroom instruction and limit his time at the range to a few days a year to maintain his qualifications.

Over the next 6 months, Mr. B.'s blood lead level decreased to the mid-30s. His physician continued to monitor his sperm count, which rose as his blood level dropped. One year later, Mr. B.'s wife gave birth to a healthy baby [32].

Table 1.1 Selected occupational exposures known to cause adverse male reproductive health effects

Exposure	Observed effects	Occupations/industries where exposure may be found
Chemicals		
Carbon disulfide	Reduced sperm motility and viability; abnormal sperm morphology; erectile dysfunction	Manufacture of rayon; synthesis of some chemicals and pesticides; rubber manufacture
Ethylene glycol	Reduced sperm count	Chemical manufacturing; use of antifreeze
Phthalates	Decreased sperm motility; abnormal sperm morphology; hormonal abnormalities	Plastics and glue manufacturing
Solvents (i.e., benzene, styrene, trichloroethylene)	Reduced sperm count and motility; abnormal sperm morphology; genotoxicity; erectile dysfunction	Petrochemical industry; plastics manufacturing; dry cleaning; degreasing operations

(continued)

Table 1.1 (continued)

Exposure	Observed effects	Occupations/industries where exposure may be found
Metals		
Cadmium	Reduced sperm motility	Manufacture of batteries, solar cells, alloys, pigments, plastics; electroplating; recycling and hazardous waste operations
Chromium	Abnormal sperm morphology; reduced semen quality; hormonal abnormalities	Manufacture of stainless steel, pigments, batteries; chrome plating; tanning and glassmaking; wood preservation; painters, cement workers, welders
Lead	Reduced sperm count, motility, and viability; abnormal sperm morphology; reduced semen quality; infertility	Brass/bronze foundries; manufacture of car batteries; residential and commercial remodeling (construction before the 1980s); sandblasters; firing range instructors
Pesticides		
Dibromochloropropane (DBCP)	Reduced sperm count; hormonal abnormalities; testicular atrophy; infertility	Agricultural fumigant, now banned in the United States
Organophosphates	Reduced sperm count; reduced semen quality; hormonal abnormalities; genotoxicity	Pesticide manufacture; insecticide sprayers; farmers; pharmaceutical manufacture; military
Multiple pesticides	Reduced sperm count and motility; abnormal sperm morphology; erectile dysfunction; hormonal abnormalities; spontaneous abortion; birth defects	Pesticide manufacture; insecticide sprayers; farmers; greenhouse workers
Physical agents		
Heat	Reduced sperm counts and semen quality; abnormal sperm morphology; hormonal abnormalities; infertility	Work near large furnaces (ceramic industry) and other heat sources; welders
Mechanical pressure, i.e., bicycle saddles	Erectile dysfunction, penis sensitivity	Bicycle patrol officers; bicycle messengers
Radiation ionizing	Reduced sperm count; infertility	Nuclear power plant workers; healthcare workers; researchers; military
Radiation nonionizing (radar, microwave)	Reduced sperm count and motility; abnormal sperm morphology	Power line, cell tower, and radio tower workers; use of lasers; welders

the testes, accessory sex glands, or neuroendocrine (hormonal) system, resulting in one or more of the following outcomes: reduced sperm counts, motility, and viability; abnormal sperm morphology; reduced semen quality; abnormal neuroendocrine hormone profiles; reduced sexual function; and adverse birth outcomes, such as low birth weights, spontaneous abortions, and birth defects [34, 35].

Despite the list in Table 1.1, many chemicals encountered in the workplace have never been tested for reproductive toxicity, and signs and symptoms of impairment to male reproductive health can be difficult to identify [36]. For instance, dibromochloropropane (DBCP), an agricultural fumigant used in the 1970s, was only discovered to be a potent testicular toxin after the wives of employees of a DBCP-manufacturing company, talking at a company softball game, discovered that they were all having trouble conceiving children. DBCP was subsequently banned in 1977. Alert clinicians may be the first to discover such a sentinel event.

1.6 Prevention in Occupational Health

Clinicians can play a major role in preventing work-related injuries, illnesses, and fatalities. Since toxicology is fundamentally an aspect of pharmacology, exploring patient exposures to toxic substances, whether in the workplace or at home, uses the same approach. Contact irritant or allergic dermatitis, urticaria, phototoxicity, or other skin disorders trigger a search for work or home exposures or for prescription, over-the-counter, or traditional medications. Similarly, liver disease, renal disease, or neurologic disorders may warrant consideration of potential exposures in the workplace, home or community environment, in addition to a review of personal habits, diet, and medication usage. Occupational and toxicology textbooks organized by organ system as well as by a class of toxicants provide useful information, and each region of the United States is served by a NIOSH-funded Education and Research Center that includes occupational medicine expertise. The OSHA's Office of Occupational Medicine launched a *Clinicians* webpage (http://www.osha.gov/dts/oom/clinicians/index.html) to assist primary care clinicians and others caring for patients who work. Since one of the first steps in assessing exposure is to identify what the worker uses at work, the webpage includes a link to the OSHA Hazard Communication Standard and information on how to obtain a safety data sheet (SDS, formerly referred to as MSDS). All employers are required to have the SDS available for each potentially hazardous chemical in the worksite. The SDS contains the chemical name of the components and a listing of toxicological information, including both acute and chronic health effects.

Workplace injuries and illnesses are the result of safety and health hazards that can be anticipated, identified, and remediated. Each instance of fatal or nonfatal disease or injury is, by definition, preventable. Primary prevention starts with a general understanding of the work the patient does and potential hazards encountered. As the story in Box 1.2 shows, workers routinely exposed to heat (and their clinicians) should understand preventive measures, know the signs of heat-related illness, understand the potentially fatal risk from heat stroke, and be aware of underlying health conditions, medications, or habits that may increase the risk [37]. Clinicians can play an important role in educating both their patients and employers regarding heat-related illness. For helpful information, see OSHA's Water, Shade, Rest Heat Campaign link under Resources at the end of this chapter.

1.7   Screening for Occupational Health Concerns

Asking about work can be challenging for clinicians, not only in terms of the time crunch in clinical practice but also because it involves ceding the role of "expert" to the patient, who has a body of knowledge that is not immediately available to us. Both patients and clinicians may have the tendency to "medicalize" workplace issues, seeking to provide medical or surgical interventions when actual prevention would require changes in work practices, labor-management negotiation, safety or industrial hygiene interventions, or regulatory enforcement. Clinicians may be asked to "fix" problems by providing written evaluations or requests for accommodation and other documents, often, it seems, to nobody's satisfaction. Breaking down these issues into components can help, along with identifying useful sources of information and referral patterns, some of which are included at the end of this chapter. It may help to keep the big picture in mind. Asking your patient about his work establishes respect and rapport, giving you a better insight into how he spends his time and what matters to him [38]. These two screening questions can be helpful in determining whether more time should be set aside for a detailed history:

• What do you do?
• Do you have any concerns about exposures at work?

Table 1.2 provides a list of situations that should trigger obtaining a more complete occupational and environmental exposure history.

Table 1.2 Reasons to take an occupational and environmental exposure history

• To determine and document mechanisms of work-related injuries
• To determine work-relatedness of injuries and illnesses (or to document reasoning for referral to a specialist for consultation regarding work-relatedness)
• To explore possible causes of illnesses of unknown origin, especially those of the skin, lungs, central nervous system, peripheral nervous system, liver, and kidneys
• To aid in management and return to work decisions regarding both work-related and non-work-related injuries and illnesses
• To determine whether or not illnesses are aggravated by work factors
• To explore causes of unexpected decline in clinical course or lack of treatment efficacy
• To provide patient education regarding the interaction between workplace hazards and health (i.e., asbestos workers and cigarettes; sleep apnea and truck driving)

1.8 Responding to Identified Occupational Concerns

When evaluating a possible work-related injury, clinicians must determine the mechanism(s) of injury, including the specific work tasks and ergonomic factors that may have contributed to the injury. Important factors include the number of hours worked per day, overtime, recent changes in job tasks or processes, tools used, environmental factors (such as temperature), previous work injuries, and exposures to chemical, biological, physical, biomechanical and psychosocial hazards. Cultural factors within the workplace and the worker including his or her primary language should be recorded. This information is important not only in establishing the cause of the injury for workers' compensation cases but also in making decisions on treatment, management, work restrictions, and return to work. Occupational diseases with long latencies require asking about previous jobs and exposures. Work activities and exposures should be considered when the usual medical management does not result in the expected improvement of a patient's illness, such as in work-exacerbated asthma, or when the etiology is unclear, especially for common target organs such as the lungs, skin, liver, kidneys, and central nervous system.

Because of its significant economic, social, and legal impact on workers and employers alike, the decision of work-relatedness for both injuries and illnesses should be based on as much information as possible. Helpful resources include OSHA's Clinicians' webpage and the Agency for Toxic Substances and Disease Registry (ATSDR)'s "Taking an Exposure History," which has a sample exposure history form, along with discussion and case studies. These and other tools and links can be found in the Resources section of this chapter.

1.9 Ethical Issues in Occupational Health

Ethical issues arise commonly in the field of occupational health. What information is an employer allowed to receive when paying for a preplacement or medical surveillance exam? What should a physician do when he or she is concerned about a dangerous workplace? How should a physician respond to an employer who is pressuring the physician to act in a way that is uncomfortable? The fundamentals of bioethics, beneficence, autonomy, justice, and non-maleficence apply in occupational health as they do in any other field of medicine. The American College of Occupational and Environmental Medicine (ACOEM)'s Code of Ethics [39] provides a good starting point for tackling these issues. Table 1.3 lists the guiding principles of ACOEM's Code of Ethics.

Maintaining confidentiality of a patient's personal health information is second nature to physicians, who are well versed in the Health Insurance Portability and Accountability Act (HIPAA). However, laws, such as State Workers' Compensation regulations or federal OSHA standards that include medical surveillance, create significant confusion in this regard. In general, physicians should follow usual practice, keeping medical information confidential, and only release information with

Table 1.3 Seven principles of ACOEM's code of ethics

1	An obligation to enhance a safe and healthy workplace environment
2	An obligation to maintain ethical standards
3	An obligation to avoid discrimination
4	An obligation to maintain professional competence
5	An obligation to maintain patient confidentiality
6	An obligation to advise and report
7	An obligation to address conflict of interest

patient authorization. Physicians should become familiar with their State Workers' Compensation laws and understand their roles and responsibilities when performing industrial examinations, such as fitness for duty and medical surveillance exams. OSHA's Clinicians' webpage includes a link to state and federal workers' compensation agencies.

In the situation where a clinician becomes aware of a dangerous workplace, the ethical challenges are to intervene and prevent further illness or injury while respecting the autonomy of the patient. Depending on the situation, a clinician may gain permission from the patient to speak with the employer in an effort to advise the employer and remove the exposure. It may be possible, for example, to engage the employer's workers' compensation insurance carrier, which should be able to mobilize resources such as safety and industrial hygiene consultation that can identify hazards in the worksite and advise on approaches to remediation. OSHA also offers small business consultations separate from its enforcement activities (see OSHA links in the Resources section of this chapter). When the hazard or the illness is new or unexpected, for example, when workers in a popcorn manufacturing facility developed bronchiolitis obliterans [40] or when workers in a swine processing facility developed progressive neuropathy [41], the NIOSH Health Hazard Evaluation (HHE) program is more suited to evaluate emerging issues. More information on the NIOSH HHE program can be found in the Resources section of this chapter.

When the employer is unwilling to investigate and reduce exposures, you or your patient may wish to contact OSHA to determine whether a complaint should be filed. OSHA enforcement activities are highly structured and the best information comes from the local area office. OSHA inspections can reduce hazards and adverse health outcomes. Levine et al. reported that randomly inspected worksites subsequently experienced a 9.4 % decline in injury rates [95 % CI −0.177 to −0.21] compared with worksites that had been randomly selected on the same criteria but not inspected [42]. However, with fewer than 2000 inspectors nationwide for private workplace enforcement activity, even the most efficient targeting systems can address only a fraction of hazardous worksites. For information on contacting OSHA, worker rights, and clinicians' role, see the Resources section of this chapter.

1.10   Summary

Despite the frustrations and challenges, attention to occupational safety and health offers unique insights into patients' emotional and physical well-being and provides patients an opportunity to take ownership of important aspects of health promotion and injury prevention. Acknowledging the centrality of the patient's role in creating and ensuring a safe, healthy and fulfilling work environment helps establish respect and honors the dignity of his calling.

1.11   Resources

The Occupational Safety and Health Administration (OSHA) [http://www.osha.gov/] is charged with creating and enforcing regulations for safe and healthy workplaces. OSHA has a webpage for workers, detailing their rights for a safe and healthy workplace: http://www.osha.gov/workers/index.html. Employers can learn about their responsibilities and how to obtain assistance from OSHA at this link: http://www.osha.gov/employers/index.html

- Occupational Safety and Health Administration (OSHA). Heat Campaign: Water Rest Shade. Accessed at: http://www.osha.gov/SLTC/heatillness/index.html. It has many resources for employers and workers, including low-literacy information and a smartphone app that calculates the heat index and provides reminders about workplace protective measures.
- OSHA's Clinicians' webpage: http://www.osha.gov/dts/oom/clinicians/index.html. It provides information, resources, and links to help clinicians navigate OSHA's web site and aid clinicians in caring for workers. Key sections of the Clinicians' webpage include:
  - Ethics and Confidentiality in Occupational Health
  - Evaluating Occupational Exposures and Injuries
  - Medical Records—Laws and Confidentiality
  - Reporting a Dangerous Workplace
  - Setting up a Safe Outpatient Office
  - Workers' Compensation

The National Institute for Occupational Safety and Health (NIOSH) [http://www.cdc.gov/NIOSH/] is the US federal agency that conducts research, provides education, and makes recommendations to prevent worker injury and illness. NIOSH webpages of particular interest:

- Men's Reproductive Health in the Workplace: http://www.cdc.gov/niosh/topics/repro/mensWorkplace.html.
- NIOSH's Education and Research Centers [http://www.cdc.gov/niosh/oep/erc.html] are university-based programs located around the country. The centers provide clinical services, train occupational health professionals, and do research.

- NIOSH Health Hazard Evaluation [http://www.cdc.gov/niosh/hhe/] is a worksite evaluation that can be obtained through a request by an employer or three or more employees.
- NIOSHTIC-2 [http://www2a.cdc.gov/nioshtic-2/] is a searchable bibliographic database of occupational safety and health publications, documents, grant reports, and journal articles supported in whole or in part by NIOSH.

The Agency for Toxic Substances and Disease Registry (ATSDR) is a federal public health agency of the US Department of Health and Human Services tasked with providing evaluation and education regarding environmental health hazards. ATSDR's Case Studies in Environmental Medicine include "Taking an Environmental History": http://www.atsdr.cdc.gov/csem/exphistory/docs/exposure_history.pdf.

The Association of Occupational and Environmental Clinics (AOEC) [http://www.aoec.org/] is a nonprofit organization committed to improving the practice of occupational and environmental health through information sharing and collaborative research. AOEC has a network of over 60 clinics and 250 individual members across the United States and in some other countries. AOEC's clinic directory is a helpful resource: http://www.aoec.org/directory.htm.

The American College of Occupational and Environmental Medicine (ACOEM) [http://www.acoem.org/] is the professional organization of physicians specializing in the field of occupational and environmental medicine. ACOEM conducts continuing educational training for physicians, produces clinical guidelines and policies, and is a source for locating an occupational medicine specialist.

The American Public Health Association (APHA) [https://www.apha.org/] is the largest organization of public health professionals in the United States. APHA is comprised of multiple interest groups, including an Occupational Safety and Health section [https://www.apha.org/apha-communities/member-sections/occupational-health-and-safety] and a Men's Health Caucus [https://www.apha.org/apha-communities/caucuses/mens-health-caucus].

References

1. International Labour Organization. Decent Work Agenda. 2015. http://www.ilo.org/global/about-the-ilo/decent-work-agenda/lang--de/index.htm. Accessed 2 Mar 2015.
2. Perlman F, Bobak M. Assessing the contribution of unstable employment to mortality in post-transition Russia: prospective individual-level analyses from the Russian longitudinal monitoring survey. Am J Public Health. 2009;99:1818–25.
3. Gerdtham UG, Johannesson M. A note on the effect of unemployment on mortality. J Health Econ. 2003;22:505–18.
4. Garcy AM, Vagero D. The length of unemployment predicts mortality differently in men and women and by cause of death: a six year mortality follow-up of the Swedish 1992–1996 recession. Soc Sci Med. 2012;74:1911–20.
5. Milner A, Page A, LaMontagne AD. Long-term unemployment and suicide: a systematic review and meta-analysis. PLoS One. 2013;8(1):e51333. doi:10.1371/journal.pone.0051333. http://www.plosone.org/article/info:doi/10.1371/journal.pone.0051333.

6. Dupre ME, George LK, Liu G, Peterson ED. The cumulative effect of unemployment on risks for acute myocardial infarction. Arch Intern Med. 2012;172:1731–7.

7. U.S. Department of Labor, Bureau of Labor Statistics. 2012 census of fatal occupational injuries (revised data): worker characteristic by event or exposure. http://www.bls.gov/iif/oshwc/cfoi/cftb0274.pdf. Accessed 2 Mar 2015.

8. Amick BC, McDonough P, Chang H, Rogers WH, Pieper CF, Duncan G. Relationship between all-cause mortality and cumulative working life course: psychosocial and physical exposures in the United States labor market from 1968 to 1992. Psychosom Med. 2002;64:370–81.

9. Gimeno D, Tabak AG, Ferrie JE, Shipley MJ, De Vogli R, Elovainio M, Vahtera J, Marmot MG, Kivimaki M. Organizational justice and metabolic syndrome: the Whitehall II study. Occup Environ Med. 2010;67:256–62.

10. Virtanen M, Ferrie JE, Singh-Manoux A, Shipley MJ, Vahtera J, Marmot MG, Kivimaki M. Overtime work and incident coronary heart disease: the Whitehall II prospective cohort study. Eur Heart J. 2010;31:1737–44.

11. Kivimaki M, Ferrie JE, Brunner E, Head J, Shipley MJ, Vhtera J, Marmot MG. Justice at work and reduced risk of coronary heart disease among employees. Arch Int Med. 2005;165:2245–51.

12. Elovainio M, Ferrie JE, Singh-Manoux S, Gimeno D, Do Vogli R, Shipley M, Vahtera J, Brunner E, Marmot MG, Kivimaki M. Organizational justice and markers of inflammation: the Whitehall II study. Occup Environ Med. 2010;67:78–83.

13. Elovainio M, Singh-Manoux A, Ferrie JE, Shipley M, Gimeno D, De Vogli R, Vahtera J, Virtanen M, Jokela M, Marmot MG, Kivimaki M. Organizational justice and cognitive function in middle-aged employees: the Whitehall II study. J Epidemiol Community Health. 2012;66:552–6.

14. U.S. Department of Labor, Bureau of Labor Statistics. Employer-reported workplace injuries and illnesses-2013. 2014. http://www.bls.gov/iif/. 4 December 2014. Accessed 8 Feb 2015.

15. Leigh JP, Marcin JP. Workers' compensation benefits and shifting costs for occupational injury and illness. J Occup Environ Med. 2012;54:445–50.

16. U.S. Department of Labor, Bureau of Labor Statistics. Nonfatal occupational injuries and illnesses requiring days away from work. 2013. http://www.bls.gov/iif/. 16 December 2014. Accessed 8 Feb 2015.

17. Gerr F, Fethke NB, Merlino L, Anton D, Rosecrance J, Jones MP, Marcus M, Meyers AR. A prospective study of musculoskeletal outcomes among manufacturing workers: I. Effects of physical risk factors. Hum Factors. 2014;56(1):112–30.

18. National Institute for Occupational Safety and Health. Ergonomics and musculoskeletal disorders. 2014. http://www.cdc.gov/niosh/topics/ergonomics/. Last updated 17 July 2014. Accessed 8 Feb 2015.

19. Occupational Safety and Health Administration. Ergonomics. http://www.osha.gov/SLTC/ergonomics/index.html. Accessed 8 Feb 2015.

20. Centers for Disease Control and Prevention. Asthma. http://www.cdc.gov/asthma/default.htm. Last updated November 25, 2014. Accessed 17 Feb 2015.

21. Toren K, Blanc PD. Asthma caused by occupational exposures is common – a systematic analysis of estimates of the population-attributable fraction. BMC Pulm Med. 2009;9:7. doi:10.1186/1471-2466-9-7.

22. Tarlo SM, Lemiere C. Occupational asthma. NEJM. 2014;370:640–922.

23. Henneberger PK, Redlich CA, Callahan DB, Harber P, Lemiere C, Martin J, Tarlo SM, Vendenplas O, Toren K. An Official American Thoracic Society statement: work-exacerbated asthma. Am J Respir Crit Care Med. 2011;184:368–78.

24. Heederik D, Henneberger PK, Redlich CA. Primary prevention: exposure reduction, skin exposure and respiratory protection. Eur Respir Rev. 2012;21:112–24.

25. Baur X, Sigsgaard T, Aasen TB, Burge PS, Heederik D, Henneberger P, Maestrelli P, Rooyackers J, Schlunssen V, Vandenplas O, Wilken D. Guidelines for the management of work-related asthma. Eur Respir J. 2012;39:529–45.

26. National Institute for Occupational Safety and Health. Noise and hearing loss prevention. http://www.cdc.gov/niosh/topics/noise/. Last updated 5 December 2014. Accessed 2 Mar 2015.
27. Levy BL, Sider VW. Adverse health consequences of the Iraq War. Lancet. 2013;381: 949–58.
28. Schoenbaum M, Kessler RC, Gilman SE, Colpe LJ, Heeringa SG, Stein MB, Ursano RJ, Cox KL. Predictors of suicide and accident death in the army study to assess risk and resilience in servicemembers (Army STARRS). JAMA Psychiatry. 2014;71:493–503.
29. Nock MK, Stein MB, Heeringa SG, Ursano RJ, Colpe LJ, Fullerton CS, Hwang I, Naifeh JA, Sampson NA, Schoenbaum M, Zaslavsky AM, Kessler RC. Prevalence and correlates of suicidal behavior among soldiers – results from the army study to assess risk and resilience in servicemembers (Army STARRS). JAMA Psychiatry. 2014;71:514–22.
30. Occupational Safety and Health Administration. Workplace violence. http://www.osha.gov/SLTC/workplaceviolence/index.html. Accessed 1 Mar 2015.
31. National Institute for Occupational Safety and Health. Stress at work. http://www.cdc.gov/niosh/topics/stress/. Last updated 29 August 2013. Accessed 1 Mar 2015.
32. Fisher-Fischbein J, Fischbein A, Melnick HD, Bardin W. Correlation between biochemical indicators of lead exposure and semen quality in a lead-poisoning firearms instructor. JAMA. 1987;257:803–5.
33. National Institute for Occupational Safety and Health (NIOSH). Cancer, reproductive, and cardiovascular diseases. 2009. http://www.cdc.gov/niosh/programs/crcd/default.html. Last updated 18 June 2009. Accessed 14 Feb 2015.
34. Kumar S. Occupational exposure associated with reproductive dysfunction. J Occup Health. 2004;46:1–19.
35. Burnett AL. Environmental erectile dysfunction: can the environment really be hazardous to your erectile health? J Androl. 2008;29:229–36.
36. Schrader SM, Marlow KL. Assessing the reproductive health of men with occupational exposures. Asian J Androl. 2014;16:23–30.
37. Bray P, Sokas R, Ahluwalia J. Heat-related illnesses: opportunities for prevention. J Occup Environ Med. 2010;52:844–5.
38. Possner A. Trying not to miss the point. JAMA. 2008;300(24):2836.
39. American College of Occupational and Environmental Medicine (ACOEM). Code of ethics. 2010. http://www.acoem.org/codeofconduct.aspx. Accessed 15 Feb 2015.
40. Kreiss K, Gomaa A, Kullman G, Fedan K, Simoes EJ, Enright PL. Clinical bronchiolitis obliterans in workers at a microwave-popcorn. N Engl J Med. 2002;347(5):330–8.
41. Holzbauer SM, DeVries AS, Sejvar JJ, Lees CH, Adjemian J, McQuiston JH, Medus C, Lexau CA, Harris JR, Recuenco SE, Belay ED, Howell JF, Buss BF, Hornig M, Gibbins JD, Brueck SE, Smith KE, Danila RN, Lipkin WI, Lachance DH, Dyck PJ, Lynfield R. Epidemiologic investigation of immune-mediated polyradiculoneuropathy among abattoir workers exposed to porcine brain. PLoS One. 2010;5(3), e9782. doi:10.1371/journal.pone.0009782.
42. Levine DI, Toffel MW, Johnson MS. Randomized government safety inspections reduce worker injuries with no detectable job loss. Science. 2012;336:907–11.43.
43. National Oceanic and Atmospheric Administration (NOAA). National Weather Service, Heat Index, online at: http://www.nws.noaa.gov/om/heat/heat_index.shtml

Sunscreens and Ultraviolet Light: What You Need to Know

2

Shilpi Khetarpal and Kenneth J. Tomecki

Abbreviations

UV   Ultraviolet
UVR   Ultraviolet radiation
CPD   Cyclopyrimidine dimers
BCC   Basal cell carcinoma
SCC   Squamous cell carcinoma
AK   Actinic keratosis
FDA   Food and Drug Administration
SPF   Sun protection factor

2.1 Ultraviolet Light

Ultraviolet radiation (UVR) from the sun is strongest between the hours of 10:00 A.M. and 4:00 P.M. and stronger at latitudes near the equator especially during the summer months. Acute and chronic exposure to UV radiation leads to cellular and clinical changes that promote the unregulated growth of skin cells that can lead to nonmelanoma skin cancer (NMSC) [1]. UV radiation consists of wavelengths of light from 200 to 400 nm and classified into three bands: UVC (200–290 nm), UVB (290–320 nm), and UVA (320–400 nm). UVA and UVB wavelengths are most damaging to human skin and directly contribute to the development of skin cancer [1]. The UVC spectrum and other subdivisions are less likely to contribute to carcinogenesis. Due to its short wavelength, UVC rays do not reach the earth's surface and

S. Khetarpal, M.D. (✉) • K.J. Tomecki, M.D.
Department of Dermatology, Cleveland Clinic Foundation,
9500 Euclid Ave Desk A61, Cleveland, OH 44195, USA
e-mail: shilpikhetarpal@gmail.com; tomeckk@ccf.org

© Springer Science+Business Media New York 2016
J.M. Potts (ed.), *Men's Health*, DOI 10.1007/978-1-4939-3237-5_2

contribute minimally to carcinogenesis. UVA accounts for more than 90 % of the radiation that reaches the earth's surface; UVB accounts for the rest. Much of the UVB radiation is scattered by the ozone layer, clouds, and glass. UVA with its longer wavelength is able to penetrate more deeply into the skin and has greater potential to damage the skin [2]. Both UVA and UVB cause cutaneous immunosuppression in the skin causing changes in DNA, specifically the formation of cyclopyrimidine dimers (CPD); these mutations block replication which negates progression to the S phase checkpoint causing apoptosis of mutated cells. UVR causes more than 90 % of the visible sun-induced aging changes in the skin [3]. Approximately 25 % of lifetime sun exposure occurs by age 18; an individual has a third of their sun exposure between the ages of 40 and 60, based on a 78-year lifespan [3].

2.2   Skin Cancer

Skin cancer is the most common type of cancer in the United States affecting approximately five million individuals each year; its incidence continues to rise [4]. Basal cell carcinoma (BCC) is the most common type of skin cancer accounting for approximately 80 % of all skin cancer, followed by squamous cell carcinoma (SCC). One in five Americans will develop a skin cancer in their lifetime [4]. The annual cost of treating skin cancer in the United States is over $8 billion. Exposure to UV radiation is the main environmental risk factor for NMSC.

2.3   Tanning

The skin darkens or "tans" after UVR as a protective response. UVA and UVB rays affect the skin in different ways. UVA rays cause immediate pigment darkening, within seconds, due to the oxidation of pre-existing melanin and the darkening fades within hours. UVB rays cause delayed pigment darkening, a protective response that occurs 72 h after UV exposure [5]. Darkening develops from increased melanocyte activity and new melanin production. Sunburn occurs from UVB exposure causing vasodilation, redness, and edema; changes occur immediately and peak within 24–48 h. Mild sunburn is equivalent to a first-degree burn; more severe sunburn can cause blistering and extensive peeling similar to a second-degree burn [5].

2.4   Photoaging

Chronic UV exposure leads to photoaging changes in the skin. Data suggest that UVA is primarily responsible for photoaging, while UVB is responsible for sunburn. Photoaging includes a variety of changes such as loss of the extracellular matrix that supports collagen leading to wrinkles, loss of elasticity, decreased subcutaneous fat, and prominence of telangiectasia [6]. Histologically, the accumulation of degraded elastic tissue, known as solar elastosis, is the main feature of photoaged skin.

2.5 Sunscreens

Sunscreens are compounds that interact with UV wavelengths that would normally interact with molecules in the skin leading to change. Sunscreens were first developed in the 1940s and were developed to prevent sunburn; today they have been refined to prevent other aspects of the sun exposure including photoaging and skin cancer. Sunscreens are composed of either inorganic (physical agents) or organic compounds (chemical sunscreens) with different ranges of activity in the UVA and UVB spectrum.

2.5.1 Mechanism of Action

Sunscreens form a film or coating on the outer layer of skin (stratum corneum) preventing UVR from penetrating the epidermis and dermis. The active ingredients work by absorbing or scattering radiation then reflecting the light particles [7]. Chemical agents, or inorganic compounds, include zinc oxide and titanium dioxide and work by absorbing radiation then scattering the light particles, based on their size. Such compounds are called sunblocks and provide protection in both the UVA and UVB ranges. Physical sunscreens, or organic agents, absorb energy from the sun then dissipate the light particles as heat. Physical agents have most of their activity in the UVB range. Most sunscreens contain a combination of chemical and physical agents and protect the skin against both UVA and UVB wavelengths. Table 2.1 shows a list of FDA-approved sunscreen ingredients and corresponding wavelengths of activity for each agent.

Table 2.1 FDA-approved sunscreen active ingredients with activity shown in UVB and UVA spectrum

Chemical Category	Compound	UVB (290-320 nm)	UVA2 (320-340 nm)	UVA1 (240-400 nm)
Organic	PABA (para-aminobenzoic acid)	■		
	Padmiate O	■		
	Octinoxate	■		
	Cinoxate	■		
	Homosalate	■		
	Octisalate	■		
	Trolamine	■		
	Octrocrylene	■		
	Ensulizole	■		
	Dioxybenzone	■	■	■
	Oxybenzone	■	■	■
	Sulibenzone	■	■	■
	Ecamsule		■	
	Meradimate		■	
	Avobenzone		■	■
Inorganic	Titanium Dioxide	■		■
	Zinc Oxide	■		■

2.5.2   Sunscreens and Skin Cancer

Actinic keratosis (AK) is a marker for high levels of cumulative UV exposure. AK is a true pre-cancer and their presence is associated with a higher risk of BCC, SCC, and melanoma [8]. The use of sunscreen on a regular basis is effective in preventing AK and squamous cell carcinoma [9]. Thompson et al. showed that regular sunscreen use reduced the occurrence of new AKs, and after 7 months the average number of new AKs decreased by more than half [10]. The use of sunscreen may help to prevent the development of basal cell carcinoma and melanoma, but data are inconclusive nonetheless; sunscreen use is recommended for any individual, regardless of his/her skin cancer history, especially for prolonged outdoor activity.

2.6   Sunscreen and Photoaging

Photoaging is a result of excessive solar UV exposure. Sun-induced skin changes are different both clinically and histologically from natural aging changes in the skin [9]. Other factors like smoking can affect photoaging, but UV exposure is the main cause. Minimizing sun exposure can help prevent both skin cancer and photoaging, a fact confirmed in individuals with similar genetic backgrounds living in different latitudes who experience different levels of UVR [9].

2.7   Regulation

Sunscreens are commonly available and are regulated by the Food and Drug Administration (FDA). Regulations include the concentration of active ingredients, sun protection factor (SPF), and safety labeling. Efficacy is measured by the SPF and calculated by the percent of blocked radiation. Current FDA labeling guidelines are illustrated in Fig. 2.1. Two recent changes include an SPF maximum of 50+ and maximum-time-claimed water resistance (either 40 or 80 min). In order to be water resistant, the product must maintain the indicated protection after either 40 or 80 min of water immersion.

2.8   How to Apply Sunscreen

Proper use and reapplication of sunscreen is essential for maximum protection [9]. Childhood sunscreen use ideally should be coupled with sun avoidance during peak hours (11 A.M. to 3 P.M.) and use of protective clothing. Working guidelines for all individuals should entail a healthy respect for the sun and its potential side effects.

Sunscreen Labeling According to 2011 Final Rule
These products have not been shown to protect against skin cancer and early skin aging. They have been shown only to help prevent sunburn.

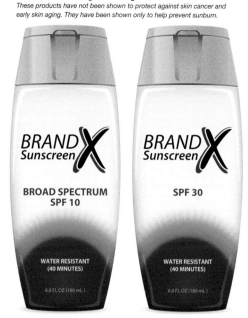

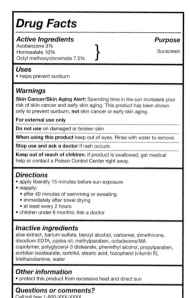

Fig. 2.1   2011 FDA sunscreen regulations. *Source*: US Food and Drug Administration

---

References

1. Mancebo SE, Wang SQ. Skin cancer: role of ultraviolet radiation in carcinogenesis. Rev Environ Health. 2014;29(3):265–73.
2. Miyamura Y, Coelho SG, Schlenz K, et al. The deceptive nature of UVA tanning versus the modest protective effects of UVB tanning on human skin. Pigment Cell Melanoma Res. 2011;24:136–47.
3. Skin Cancer Foundation. Skin cancer information: what are the facts? http://www.skincancer.org/skin-cancer-information/skin-cancer-facts#general. Accessed 10 Nov 2014.
4. Rogers HW, et al. Incidence estimate of nonmelanoma skin cancer in the United States, 2006. Arch Dermatol. 2010;146(3):283–7.
5. Wolber R, et al. Pigmentation effects of solar-stimulated radiation as compared with UVA and UVB radiation. Pigment Cell Melanoma Res. 2008;21:487–91.
6. Yano K, et al. Ultraviolet B irradiation of human skin induces an angiogenic switch that is mediated by upregulation of vascular endothelial growth factor and by downregulation of thrombospondin-1. Br J Dermatol. 2005;152:115–21.
7. Burnett ME, Wang SQ. Current sunscreen controversies: a critical review. Photodermatol Photoimmunol Photomed. 2011;27(2):58–67.
8. Jou PC, Feldman RJ, Tomecki KJ. UV protection and sunscreens: what to tell patients. Cleve Clin J Med. 2012;79(6):427–36.
9. Iannacone MR, Hughes MC, Green AC. Effects of sunscreen on skin cancer and photoaging. Photodermatol Photoimmunol. 2014;30:55–61.
10. Thompson SC, Jolley D, Marks R. Reduction of solar keratoses by regular sunscreen use. N Engl J Med. 1993;329:1147–51.

His Mouth

3

Gary K. Roberts

As adopted by the 1997 American Dental Association House of Delegates, dentistry is defined as the evaluation, diagnosis, prevention, and/or treatment (*nonsurgical, surgical, or related procedures*) of diseases, disorders, and/or conditions of the oral cavity, maxillofacial area, and/or the adjacent and associated structures and their impact on the human body, provided by a dentist, within the scope of his/her education, training, and experience, in accordance with the ethics of the profession and applicable law. In addition to general dentistry, the American Dental Association (ADA) currently recognizes the following dental specialties:

1. Pedodontics (*children*)
2. Orthodontics and dentofacial orthopedics (*braces*)
3. Endodontics (*root canals*)
4. Periodontics (*gums*)
5. Prosthodontics (*fixed and removable dentures*)
6. Oral and maxillofacial surgery (*OMFS*)
7. Oral and maxillofacial radiology
8. Oral and maxillofacial pathology
9. Dental public health (*dental epidemiology and community health policies*)

Note that "cosmetic dentistry" is NOT a recognized dental specialty!

While that definition seems relatively straightforward in print, in actual practice it can be a confusing miasma for both patients and healthcare providers to determine when an oropharyngeal condition is best treated by a dentist or physician. Equally important is the confusing issue of whether treatment should be paid for by dental or medical insurance.

G.K. Roberts, D.D.S. (✉)
Oral Medicine and Maxillofacial Surgery, Department of Surgery, Stanford University Medical Center and Lucille Packard Children's Hospital, 750 Welch Road #118, Palo Alto, CA 94304, USA
e-mail: groberts@stanford.edu

© Springer Science+Business Media New York 2016
J.M. Potts (ed.), *Men's Health*, DOI 10.1007/978-1-4939-3237-5_3

For example, a patient is in a bicycle accident not protected by a helmet and sustains Le Fort II fx, nasal fx, midline AP palatal fx, mandibular condylar fx, mandibular angle fx, mandibular midline symphysis fx, maxillary and mandibular alveolar ridge fx's, several tooth avulsions, multiple coronal fractures into dentin and pulp of various teeth, and extensive facial and perioral lacerations. Treatment includes an initial major multi-hour surgery to reduce and stabilize the bone fractures, repair soft tissue lacerations, as well as extract all non-restorable teeth. A couple of weeks after the initial surgery, endodontic treatment is performed on the teeth with exposed pulps; dental restorations are placed to cover dentin and repair coronal fractures, along with interim fixed and removable partial dentures to restore some oral function and aesthetics. Several months later, implants are inserted to more definitively replace the missing teeth, followed by implant-supported crowns and bridges after several additional months of healing. Over the course of recovery, this patient also benefited from the care of a physical therapist well versed in head and neck injuries, as well as an orthodontist. Certainly an OHNS/ENT physician, facial plastics surgeon, or OMFS could provide the initial acute surgical care, but which provider is going to coordinate and provide the requisite follow-up reconstructive care that may take up to 24 months to complete in such situations? Will medical or dental insurance pay for all these very expensive services?

Another patient had oropharyngeal cancer treated with surgical resection of the tumor and extraction of all nonviable teeth, head and neck radiation therapy, and chemotherapy. The patient was advised to have professional dental prophylaxis every 2–3 months due to the radiation-induced xerostomia, but unfortunately the patient's dental insurance plan only covered two dental cleanings a year, and the patient did not have sufficient disposable income to afford the additional suggested cleanings. Several dozen months after surviving cancer, the patient developed multiple painful dental caries extending the pulp, resulting in dental abscesses and requires endodontic treatment on 17 teeth along with 21 crowns. The patient's medical insurance carrier stated these were dental problems and refused to offer coverage. The patient's dental insurance provider stated the problem was a result of the patient's cancer, so treatment should be covered by the medical insurance; complicating the issue is the fact that the patient only had a $1500 maximum dental benefit per year which would not adequately cover the necessary costs in any event. Unfortunately the patient did not have $50,000 lying around to pay for this care. How will this patient be able to afford the necessary care to get out of pain and restore normal oral function?

Since the teeth are part of the maxilla and mandible—which incidentally are anatomically attached to and physiologically part of the rest of the body—it would seem much more logical and efficient if all healthcare needs, including those of an odontogenic origin, would be covered by a patient's health insurance. The current system of having dental insurance separate and not integrated with overall healthcare insurance does not make any logical sense.

This chapter will provide a brief overview of many common oral issues that we have seen in both our hospital dental clinic and the author's private practice; it is not meant to be a comprehensive source for dental research, but rather a practical overview. It was primarily extracted from a series of lectures on oral health concerns given annually at Stanford Medical School by the author.

What can a person do to help ensure a lifetime of healthy teeth? Like many other aspects of healthcare, most dental problems can be broken down to those injuries caused by outside factors, such as trauma and those problems caused by lifestyle choices. It turns out that most dental problems are *PREVENTABLE* with a modicum of daily care! A man's journey to dental health starts at a young age; parents can help their children develop healthy teeth by establishing a daily home care regimen once the teeth begin erupting, encouraging a diet that is low in sugar and acids, implementing biannual visits to the dentist beginning around age 3–4 years old for professional care including placement of sealants as posterior adult teeth erupt, initiating orthodontic care to ideally align teeth if needed, and modeling healthy lifestyle choices.

Good daily home dental hygiene care includes:

- Carefully brushing all the teeth for at least 2 min with a manual or powered brush with soft, compact bristles, at least once and preferably twice per day—also be sure to replace the toothbrush/brush head every 3 months or so
- Meticulous daily flossing of all teeth
- Use of a non-alcohol fluoride rinse or gel each day
- Use of a antibacterial mouth rinse, if needed
- Adherence to a healthy diet low in sugars and acids

Recommended periodic professional dental care includes:

- Routine radiographic studies (*full mouth X-ray (FMX) q/5 years, bitewings (BW) q/12–30 months*)
- Routine clinical examination (*q12 months*)
- Routine dental prophylaxis (*q3–6 months*)
- Sealants and preventive resin restorations (PRN)

Sadly, most research and surveys on oral health by organizations such as the ADA and CDC demonstrate that men are at higher risk for intraoral problems and also fail to care for their dentition as well as women. Men frequently make lifestyle choices that can place the mouth at risk: contact sports, tobacco chewing, excess alcohol intake, smoking various substances, and over working—all of which can lead to systemic medical issues and oral health problems. For example, men have higher rates of oral cancer, as well as increased likelihood of cardiovascular disease, both of which are often treated with medications that can cause xerostomia. According to the American Academy of Periodontology, females are twice as likely to seek routine professional dental examinations compared to males and are 26 % more likely to perform recommended daily home care; in addition, men are much less likely to follow through with completing proposed treatment.

Note that home oral healthcare can become more problematic in disabled and elderly patients. Decreased visual acuity associated with normal aging can limit the ability of older patients to see plaque and tarter. Reduced manual dexterity can also be a significant issue with disabled and geriatric patients, as problems such as arthritis, Parkinson's, and stroke can interfere with the ability to properly brush and floss. Powered toothbrushes are often beneficial at improving plaque removal; flossing tools can also be helpful. Cognitive changes associated with mental illness as well as aging frequently impact home oral healthcare. Older patients may exhibit short-term memory loss; these patients may simply forget to brush and floss. Depression can also impact home care. More serious cognitive functional challenges such as severe autism, schizophrenia, senility, dementia, and Alzheimer's can preclude patients from being able to care for themselves, cause difficulty for in-home caregivers, and limit the ability of these patients to receive dental care in a routine outpatient setting.

Access to dental care can also become an issue. During the majority of their lives, most adults exercise a great deal of control over their oral health status and retain full responsibility for their home healthcare. However, in times of disability and when reaching geriatric stages of life, some patients may no longer be able to drive themselves to dental appointments, may have reduced mobility, may frequently become dependent upon others for their daily living needs, and may often feel they have lost their ability to influence and control their dental health status. Currently in America, many caregivers assisting disabled and elderly patients are immigrants that speak English as a second language. Dental care may not have been a cultural priority in many caregivers' homelands, so caregivers may need to be educated on the expected standards of dental care in the United States, so they may properly assist with the required routine dental needs and daily home care regimen necessary to maintain the oral health of their elderly patients. Over 1.5 million elderly Americans are living in assisted care facilities. Over 60 % of these facilities do NOT have a dentist either on staff or on call to treat inpatients. A survey of skilled nursing facilities in California found that over 30 % of patients were in need of emergency dental care, and over 90 % of nursing home residents required some form of dental therapy. Financial barriers blocking appropriate dental care are also a significant concern for disabled and geriatric patients. Many adults lose their dental insurance benefits upon retiring from work and Medicare does NOT cover dental procedures. Likewise, during times of temporary or permanent disability, disposable income may be reduced. Many disabled and elderly patients present with challenging oral health conditions that require costly, complex, multidisciplinary care to resolve. Unfortunately many such patients no longer have the financial resources to fund such efforts and are forced to defer comprehensive dental care.

Obviously avoiding tobacco products, limiting alcohol intake, not placing very high temperature items in the mouth (*including smoke, liquids, and food*), not engaging in tooth damaging habits or body modifications (*such as tongue piercings and cheek gauging*), and skipping other behaviors potentially injurious to the dentition can all be of help in preserving a healthy oral environment. Likewise, given the high incidence of head and maxillofacial trauma, the severe potential risks, along with enormous personal and societal costs, taking a basic protective step like wearing a helmet is appropriate for ANY activity involving motion and the risk of falling or being struck, particularly common activities like—bicycling, rollerblading, skate boarding, skiing, snowboarding, etc. In addition to a helmet, wearing protective eyewear and an athletic mouth guard can also be prudent for many other activities and sports.

Numerous systemic medical problems impact oral health, particularly as patients age:

- Diabetes
- Cancer
- Hypertension
- Cardiovascular disease
- Pulmonary problems
- Organ transplant
- Osteoporosis
- Joint replacement
- Alzheimer's
- Parkinson's
- Depression and other mental health conditions
- Sleep apnea
- Vision issues
- Arthritis
- Sjögren's syndrome

Orofacial pain can be placed into two categories: odontogenic pain that arises from the teeth or supporting structures and non-odontogenic pain. Diagnosis can be complicated by pain referral and other factors; however, in most cases of odontogenic discomfort, the dental cause can eventually be found with careful history, thorough exam, appropriate imaging, and a degree of patience.

Common odontogenic causes of orofacial discomfort:

- Caries/cavities/decay
- Broken or lost dental restorations
- Dentin exposure
- Attrition/erosion of teeth
- Pulpitis/abscesses
- Periodontal problems
- Cracked tooth syndrome
- Gross tooth fracture
- Vertical and horizontal root fractures
- Malocclusion
- Congenital malformation of teeth
- Tooth displacement trauma

Examples of non-odontogenic causes of orofacial discomfort:

- Sinusitis/allergic rhinitis
- Myofascial pain dysfunction of the muscles of mastication (*MPD*)
- Temporomandibular disorders (*TMD/TMJ disorders*)

- Recurrent aphthous ulcers
- Herpetic gingivostomatitis
- Herpes zoster (*shingles*)
- Maxillofacial trauma
- Sialadenitis
- Maxillofacial pathology
- Neuralgia and headaches
- Angina pectoris (*radiating to left posterior mandible*)

Note that patients receiving immunosuppressive therapy are at considerable risk for sepsis if active odontogenic disease is not identified and treated before initiation of care. Patients requiring dental screening prior to medical care include those having:

- Chemotherapy
- Radiation therapy to head and neck
- Bone marrow transplant (*BMT*)
- Solid organ transplant (e.g., *heart, kidney, liver*)
- Cardiac prostheses (e.g., *valve replacement, LVAD*)
- Orthopedic appliances (e.g., *total joints*)

Dental caries is a complex disease with many contributing factors. It is a transmissible bacterial infection, caused primarily by *Streptococcus mutans, Streptococcus sobrinus*, and *Lactobacilli*, as well as *Actinomyces viscosus* and *Nocardia* spp. The enamel and dentin are demineralized and destroyed by acid, primarily through bacterial fermentation of food debris—principally carbohydrates. When the oral pH drops below 5, then demineralization exceeds the natural remineralization, resulting in caries formation. Caries confined to the enamel may remineralize in the right circumstances, but once caries extends into the dentin, a dental restoration is required to restore the tooth and prevent the caries from reaching the pulp. Once the caries reaches the pulp, the only treatment options are endodontic therapy or tooth extraction. Fortunately dental caries is completely preventable with good home care and regular professional dental visits. One of the best clinical tools available for limiting dental disease is the Caries Management by Risk Assessment (CAMBRA) protocols developed over the last decade or so.

Periodontitis is a bacterially induced, localized, chronic inflammatory disease that destroys the connective tissue and bone that support the teeth. With good home care, it is completely preventable. Periodontal disease is the most common reason adults over the age of 30 lose teeth; approximately 50 % of older adults suffer from periodontal disease. Common periodontal problems include:

- Gingivitis
- Necrotizing ulcerative gingivitis (*NUG*)
- Periodontitis
- Periodontal abscess

- Pericoronitis
- Gingival recession/root exposure
- Recurrent aphthous ulcers
- Herpetic stomatitis

Once it progresses, periodontitis can be difficult to treat, so the key is prevention and early intervention!

Fortunately most odontogenic infections still respond to penicillin (*Pen VK 500 mg, po qid for 5–7 days*). Metronidazole (*500 mg, po qid for 7–10 days*) can be added for more virulent mixed infections. For more severe odontogenic infections, Augmentin (*875 mg, po bid for 7–10 days*) also works well. If allergic to penicillin, then clindamycin (*300 mg, po tid for 5–7 days*) is a good choice. Other common options include azithromycin and clarithromycin. Be sure to review current guidelines from the American Dental Association, American Heart Association, and the American Academy of Orthopedic Surgeons, as routine antibiotic prophylaxis for dental treatment for patients with heart murmurs and prosthetic joints are no longer recommended.

Edentulism refers to the loss of adult teeth and can be either partial or complete. Partial edentulism can place patients at risk for collapse of the dental arch form, increase the risk of periodontal disease, and result in higher dental decay rates. Both partial and complete edentulism can cause difficulties with eating and nutritional intake, interfere with normal speech and phonation, precipitate jaw bone resorption, cause problems with the TMJ and muscles of mastication, and alter normal facial appearance resulting in negative psychosocial effects, poor self-image, and depression. Edentulous patients can be treated using a traditional removable prosthesis for far less cost than with implant prosthetics or fixed crown and bridge restorations. A complete denture (*CD*) or partial removable denture (*RPD*) can cost $2500 or less. Although offering a reduced cost, removable prostheses are unfortunately not a panacea, as they result in other sequela. Most edentulous patients prefer the stability and security of implant-supported prostheses whenever possible—particularly on the mandible. Implants also have the added advantage of preserving residual bone. However, implants are more invasive, costly, and time consuming than removable prostheses. Looked at in aggregate, implant-retained prosthesis are clearly the best current option for restoring function in most patients suffering from tooth loss. Unfortunately, patients who have received radiation treatment for oropharyngeal cancer and those who have had bisphosphonate treatment may not be candidates for implants. After oropharyngeal radiation therapy, treatment of edentulism should be deferred for several months. In addition, post-cancer treatment sequelae can significantly impact prosthetic options due to limited mouth opening, insufficient residual tissue to support prosthesis, mucositis preventing use of removable prostheses, and radiation damage limiting reconstructive surgical options—including placement of dental implants. In some cases functional limitations occurring in the oral cavity as a result of oropharyngeal cancer treatment may prevent ANY dental prostheses from being successfully utilized.

Recurrent aphthous ulcers often occur in response to stress and appear as discrete, shallow ulcerations that are often quite painful. They are usually located on moveable, unattached intraoral mucosa surfaces—initially presenting with an erythematous halo then turning while. They are typically at a different location each episode and are usually self-limiting in 7–10 days. There is no effective treatment, just palliative care using topical medications.

In contrast, herpetic gingivostomatitis is caused by the HSV (herpes simplex virus). A brief period of prodromal tingling and itching may occur. The primary form is accompanied by fever and pharyngitis, followed by the eruption of small irritating vesicles on the oral mucosa, especially the tongue, gums, and cheeks. Ninety percent of the population has HSV ABs; 40 % develop secondary HSV infection. The secondary form repeats in the same location and generally manifests only as pain and vesicles. These diffuse vesicles form on the attached (*bound down*) mucosa and then rupture, leaving painful ulcers, followed by a yellowish crust. Other findings can include submaxillary lymphadenopathy, increased salivation, halitosis, anorexia, and keratoconjunctivitis. Treatment includes topical and systemic antiviral agents, no steroids.

Herpes zoster or shingles is another virus that can occasionally manifest as pain or sores in the mouth, typically in older adults. Before cutaneous signs emerge, it can present a confusing mix of symptoms that can mimic odontogenic disease. Herpes zoster classically presents as small red nodules erupting unilaterally around the thorax or vertically on the arms and legs, which rapidly become vesicles filled with clear fluid or pus; these vesicles dry and form scabs about 10 days after eruption. However, herpes zoster may produce painful vesicles in the oral cavity on the buccal mucosa, tongue, uvula, pharynx, or larynx. Fever and general malaise accompany pruritus, paresthesia or hyperesthesia, and tenderness along the course of the involved sensory nerve. Treatment includes supportive therapy and systemic antiviral agents.

Candidiasis can afflict many people and is a common infection during chemotherapy. It characteristically produces soft, elevated plaques on the buccal mucosa, tongue, and sometimes the palate, gingivae, and floor of the mouth; the plaques may be wiped away. The lesions of acute atrophic candidiasis are red and painful. The lesions of chronic hyperplastic candidiasis are white and firm. Localized areas of redness, pruritus, and a foul odor may be present. *Treatment includes topical and systemic antifungal agents.* Do NOT use the destructive sugar containing oral troches and rinses! Finding nonsugar-containing oral medications can be challenging. For years the best option for a nonsugar-containing oral antifungal preparation was for patients to place nystatin vaginal pastilles in their mouth and let them dissolve. Unfortunately, this formulation is no longer available. Sadly the current nystatin suspension and clotrimazole oral troches contain sugar compounds which in debilitated and immune-compromised patients can rapidly decay teeth in a matter of weeks. The best currently available sugar-free options are to prescribe either:

– Nystatin USP powder and allow patients to mix it with water prior to each use (*RX: dispense 60 g powder, have patients dissolve 1 tsp of powder into 2–4 oz water, and swish for 60 s QID*).
– Miconazole seven vaginal suppository dissolved in the mouth QID.

Xerostomia (*chronic dry mouth*) affects numerous people, including approximately 30 % of persons over the age of 65. Xerostomia can lead to a variety of problems including dysphasia (*difficulty in swallowing*), dysgeusia (*inability to taste*), dysphonia (*difficulty in speaking*), halitosis (*bad breath*), rampant ectopic tooth decay, inability to wear dentures, and an increase in oral infections, especially yeast (*thrush caused by Candida albicans*).

Xerostomia can be caused by a variety of medications, including some antihistamines and decongestants, certain antidepressants, anticholinergics, anorexiants, antihypertensives, antipsychotics, anti-Parkinson agents, diuretics, and some sedatives, along with some illegal recreational drugs including methamphetamine, cocaine, and ecstasy. A variety of medical conditions can also induce xerostomia, including radiation therapy for the treatment of head and neck cancer, chemotherapy for cancer, poorly controlled diabetes, sarcoidosis, Sjögren's syndrome, systemic lupus erythematosus (*SLE*), obstructive sleep apnea (*OSA*), and rheumatoid arthritis (*RA*).

There is no definitive treatment for xerostomia; however, multifocal palliative care includes:

- Increased intake of cold, nonsugar-containing fluids, including water.
- Chewing/sucking on sugarless gum or candy (*particularly those with xylitol*).
- Hourly use of saliva substitutes and moisturizing agents (*Biotene, Oasis, etc.*) as needed.
- Daily application of non-alcohol topical fluoride preparations (*ACT, Phos-Flur, Gel Kam, Prevident, Natural Dentist, etc.*); consider fluoride tray use.
- Daily use of alcohol-free antibacterial rinses (*0.12 % chlorhexidine gluconate USP: NDC 052376-021-02*).
- Salivary gland inductive medications (*pilocarpine and cevimeline HCl*).
- Meticulous daily home oral hygiene care with flossing and brushing:
  - Consider power brush (Oral B-Braun or Philips Sonicare) with small compact soft heads changed q3 months or extra soft compact manual brush (e.g., Nimbus).
  - Consider flossing tool (Johnson & Johnson Reach Access).
  - Use dry cotton swabs (Q-tips) to clean sensitive areas.
- Increased frequency of dental prophylaxis (*q3 months*).
- Low-sugar/low-acid diet.

It is critical for patients with xerostomia to avoid food with high sugar and high acid. Beware of hidden sources (*simple carbohydrates, corn syrup, low pH, etc.*). For example, 20 oz of one of the most common sports drinks has a pH of 3.3 and 34 g of sugar; soft drinks are even worse—20 oz of an average cola has a pH of 2.46 and 69 g of sugar. Likewise, some common nutrition beverages used in healthcare have 20 g of sugar, while others only contain only 1 g; patients and providers need to be vigilant.

Oral mucositis is a painful condition that can severely compromise oral and pharyngeal function, inhibit adequate nutrition and hydration, as well as lead to local and systemic infections. It effects 40 % of chemotherapy patients and 80 % of head and neck radiation therapy patients. It can make oral tissue so painful and friable that removable prosthetic devices cannot be tolerated. Treatment includes aphthous ulcer rinse, alcohol-free CHG rinse, viscous lidocaine, 0.1 % hydrocortisone rinse, Caphosol rinse, MuGard rinse, NeutraSal rinse, GelClair, and Palifermin KGF.

Patients are often referred to our clinic after being told they have TMJ. My response is typically yes, you have two of them, which often leaves the patient somewhat baffled until they are informed that TMJ actually means temporomandibular joint—kind of like saying you have a knee or elbow joint. Temporomandibular disorder (TMD) is the more accurate designation for discomfort emanating from the TMJ; TMD is typically caused by either injury to the supporting soft tissue or damage to the actual joint. The vast majority of patients we see for purported TMJ problems actually have very little issues with their joint but in fact have problems with the muscles of mastication—referred to as myofascial pain dysfunction syndrome (MPD). Clenching and bruxism are associated with MPD and situational stress is often a contributing factor. MPD treatment is almost always NONSURGICAL and includes:

- NSAIDs and short-duration muscle relaxants—benzodiazepines work well for this role (e.g., *Temazepam 30 mg po QHS for 7 days*).
- Moist heat alternating with ice to affected muscles.
- Limit opening and unnecessary function.
- Soft diet.
- Bite splint/night guard.
- Physical therapy with a provider well versed in head and neck problems.
- Steroid, local anesthetic, or Botox injections in muscles.

Conversely, damage can occur to the actual TMJ resulting in temporomandibular joint internal derangement, including intra-articular damage, with disk displacement, joint capsule rupture, or other pathologic changes in the TMJ. These are frequently associated with traumatic injury or blow. Another major cause is degenerative joint disease (DJD). Asymptomatic joint noises are typically not a cause for concern and are not always predictive of future problems. Note that temporomandibular joint internal derangement therapy is frequently SURGICAL:

- Initially may be treated as MPD; if no resolution, then surgery
- Arthrocentesis, steroid injection, manipulation under sedation or GA
- Arthroscopy
- Arthroplasty: disk repositioning, diskectomy, articular eminence recontouring, and total joint replacement
- Fracture repair with MMF, rigid fixation

Osteonecrosis of the jaw results in jaw bones being unable to meet increased repair needs following tooth removal, infection, and even the simple day-to-day physiological stress of mastication. ONJ leads to bone pain, bone destruction, and overlying tissue loss and results in various conditions that result in the impairment of blood supply to bone. ONJ is defined as an area of exposed bone in the jaw region that does not heal within 8 weeks of identification. During the past century, the primary cause of ONJ was vascular disturbances in the jaws following radiation therapy for cancer treatment. These cases of osteoradionecrosis generally respond to hyperbaric oxygen treatment, antibiotics, and non-alcohol chlorhexidine gluconate rinses to prevent the onset of osteomyelitis. In the last decade, there has been a dramatic surge of ONJ in patients that have NOT received radiation treatment. Beginning in 2003, the first case studies linking bisphosphonate use to the increased incidence of non-radiation related ONJ cases were published. Since then, several antiresorptive and anti-angiogenic therapies have been linked to medication-related osteonecrosis of the jaw (MRONJ). MRONJ typically affects the mandible twice as frequently as the maxilla; however, both jaws can be involved. Concomitant corticosteroid use, poor oral hygiene, and smoking seem to increase the risk of MRONJ. There is NO current consistent effective treatment for MRONJ; classic ONJ treatments tend to be ineffective for MRONJ, and cessation of antiresorptive and anti-angiogenic therapy prior to oral surgery does not seem to reduce the incidence of MRONJ. Thus, it is CRITICAL that any patient in need of antiresorptive and anti-angiogenic treatments that are linked with MRONJ receive a thorough clinical and radiographic dental examination, along with any required dental surgical care prior to the initiation of such treatment.

Suggested Reading

Diringer JD, Phipps K, Carsel B. Critical trends affecting the future of dentistry: assessing the shifting landscape. ADA; 2013.
Young DA, Featherstone JDB, Roth JR. Curing the silent epidemic: caries management in the 21st century and beyond. CDA J. 2007;35(10):681–5.
Regezi JA, Sciubba JJ, Jordan RCK. Oral pathology–clinical pathological correlations. Saunders; 2008.
Sollecito TP, et al. The use of prophylactic antibiotics prior to dental procedures in patients with prosthetic joints: evidence-based clinical practice guideline for dental practitioners—a report of the American Dental Association Council on Scientific Affairs. JADA. 2015;146(1).
AAOMS. Position Paper: Medication related osteonecrosis of the jaw—2014 update.

Screening and Management for Pulmonary and Sleep Issues

4

Loutfi S. Aboussouan

4.1 Introduction

The morbidity and mortality consequence of various pulmonary and sleep conditions may disproportionately affect men. The pulmonary sections covered in this chapter include smoking, COPD, lung cancer screening, and asthma, and the sleep sections include sleep deprivation, obstructive sleep apnea, insomnia, and the restless legs syndrome. Together, these conditions should be representative of the majority of the pulmonary or sleep issues that may be encountered in a clinical practice. This chapter will review the prevalence, morbidity, available screening tools, and therapeutic options for these conditions. Where applicable, the potential gender differences will be covered as well.

4.2 Pulmonary Conditions

4.2.1 Smoking and Smoking Cessation

Global tobacco smoking rates predominantly affect men. For instance, global declines in the prevalence of smoking between 1980 and 2012 are smaller for men (41.2–31.1 % over that period of time, a 25 % decrease) relative to women (10.6–6.2 %, a 42 % decrease) [1]. Despite the declining prevalence, because of an overall increase in the total population, the number of male daily smokers has increased by 41 % over that period of time, relative to a 7 % increase in the number of female daily smokers [1, 2]. The United States experienced a steady decrease in the

L.S. Aboussouan, M.D. (✉)
Cleveland Clinic, Respiratory Institute, Desk A90, 9500 Euclid Avenue,
Cleveland, OH 44195, USA
e-mail: aboussl@ccf.org

© Springer Science+Business Media New York 2016
J.M. Potts (ed.), *Men's Health*, DOI 10.1007/978-1-4939-3237-5_4

prevalence of smoking from more than 40 % in the 1950s to 18.1 % in 2012, along with a decrease in the cigarettes consumed per day from 16.7 in 2005 to 14.6 in 2012 [3, 4].

Of the available pharmacologic interventions available for smoking cessation, the rates of continuous abstinence for 6 months or more were 10 % for placebo compared to 18 % for nicotine replacement therapy, 19 % with bupropion, and 27.6 % for varenicline [5]. Viewed differently, for every 10 individuals who quit with placebo, 18 would be expected to quit with the use of nicotine replacement therapy or bupropion and 28 with the use of varenicline [6]. For every 10 people quitting with the use of nicotine replacement, 15 would be expected to quit with varenicline [6]. Combination techniques are also more effective: A combination of two types of nicotine replacement therapy (such as patch with inhaler) is as effective as varenicline, and a combination of nicotine replacement therapy with nortriptyline or bupropion was more effective than nicotine replacement therapy alone [6].

In looking at gender differences, abstinence rates were not affected by gender for varenicline [7]. However, males had more success in quitting smoking with bupropion than females [8]. Cytisine, like varenicline, is a nicotine receptor partial agonist, available in Eastern Europe, which has 1-month continuous smoking abstinence rates of 40 % relative to 31 % for nicotine replacement, with significantly higher abstinence rates in women [9]. The benefits of electronic cigarettes (e-cigarettes), which deliver an aerosol (vapor) of nicotine, in achieving smoking cessation are controversial. In controlled trials, the use of e-cigarettes with nicotine cartridges was associated with a 6-month continuous abstinence rate of 7.3 % similar to that of nicotine patches [10]. However, there is also significant concern that it may promote dual use with cigarettes, normalize smoking behavior, increase initiation of young individuals to nicotine, and delay or deter quitting [11].

4.2.2 Chronic Obstructive Pulmonary Disease

The overall prevalence of COPD in the United states is 6.2 % (5.2 % in males and 7.2 % in females) [12]. Because of the long clinical prodrome of COPD, trends in the morbidity of mortality of COPD may not track with the declining smoking prevalence [13]. As a demonstration of that concept, the mortality from COPD in the United States has been steadily rising, and COPD is currently ranking third among the most common causes of death and outstripping cerebrovascular disease deaths since 2010 [2]. There were 138,000 deaths from COPD in 2010, and 52.3 % of those deaths were in women. The number of deaths from COPD has been consistently higher in women relative to men since 1999 [2, 12].

Significant gender differences exist in the phenotype of COPD. Men tend to have less perception of dyspnea relative to women even after adjustment for age [14]. Subtle physiologic variability may account for this difference. For instance, dyspnea with exercise was better accounted for by respiratory factors such as the diffusion capacity and the arterial oxygen tension in men and by central factors such as the central respiratory drive (P100) in women [15]. There may also be difference in the pathology of COPD, with evidence from histologic samples obtained in the course of lung volume reduction surgery, as well from computed tomography studies, indicating that men tend to have more emphysema, whereas women may have increased airway thickness [16–18].

Data from the National Health and Nutrition Examination Survey suggest that 40 % of patients with COPD may be undiagnosed [19]. Although a spirometry is an essential tool for the diagnosis of COPD [20], routine screening of the general population is not indicated [21, 22]. Additionally, while current standards support a fixed $FEV_1/FVC < 0.70$ for the definition of COPD [20], this approach may overdiagnose COPD in the elderly because the FEV_1/FVC decreases with age. As a result, 35 % of healthy never smokers over the age of 70 and 50 % of those over 80 will have an FEV_1/FVC less than 0.7 [23]. Therefore, screening is best indicated for adults who have symptoms suggestive of COPD such as dyspnea, progressive exercise intolerance, cough, or sputum production. The COPD Population Screener ™ is a validated screening tool which incorporates symptoms, smoking history, and age (available at http://www.chestnet.org/Foundation/Patient-Education-Resources/COPD). A score greater than 5 on the screener indicates that spirometry testing may be appropriate.

Treatment of COPD can be based on a combined assessment of symptom severity and risk (see Table 4.1). General principles of management indicate that

Table 4.1 COPD assessment and management

Combined COPD assessment	Symptoms	Risk	Treatment options
Category A Less symptoms, low risk	mMRC 0–1 or CAT < 10	GOLD I (FEV_1 > 80 %) or GOLD II (50 % ≤ FEV_1 < 80 %) AND ≤1 exacerbation in the past year	First choice: SAMA or SABA prn Second choice: LAMA, LABA, SABA, and SAMA prn Alternatives: theophylline
Category B More symptoms, low risk	mMRC 2–4 or CAT ≥ 10	GOLD I (FEV_1 > 80 %) or GOLD II (50 % ≤ FEV_1 < 80 %) AND ≤1 exacerbation in the past year	First choice: LAMA or LABA Second choice: LAMA and LABA Alternatives: SABA and/or SAMA, theophylline All regimens should also include SAMA or SABA prn
Category C Less symptoms, high risk	mMRC 0–1 or CAT < 10	GOLD III (30 % ≤ FEV_1 ≤ 50 %) or GOLD IV (FEV_1 < 30 %) OR ≥ 2 exacerbations per year or hospitalization for exacerbation	First choice: LABA/ICS or LAMA Second choice: LAMA and LABA Alternatives: PDE4 inhibitor, SABA±SAMA, theophylline All regimens should also include SAMA or SABA prn

(continued)

Table 4.1 (continued)

Combined COPD assessment	Symptoms	Risk	Treatment options
Category D More symptoms, high risk	mMRC 2–4 or CAT ≥ 10	GOLD III (30 % ≤ FEV$_1$ ≤ 50 %) or GOLD IV (FEV$_1$ < 30 %) OR ≥ 2 exacerbations per year or hospitalization for exacerbation	First choice: LABA/ICS or LAMA Second choice: LABA/ICS and LAMA, LABA/ICS and PDE4 inhibitors, LAMA and LABA, LAMA and PDE4 inhibitor Alternatives: carbocysteine[a], SABA±SAMA, theophylline All regimens should also include SAMA or SABA prn

Alternative choices can be used alone or in combination with first or second choice options. mMRC 2–4 indicates that the level of dyspnea is at least such that the subject walks slower than people of the same age on the level because of breathlessness or has to stop for breath when walking at his/her own pace on the level. COPD Assessment Test (CAT): http://www.catestonline.org/. Adapted from www.goldcopd.com
(S/L)AMA short-/long-acting muscarinic antagonist, *(S/L)ABA* short-/long-acting beta-agonist, *ICS* inhaled corticosteroids, *PDE4* phosphodiesterase 4
[a]Carbocysteine is not available in the United States but may be replaced with N-acetylcysteine

patients at higher risk (groups C and D in the table) will require therapeutic options that can favorably modify the risk of exacerbations (including a combination of long-acting beta-agonists with inhaled corticosteroids and/or long-acting muscarinic antagonists).

4.2.3 Lung Cancer Screening

The National Lung Screening Trial (NSLT) was a trial of 53,454 previous or current smokers ages 55–74, with at least a 30-pack-year smoking history. The participants were randomized to annual screening for 2 years either with a low-dose helical CT (LDCT) or a chest radiograph. After 6–8 years, there were 442 lung cancer deaths in the chest radiograph arm compared to 354 in the LDCT arm. Screening of 320 patients with LDCT would be required in order to avoid one lung cancer death over an observation period of 7 years [24].

In follow-up to this study, the US Preventive Services Task Force (USPSTF) has issued recommendations for annual lung cancer screening with low-dose helical computed tomography in adults aged 55–80 years who have a 30-pack-year smoking history and either smoke or have quit only within the past 15 years. Screening is discontinued once a person has not smoked for 15 or more years or develops a health problem that limits life expectancy or the ability to have curative lung surgery [25].

Yearly screening carries the risk of having unnecessary follow-up procedures and possibly surgery for benign lesions. In a systematic review, 20 % of individuals screened had findings on LDCT which required follow-up, while only 1 % had lung cancer [26]. Additionally, 18.5 % of lung cancer detected by LDCT were considered to be indolent and therefore overdiagnosed [27]. LDCT also carries a risk of cancer death due to radiation exposure, with modeling based on the NSLT data suggesting that there may be one cancer death for each of the 2500 persons screened, with that risk manifesting 10–20 years later [26]. These data emphasize the importance of selection of appropriate candidates for LDCT screening, along the age and smoking history guidelines of the NSLT or USPSTF, to maintain the favorable balance between prevention of lung cancer death and radiation risk.

4.2.4 Asthma

The prevalence of asthma in the United States is 72 per 1000 males and 97 per 1000 females. In children under the age of 18, the prevalence is higher in males (102 per 1000 males vs. 88 per 1000 females) and the reversal in prevalence by gender at older age may be hormonal [28]. Between 2001 and 2003, an average of 4210 asthma deaths occurred each year, with half of those deaths occurring in individuals over the age of 65 and 64 % of those deaths being in women [29]. However, mortality increases with age, and for most age groups under age 65, males had higher mortality rates than females [29]. Specifically, the highest mortality from asthma was in men 35 or less years of age [30].

Treatment of asthma is based on the National Asthma Education and Prevention Program Expert Panel Report (NAEPP-EP3) which requires separate identification of disease severity and of disease control. Patients with low asthma severity (i.e., intermittent asthma) may only require as needed short-acting beta-agonists (such as albuterol), whereas persistent asthma may require a stepwise approach based on asthma control, initially starting with inhaled corticosteroids and stepping up to increase inhaled corticosteroid strength and addition of long-acting beta-agonists. Alternative or supplemental treatment options include cromolyn, leukotriene modifiers, or theophylline. Persistence of poor control despite optimal therapy in patients with an atopic state and with an elevated IgE level may require the addition of the anti-IgE agent (omalizumab) [31].

4.3 Sleep Disorders

4.3.1 Sleep Deprivation and Attitudes Toward Sleep

Sleep loss usually indicates an average sleep duration of less than 7–8 h/night [32]. In that context, the Centers for Disease Control reports that 35.3 % of adults sleep less than 7 h on the average, without a significant difference between genders in that prevalence [33]. Moreover, a reported sleep duration of less than 6 h and 45 min was associated with a 94 % probability of falling asleep within 20 min on one or more of four nap opportunities in the setting of a multiple sleep latency testing [34].

Sleep deprivation affects the performance of men much more significantly than women. For instance, 5.8 % of men (compared to 3.5 % of women) reported nodding off while driving in the 30 days preceding a survey [33]. Similarly, sleep-deprived men perform worse than sleep-deprived women on vigilance, verbal, and visual tasks, and there is more sleep EEG activity in sleep-deprived men during rest and cognitive performance tests [35, 36]. Men are also at increased risk of falling asleep during a multiple sleep latency test [34].

In contrast, there is a stronger relationship between sleep deprivation and hypertension or diabetes in women relative to men [37, 38], perhaps in part because men appear to have a reduced muscle sympathetic nervous activity following total sleep deprivation which was not present in women [39].

Despite the loss of performance associated with sleep deprivations, sociologic studies indicate that men consider sleep as a necessity of the body which is pliable to some extent and linked to employment, as opposed to women's attitudes that sleep is viewed within the context of healthy behavior and a corporeal pleasure they would want [40, 41]. As such, men view sleep as something they need to suffer through for the demands of their body, with the need and duration of sleep assessed by how they felt and how they functioned the next day [40, 41].

4.3.2 Obstructive Sleep Apnea

Obstructive sleep apnea is common in men. The prevalence of undiagnosed sleep-disordered breathing (apnea-hypopnea index ≥ 5) was estimated to be as high as 24 % in middle-aged males (compared to 9 % in women) [42]. In cohort studies, the prevalence of sleep apnea syndrome (apnea-hypopnea index ≥ 5–10 in association with daytime sleepiness) was 4 % in men compared to 1–2 % in women [42, 43]. Severe sleep apnea with an index ≥ 50 events per hour is even more skewed toward men with an 8:1 male to female ratio [44].

Short-term consequences of obstructive sleep apnea include excessive daytime sleepiness and motor vehicular accidents, whereas long-term consequences include cardiovascular disease. Men with obstructive sleep apnea have significantly more sleepiness relative to women [45]. A progressive increase in the risk of motor vehicular accidents is seen with increase sleep apnea severity in men but not in women (though the amount of driving was not controlled in this study) [46].

The polysomnographic patterns of obstructive sleep apnea are also different in men compared to women, with women having milder sleep apnea in NREM and more common REM sleep apnea and men having more severe supine sleep apnea [44]. Obesity also affects men separately than women, with a greater variance in the apnea-hypopnea index being explained by neck circumference in women and by abdominal obesity in men [47].

There is also an association between obstructive sleep apnea and sleepiness, inflammatory markers (such as CRP and IL-6), and insulin resistance which is

Table 4.2 STOP-BANG questionnaire

1.	Do you *S*nore loudly (louder than talking or loud enough to be heard through closed doors)?
2.	Do you often feel *T*ired, fatigued, or sleepy during daytime?
3.	Has anyone *O*bserved you stop breathing during your sleep?
4.	Do you have or are you being treated for high blood *P*ressure?
5.	*B*MI more than 35 kg/m^2?
6.	*A*ge over 50 years?
7.	*N*eck circumference greater than 40 cm/16 in.?
8.	Male *G*ender?

Three or more "yes" answers have a 93 % sensitivity for detecting moderate OSA and a 100 % sensitivity for severe OSA. Adapted from [54]

stronger in males than in females [45]. There is a progressive increase in the odds ratio for hypertension with increasing apnea-hypopnea severity, with that association being stronger in males relative to females [48]. Other cardiovascular risk factors associated with obstructive sleep apnea such as endothelial and vascular function appear to be more prominent in women relative to men [49, 50].

These subtle differences in the cardiovascular risk factors between genders may explain differences in the cardiovascular outcomes. For instance, sleep-disordered breathing is associated with coronary artery disease in men aged 40–70 years [51, 52] and with incident heart failure in men but not in women [52]. In contrast, the association between obstructive sleep apnea and incident cardiovascular disease is most prominent for cerebrovascular disease in women [53].

There are numerous screening tools for the assessment of sleep apnea such as the STOP-BANG tool (Table 4.2), which includes male gender as a risk factor, being frequently used [54].

Of the interventions that can be given for obstructive sleep apnea, the best evidence for as association with a reduction in adverse cardiovascular outcomes is with positive airway therapy for both men [55] and women [53]. Otherwise, there are several options for the management of obstructive sleep apnea including oral appliances [56], oral pressure therapy [57], nasal expiratory positive pressure therapy [58], and upper airway stimulation therapy [59]. Specific benefits, indications, and efficacy of each of those nonsurgical interventions are shown in Table 4.3. Surgical options include maxillomandibular advancement, uvulopharyngopalatoplasty, laser-assisted uvulopalatoplasty, and radiofrequency ablation, but studies of those interventions consist mainly of case series rather than controlled trials, and further research is needed to define candidate patients and better assess the efficacy and safety of these interventions [60].

Table 4.3 Comparison of options for the management of obstructive sleep apnea

	Oral appliance	Nasal EPAP (Provent®)	Oral pressure (Winx®)	Upper airway pacer (Inspire®)	CPAP
Indication	Positional, mild to moderate	Positional, mild to severe	Mild to severe	Moderate to severe, difficulty with CPAP	Mild to severe
AHI reduction (%)	22	42.7	46	68	89
% success (AHI < 10 and/or ≥ 50 % reduction)	57–81	51	32	66	84.3
Adherence (%)	48–90	88.2	84	>99	46–79
Effects on blood pressure	At 3 years: improved BP systolic (−15 mmHg) and diastolic (−10 mmHg)	No difference in BP at 2 weeks compared to placebo	NA	NA	Improved BP even in resistant hypertension
Price	$100–600	$65/month	Comparable to CPAP	$30,000–40,000	$260–550

Adapted from [56–59]

AHI apnea-hypopnea index, *BP* blood pressure, *CPAP* continuous positive airway pressure, *EPAP* expiratory positive airway pressure, *NA* not available

4.3.3 Insomnia

Chronic insomnia may affect 30 % of individuals [61]. When the definition of insomnia includes persistence of symptoms for at least on month along with daytime impairment or distress, the prevalence is estimated to be about 13 % [62]. Of note, there has been a 13 % increase in office visits for insomnia between 1999 and 2010 and a 430 % increase in benzodiazepine receptor agonists over the same period [63]. About 40 % of subjects with insomnia have underlying psychiatric issues, of which depression is most common. Insomnia in men appears to be linked to lifestyle factors such as overweight, inactivity, and alcohol use but not to aging [64]. The consequence of insomnia includes motor vehicular or industrial accidents and absenteeism [61].

There is a clear increased risk of insomnia in women with a female to male risk ratio of 1.41 (95 % confidence interval: 1.28–1.55) [65]. However, in a large cohort of patients with 13–15 years of follow-up, insomnia was associated with a higher mortality in men relative to women (hazard ratio 4.7 vs. 1.9, respectively) particularly when associated with reduced total sleep time to <6.5 h [66].

Screening suggested tool: the insomnia severity index. This screening tool assesses both the nighttime and daytime components of insomnia (Table 4.4) [67].

Table 4.4 Insomnia severity index

For each question, please CIRCLE the number that best describes your answer.

Please rate the CURRENT (i.e. LAST 2 WEEKS) SEVERITY of your insomnia problem(s).

Insomnia problem	None	Mild	Moderate	Severe	Very severe
1. Difficulty falling asleep	0	1	2	3	4
2. Difficulty staying asleep	0	1	2	3	4
3. Problem waking up too early	0	1	2	3	4

4. How SATISFIED/DISSATISFIED are you with your CURRENT sleep pattern?

Very Satisfied	Satisfied	Moderately Satisfied	Dissatisfied	Very Dissatisfied
0	1	2	3	4

5. How NOTICEABLE to others do you think your sleep problem is in terms of impairing the quality of your life?

Not at all Noticeable	A Little	Somewhat	Much	Very Much Noticeable
0	1	2	3	4

6. How WORRIED/DISTRESSED are you about your current sleep problem?

Not at all Worried	A Little	Somewhat	Much	Very Much Worried
0	1	2	3	4

7. To what extent do you consider your sleep problem to INTERFERE with your daily functioning (e.g. daytime fatigue, mood, ability to function at work/daily chores, concentration, memory, mood, etc.) CURRENTLY?

Not at all Interfering	A Little	Somewhat	Much	Very Much Interfering
0	1	2	3	4

Guidelines for Scoring/Interpretation:

Add the scores for all seven items (questions 1 + 2 + 3 + 4 + 5 +6 + 7) = _____ your total score

Total score categories:

0–7 = No clinically significant insomnia
8–14 = Subthreshold insomnia
15–21 = Clinical insomnia (moderate severity)
22–28 = Clinical insomnia (severe)

Used with permission from Charles M. Morin, Ph.D., Université Laval, Quebec, Canada

Generally, treatment of insomnia can include hypnotics, sleep hygiene and stimulus control techniques (Table 4.5), and cognitive behavioral therapy. In an NIH statement, the treatment considered to be successful in the acute management of chronic insomnia has been benzodiazepine receptor agonists (including

Table 4.5 Sleep hygiene and stimulus control techniques

Before getting into bed:
– Establish a regular routine for bedtime.
– Create a positive sleep environment.
– Relax before getting into bed.
– Avoid alcohol, smoking, and caffeine for at least a few hours before bedtime.
– Do not go to bed unless you are sleepy.
While in bed:
– Turn your clock around (or cover it) and use your alarm if needed.
– If you cannot fall asleep in 20 min (based on your internal sense of time), get out of bed, and do something relaxing or boring (reading, listening to music, etc.). Return to bed only when sleepy.
– Use your bed only for sleep and sex.
In the morning and during the daytime:
– Wake up at the same time every morning, even on weekends.
– Avoid naps during the day.
– Avoid caffeinated beverages and food in the evening.
– Exercise regularly but not within 4 h of bedtime.

benzodiazepines and non-benzodiazepine agents that act on the benzodiazepine receptor) and cognitive behavioral therapy [68]. Other frequently used treatments include antidepressants (especially trazodone and doxepin), phenobarbiturates, antipsychotics (quetiapine and olanzapine), and over-the-counter aids (such as antihistamines, melatonin, herbal supplements such as valerian, and L-tryptophan). Although these agents may be effective in select individuals, the NIH statement cautions that "little is known about the comparative benefits of these treatment, their combination, and their effects on understudied features of chronic insomnia" [68].

In a study which compared the cognitive behavioral therapy with or without zolpidem, the strategic approach which resulted in the highest remission rates was a 6-week course of combined cognitive behavioral therapy with zolpidem followed by discontinuation of zolpidem during maintenance cognitive behavioral therapy [69]. Specifically, this combined approach resulted in a 6-month remission of 68 %, compared to 42 % in those who continued zolpidem during the cognitive behavioral therapy maintenance [69].

4.3.4 Restless Legs Syndrome

The clinical diagnostic criteria from the International RLS Study Group include four essential diagnostic features including an urge to move the legs along with uncomfortable sensation in the legs (paresthesias or dysesthesias), which begin or worsen during inactivity, are at least partially relieved by movement, and are worse in the evening or at night [70].

The prevalence of the restless legs syndrome is 5–15 % with a 2–3:1 predominance in women relative to men [71]. However, this gender difference may be at least in part due to pregnancy. For instance, pregnancy was reported to account for most of the gender difference in the prevalence of familial RLS, as well as that of

RLS in the general population [72, 73]. Moreover, the prevalence of RLS is similar in men and nulliparous women [73], and there is no gender difference in the prevalence of pediatric RLS [74].

There is no significant difference in health-related quality of life between genders in subjects with the restless legs syndrome [75]. However, men with the restless legs syndrome have a 39 % increased risk of mortality, even after correction for potentially confounding risk factors [76], and restless legs may be an early manifestation of Parkinson disease in men [77].

The American Academy of Sleep Medicine considers dopaminergic agonist such as ropinirole and pramipexole as standard therapy for the treatment of restless legs [78]. At the guideline level of recommendation is treatment with levodopa with dopa decarboxylase inhibitor, opioids, gabapentin enacarbil, and cabergoline [78]. At the option level of recommendation are carbamazepine, gabapentin, pregabalin, and clonidine [78]. Supplementation with iron is also considered an option for patients with ferritin levels under 50 ng/mL [78].

4.4   Conclusions

The above discussion highlights important gender differences in the prevalence, manifestations, and morbidity of various sleep and pulmonary conditions. Of some concern, the rising mortality from COPD does not track (at least not yet) with the overall declining prevalence of smoking in the United States. Worldwide, there has been a greater increase in male relative to female smokers. There are subtle differences in the manifestations and pathology of COPD, with men experiencing less dyspnea and their pathology showing more emphysema relative to women. About 40 % of patients with COPD may be undiagnosed, and an appropriate level of suspicion needs to be maintained to obtain a diagnostic spirometry. Lung cancer screening with a low-dose CT scan is an important tool to reduce lung cancer deaths in selected smokers or ex-smokers. Asthma prevalence is generally higher in postpubertal females, but mortality is higher in men for most age groups under 65 (and higher in women beyond 65). Sleep deprivation has a greater deleterious effect on the performance of men on various mental and vigilance tasks, but is associated with a greater risk of hypertension and diabetes in women. Sleep-disordered breathing such as obstructive sleep apnea is at least twice as common in men, and cardiovascular consequences appear to be different in men, in whom sleep-disordered breathing is associated with cardiovascular disease and heart failure experience, than in women who may experience a greater risk of cerebrovascular disease. A higher prevalence of insomnias and restless legs is noted in women, but the morbidity consequences disproportionately affect men.

References

1. Ng M, Freeman MK, Fleming TD, Robinson M, Dwyer-Lindgren L, Thomson B, Wollum A, Sanman E, Wulf S, Lopez AD, Murray CJ, Gakidou E. Smoking prevalence and cigarette consumption in 187 countries, 1980–2012. JAMA. 2014;311:183–92.

2. Murphy SL, Xu J, Kochanek KD. Deaths: final data for 2010. National Vital Statistics Reports 2013;61.
3. Centers for Disease Control and Prevention (CDC). Vital signs: current cigarette smoking among adults aged ≥18 Years—United States, 2009. MMWR Morb Mortal Wkly Rep. 2010;59:1135–40.
4. Agaku IT, King BA, Dube SR. Current cigarette smoking among adults – United States, 2005–2012. MMWR Morb Mortal Wkly Rep. 2014;63:29–34.
5. Cahill K, Stevens S, Lancaster T. Pharmacological treatments for smoking cessation. JAMA. 2014;311:193–4.
6. Cahill K, Stevens S, Perera R, Lancaster T. Pharmacological interventions for smoking cessation: an overview and network meta-analysis. Cochrane Database Syst Rev. 2013;5, CD009329.
7. Nides M, Glover ED, Reus VI, Christen AG, Make BJ, Billing Jr CB, Williams KE. Varenicline versus bupropion SR or placebo for smoking cessation: a pooled analysis. Am J Health Behav. 2008;32:664–75.
8. Scharf D, Shiffman S. Are there gender differences in smoking cessation, with and without bupropion? Pooled- and meta-analyses of clinical trials of Bupropion SR. Addiction. 2004;99:1462–9.
9. Walker N, Howe C, Glover M, McRobbie H, Barnes J, Nosa V, Parag V, Bassett B, Bullen C. Cytisine versus nicotine for smoking cessation. N Engl J Med. 2014;371:2353–62.
10. Bullen C, Howe C, Laugesen M, McRobbie H, Parag V, Williman J, Walker N. Electronic cigarettes for smoking cessation: a randomised controlled trial. Lancet. 2013;382:1629–37.
11. Grana R, Benowitz N, Glantz SA. E-cigarettes: a scientific review. Circulation. 2014;129:1972–86.
12. American Lung Association. Trends in COPD (Chronic Bronchitis and Emphysema): morbidity and mortality. 2013. http://www.lung.org/finding-cures/our-research/trend-reports/copd-trend-report.pdf. Accessed 17 Mar 2015.
13. Pride NB. Smoking cessation: effects on symptoms, spirometry and future trends in COPD. Thorax. 2001;56 Suppl 2:ii7–10.
14. Tessier JF, Nejjari C, Letenneur L, Filleul L, Marty ML, Barberger GP, Dartigues JF. Dyspnea and 8-year mortality among elderly men and women: the PAQUID cohort study. Eur J Epidemiol. 2001;17:223–9.
15. de Torres JP, Casanova C, de Montejo G, Aguirre-Jaime A, Celli BR. Gender and respiratory factors associated with dyspnea in chronic obstructive pulmonary disease. Respir Res. 2007;8:18.
16. Grydeland TB, Dirksen A, Coxson HO, Pillai SG, Sharma S, Eide GE, Gulsvik A, Bakke PS. Quantitative computed tomography: emphysema and airway wall thickness by sex, age and smoking. Eur Respir J. 2009;34:858–65.
17. Dransfield MT, Washko GR, Foreman MG, Estepar RS, Reilly J, Bailey WC. Gender differences in the severity of CT emphysema in COPD. Chest. 2007;132:464–70.
18. Martinez FJ, Curtis JL, Sciurba F, Mumford J, Giardino ND, Weinmann G, Kazerooni E, Murray S, Criner GJ, Sin DD, Hogg J, Ries AL, Han M, Fishman AP, Make B, Hoffman EA, Mohsenifar Z, Wise R. Sex differences in severe pulmonary emphysema. Am J Respir Crit Care Med. 2007;176:243–52.
19. Mannino DM, Gagnon RC, Petty TL, Lydick E. Obstructive lung disease and low lung function in adults in the United States: data from the National Health and Nutrition Examination Survey, 1988–1994. Arch Intern Med. 2000;160:1683–9.
20. Vestbo J, Hurd SS, Agusti AG, Jones PW, Vogelmeier C, Anzueto A, Barnes PJ, Fabbri LM, Martinez FJ, Nishimura M, Stockley RA, Sin DD, Rodriguez-Roisin R. Global strategy for the diagnosis, management, and prevention of chronic obstructive pulmonary disease: GOLD executive summary. Am J Respir Crit Care Med. 2013;187:347–65.
21. U.S. Preventive Services Task Force recommendation statement. Screening for chronic obstructive pulmonary disease using spirometry. Ann Intern Med. 2008;148:529–34.
22. Lin K, Watkins B, Johnson T, Rodriguez JA, Barton MB. Screening for chronic obstructive pulmonary disease using spirometry: summary of the evidence for the U.S. Preventive Services Task Force. Ann Intern Med. 2008;148:535–43.

23. Hardie JA, Buist AS, Vollmer WM, Ellingsen I, Bakke PS, Morkve O. Risk of over-diagnosis of COPD in asymptomatic elderly never-smokers. Eur Respir J. 2002;20:1117–22.
24. Aberle DR, Adams AM, Berg CD, Black WC, Clapp JD, Fagerstrom RM, Gareen IF, Gatsonis C, Marcus PM, Sicks JD. Reduced lung-cancer mortality with low-dose computed tomographic screening. N Engl J Med. 2011;365:395–409.
25. Moyer VA. Screening for lung cancer: U.S. Preventive Services Task Force recommendation statement. Ann Intern Med. 2014;160:330–8.
26. Bach PB, Mirkin JN, Oliver TK, Azzoli CG, Berry DA, Brawley OW, Byers T, Colditz GA, Gould MK, Jett JR, Sabichi AL, Smith-Bindman R, Wood DE, Qaseem A, Detterbeck FC. Benefits and harms of CT screening for lung cancer: a systematic review. JAMA. 2012;307:2418–29.
27. Patz Jr EF, Pinsky P, Gatsonis C, Sicks JD, Kramer BS, Tammemagi MC, Chiles C, Black WC, Aberle DR. Overdiagnosis in low-dose computed tomography screening for lung cancer. JAMA Intern Med. 2014;174:269–74.
28. American Lung Association. Trends in asthma morbidity and mortality. 2012. http://www.lung.org/finding-cures/our-research/trend-reports/asthma-trend-report.pdf. Accessed 17 Mar 2015.
29. Moorman JE, Rudd RA, Johnson CA, King M, Minor P, Bailey C, Scalia MR, Akinbami LJ. National surveillance for asthma–United States, 1980–2004. MMWR Surveill Summ. 2007;56:1–54.
30. Getahun D, Demissie K, Rhoads GG. Recent trends in asthma hospitalization and mortality in the United States. J Asthma. 2005;42:373–8.
31. National Asthma Education and Prevention Program. Guidelines for the diagnosis and management of asthma (EPR-3). Bethesda, MD, U.S. Department of Health and Human Services: National Institutes of Health; 2007.
32. Improving awareness, diagnosis, and treatment of sleep disorders. In: Colten HR, Altevogt BM, editors. Sleep disorders and sleep deprivation: an unmet public health problem. Washington, DC: National Academies Press (US); 2006. www.ncbi.nlm.nih.gov/books/NBK19963/. Accessed 17 Mar 2015.
33. Unhealthy sleep-related behaviors–12 States, 2009. MMWR Morb Mortal Wkly Rep. 2011;60:233–8.
34. Punjabi NM, Bandeen-Roche K, Young T. Predictors of objective sleep tendency in the general population. Sleep. 2003;26:678–83.
35. Corsi-Cabrera M, Sanchez AI, Rio-Portilla Y, Villanueva Y, Perez-Garci E. Effect of 38 h of total sleep deprivation on the waking EEG in women: sex differences. Int J Psychophysiol. 2003;50:213–24.
36. Binks PG, Waters WF, Hurry M. Short-term total sleep deprivations does not selectively impair higher cortical functioning. Sleep. 1999;22:328–34.
37. Cappuccio FP, Stranges S, Kandala NB, Miller MA, Taggart FM, Kumari M, Ferrie JE, Shipley MJ, Brunner EJ, Marmot MG. Gender-specific associations of short sleep duration with prevalent and incident hypertension: the Whitehall II Study. Hypertension. 2007;50:693–700.
38. Suarez EC. Self-reported symptoms of sleep disturbance and inflammation, coagulation, insulin resistance and psychosocial distress: evidence for gender disparity. Brain Behav Immun. 2008;22:960–8.
39. Carter JR, Durocher JJ, Larson RA, DellaValla JP, Yang H. Sympathetic neural responses to 24-hour sleep deprivation in humans: sex differences. Am J Physiol Heart Circ Physiol. 2012;302:H1991–7.
40. Venn S, Meadows R, Arber S. Gender differences in approaches to self-management of poor sleep in later life. Soc Sci Med. 2013;79:117–23.
41. Meadows R, Arber S, Venn S, Hislop J. Engaging with sleep: male definitions, understandings and attitudes. Sociol Health Illn. 2008;30:696–710.
42. Young T, Palta M, Dempsey J, Skatrud J, Weber S, Badr S. The occurrence of sleep-disordered breathing among middle-aged adults. N Engl J Med. 1993;328:1230–5.

43. Bixler EO, Vgontzas AN, Lin HM, Ten Have T, Rein J, Vela-Bueno A, Kales A. Prevalence of sleep-disordered breathing in women: effects of gender. Am J Respir Crit Care Med. 2001;163:608–13.
44. O'Connor C, Thornley KS, Hanly PJ. Gender differences in the polysomnographic features of obstructive sleep apnea. Am J Respir Crit Care Med. 2000;161:1465–72.
45. Kritikou I, Basta M, Vgontzas AN, Pejovic S, Liao D, Tsaoussoglou M, Bixler EO, Stefanakis Z, Chrousos GP. Sleep apnoea, sleepiness, inflammation and insulin resistance in middle-aged males and females. Eur Respir J. 2014;43:145–55.
46. Ward KL, Hillman DR, James A, Bremner AP, Simpson L, Cooper MN, Palmer LJ, Fedson AC, Mukherjee S. Excessive daytime sleepiness increases the risk of motor vehicle crash in obstructive sleep apnea. J Clin Sleep Med. 2013;9:1013–21.
47. Simpson L, Mukherjee S, Cooper MN, Ward KL, Lee JD, Fedson AC, Potter J, Hillman DR, Eastwood P, Palmer LJ, Kirkness J. Sex differences in the association of regional fat distribution with the severity of obstructive sleep apnea. Sleep. 2010;33:467–74.
48. Hedner J, Bengtsson-Bostrom K, Peker Y, Grote L, Rastam L, Lindblad U. Hypertension prevalence in obstructive sleep apnoea and sex: a population-based case-control study. Eur Respir J. 2006;27:564–70.
49. Faulx MD, Larkin EK, Hoit BD, Aylor JE, Wright AT, Redline S. Sex influences endothelial function in sleep-disordered breathing. Sleep. 2004;27:1113–20.
50. Randby A, Namtvedt SK, Hrubos-Strom H, Einvik G, Somers VK, Omland T. Sex-dependent impact of OSA on digital vascular function. Chest. 2013;144:915–22.
51. Punjabi NM, Caffo BS, Goodwin JL, Gottlieb DJ, Newman AB, O'Connor GT, Rapoport DM, Redline S, Resnick HE, Robbins JA, Shahar E, Unruh ML, Samet JM. Sleep-disordered breathing and mortality: a prospective cohort study. PLoS Med. 2009;6:e1000132.
52. Gottlieb DJ, Yenokyan G, Newman AB, O'Connor GT, Punjabi NM, Quan SF, Redline S, Resnick HE, Tong EK, Diener-West M, Shahar E. Prospective study of obstructive sleep apnea and incident coronary heart disease and heart failure: the sleep heart health study. Circulation. 2010;122:352–60.
53. Campos-Rodriguez F, Martinez-Garcia MA, Reyes-Nunez N, Caballero-Martinez I, Catalan-Serra P, Almeida-Gonzalez CV. Role of sleep apnea and continuous positive airway pressure therapy in the incidence of stroke or coronary heart disease in women. Am J Respir Crit Care Med. 2014;189:1544–50.
54. Chung F, Yegneswaran B, Liao P, Chung SA, Vairavanathan S, Islam S, Khajehdehi A, Shapiro CM. STOP questionnaire: a tool to screen patients for obstructive sleep apnea. Anesthesiology. 2008;108:812–21.
55. Marin JM, Carrizo SJ, Vicente E, Agusti AG. Long-term cardiovascular outcomes in men with obstructive sleep apnoea-hypopnoea with or without treatment with continuous positive airway pressure: an observational study. Lancet. 2005;365:1046–53.
56. Ferguson KA, Cartwright R, Rogers R, Schmidt-Nowara W. Oral appliances for snoring and obstructive sleep apnea: a review. Sleep. 2006;29:244–62.
57. Colrain IM, Black J, Siegel LC, Bogan RK, Becker PM, Farid-Moayer M, Goldberg R, Lankford DA, Goldberg AN, Malhotra A. A multicenter evaluation of oral pressure therapy for the treatment of obstructive sleep apnea. Sleep Med. 2013;14:830–7.
58. Berry RB, Kryger MH, Massie CA. A novel nasal expiratory positive airway pressure (EPAP) device for the treatment of obstructive sleep apnea: a randomized controlled trial. Sleep. 2011;34:479–85.
59. Strollo Jr PJ, Soose RJ, Maurer JT, de Vries N, Cornelius J, Froymovich O, Hanson RD, Padhya TA, Steward DL, Gillespie MB, Woodson BT, Van de Heyning PH, Goetting MG, Vanderveken OM, Feldman N, Knaack L, Strohl KP. Upper-airway stimulation for obstructive sleep apnea. N Engl J Med. 2014;370:139–49.
60. Caples SM, Rowley JA, Prinsell JR, Pallanch JF, Elamin MB, Katz SG, Harwick JD. Surgical modifications of the upper airway for obstructive sleep apnea in adults: a systematic review and meta-analysis. Sleep. 2010;33:1396–407.

61. Roth T. Insomnia: definition, prevalence, etiology, and consequences. J Clin Sleep Med. 2007;3:S7–10.
62. Ohayon MM. Prevalence of DSM-IV diagnostic criteria of insomnia: distinguishing insomnia related to mental disorders from sleep disorders. J Psychiatr Res. 1997;31:333–46.
63. Ford ES, Wheaton AG, Cunningham TJ, Giles WH, Chapman DP, Croft JB. Trends in outpatient visits for insomnia, sleep apnea, and prescriptions for sleep medications among US adults: findings from the National Ambulatory Medical Care survey 1999–2010. Sleep. 2014;37:1283–93.
64. Janson C, Lindberg E, Gislason T, Elmasry A, Boman G. Insomnia in men–a 10-year prospective population based study. Sleep. 2001;24:425–30.
65. Zhang B, Wing YK. Sex differences in insomnia: a meta-analysis. Sleep. 2006;29:85–93.
66. Sivertsen B, Pallesen S, Glozier N, Bjorvatn B, Salo P, Tell GS, Ursin R, Overland S. Midlife insomnia and subsequent mortality: the Hordaland health study. BMC Public Health. 2014;14:720.
67. Bastien CH, Vallieres A, Morin CM. Validation of the Insomnia Severity Index as an outcome measure for insomnia research. Sleep Med. 2001;2:297–307.
68. National Institutes of Health. National Institutes of Health State of the Science Conference statement on Manifestations and Management of Chronic Insomnia in Adults, June 13–15, 2005. Sleep 2005;28:1049–57.
69. Morin CM, Vallieres A, Guay B, Ivers H, Savard J, Merette C, Bastien C, Baillargeon L. Cognitive behavioral therapy, singly and combined with medication, for persistent insomnia: a randomized controlled trial. JAMA. 2009;301:2005–15.
70. Allen RP, Picchietti D, Hening WA, Trenkwalder C, Walters AS, Montplaisi J. Restless legs syndrome: diagnostic criteria, special considerations, and epidemiology. A report from the restless legs syndrome diagnosis and epidemiology workshop at the National Institutes of Health. Sleep Med. 2003;4:101–19.
71. Manconi M, Ulfberg J, Berger K, Ghorayeb I, Wesstrom J, Fulda S, Allen RP, Pollmacher T. When gender matters: restless legs syndrome. Report of the "RLS and woman" workshop endorsed by the European RLS Study Group. Sleep Med Rev. 2012;16:297–307.
72. Pantaleo NP, Hening WA, Allen RP, Earley CJ. Pregnancy accounts for most of the gender difference in prevalence of familial RLS. Sleep Med. 2010;11:310–3.
73. Berger K, Luedemann J, Trenkwalder C, John U, Kessler C. Sex and the risk of restless legs syndrome in the general population. Arch Intern Med. 2004;164:196–202.
74. Picchietti D, Allen RP, Walters AS, Davidson JE, Myers A, Ferini-Strambi L. Restless legs syndrome: prevalence and impact in children and adolescents–the Peds REST study. Pediatrics. 2007;120:253–66.
75. Happe S, Reese JP, Stiasny-Kolster K, Peglau I, Mayer G, Klotsche J, Giani G, Geraedts M, Trenkwalder C, Dodel R. Assessing health-related quality of life in patients with restless legs syndrome. Sleep Med. 2009;10:295–305.
76. Li Y, Wang W, Winkelman JW, Malhotra A, Ma J, Gao X. Prospective study of restless legs syndrome and mortality among men. Neurology. 2013;81:52–9.
77. Wong JC, Li Y, Schwarzschild MA, Ascherio A, Gao X. Restless legs syndrome: an early clinical feature of Parkinson disease in men. Sleep. 2014;37:369–72.
78. Aurora RN, Kristo DA, Bista SR, Rowley JA, Zak RS, Casey KR, Lamm CI, Tracy SL, Rosenberg RS. The treatment of restless legs syndrome and periodic limb movement disorder in adults–an update for 2012: practice parameters with an evidence-based systematic review and meta-analyses: an American Academy of Sleep Medicine Clinical Practice Guideline. Sleep. 2012;35:1039–62.

His Upper GI Tract

5

Lyen C. Huang and Dan E. Azagury

5.1 Introduction

The upper gastrointestinal (GI) tract extends from the mouth to the esophagus and then down through the stomach to the duodenum and ends at the terminal ileum. Problems in the upper GI tract are a common source of patient complaints. In the United States, 45 % of respondents to one survey reported one or more upper GI symptoms in the previous 3 months [1]. Among men, the most common symptoms are heartburn, dysphagia, early satiety, and bloating (in descending order). These symptoms are associated with significant impact in terms of both missed work and leisure days as well as physician visits [1, 2].

Patients often present with a combination of symptoms which can make diagnosis difficult. Careful history taking is key in determining where to start the diagnostic workup and initial therapeutic treatments. It is important to note whether these symptoms are acute or chronic and how they relate to food ingestion and time of day. Dietary habits, alleviating (or worsening) factors, current medications and supplements, and the patient's previous surgical history are also critical.

Since there is no shortage of disease-specific resources available in textbooks and online, we organized this chapter by common presenting symptoms. We broke down the symptoms into five broad categories: heartburn and reflux, upper abdominal pain and discomfort, esophageal dysphagia, chronic nausea and vomiting, and bleeding. Within each category, we discuss common diseases, suggest initial

L.C. Huang, M.D., M.P.H.
Department of Surgery, Stanford University School of Medicine,
300 Pasteur Drive, Stanford, 300 Pasteur Drive, H3680A, Stanford,
CA 94305, USA
e-mail: lyenh@stanford.edu

D.E. Azagury, M.D. (✉)
Assistant Professor of Surgery, Stanford University School of Medicine,
300 Pasteur Drive, Stanford, CA 94305, USA
e-mail: dazagury@stanford.edu

© Springer Science+Business Media New York 2016
J.M. Potts (ed.), *Men's Health*, DOI 10.1007/978-1-4939-3237-5_5

diagnostic studies and therapies, note important risk factors, and review potential reasons for specialist referrals. Keep in mind that many patients will have symptoms from more than one category, so the workup needs to be tailored to individual cases.

5.2   Heartburn and Reflux

Heartburn (defined as burning chest pain occurring after eating) and regurgitation (the presence of refluxed gastric contents and acid into the mouth or hypopharynx) are among some of the most common problems reported by patients. While an initial diagnosis of gastroesophageal reflux disease (GERD) is often appropriate, non-GI etiologies should always be assessed and ruled out first. Specifically, causes such as angina often carry similar risk factors and patient profiles as GERD (e.g., obesity).

5.2.1   Gastroesophageal Reflux Disease

GERD is a chronic disorder that occurs when acid (or other GI contents, such as bile) flows backward into the esophagus. While a small amount of reflux is normal, heartburn is considered troublesome when mild symptoms occur two or more times per week or severe symptoms occur at least once per week [3]. Surveys of Western countries suggest that 8–27 % of the population experience heartburn or acid regurgitation on a weekly basis, and nearly half of these individuals have been suffering from these symptoms for 5 or more years [4]. Asian countries seem to have a lower prevalence ranging from 3 to 5 %.

While the most common symptoms of GERD are heartburn and regurgitation, other presenting symptoms may include chest pain, globus (the perception of a lump in the throat not related to swallowing), nausea, nighttime or chronic cough, hoarseness, or bitter or sour tastes in the morning. The diagnosis of GERD is usually clinical though the same symptoms are also seen in diseases such as esophagitis, peptic ulcer disease, biliary tract disease, coronary artery disease, and esophageal dysmotility disorders.

When the diagnosis of GERD is suspected, it is reasonable to start acid suppression treatment with an H2 blocker or a proton pump inhibitor (PPI). Patients can also be encouraged and counseled on weight loss (if overweight or obese), elevating the head of the bed to minimize nighttime symptoms, and eating meals 2–3 h before bedtime. Dietary experimentation can also be helpful.

Keep in mind that improvement of symptoms after starting treatment does not definitively make the diagnosis. About half of patients without GERD (as confirmed by endoscopy and other testing) will still improve on PPI treatment [5]. Clinical suspicion for other diseases and the presence of alarm symptoms or risk factors should generally prompt further workup. Some indications for further testing (generally starting with upper endoscopy) are listed in Table 5.1.

Table 5.1 Indications for upper endoscopy [6]

• Failure of twice-daily H2/PPI treatment after 4–8 weeks
• Alarm symptoms
– Pain with swallowing or difficulty swallowing
– Bleeding
– Anemia
– Involuntary weight loss or weight loss >10 %
– Previous upper GI malignancy
– Previously documented peptic ulcer disease
– Lymphadenopathy
– Abdominal mass
• History of erosive esophagitis
• Men >50 years old with one of the following:
– GERD symptoms for 5 or more years
– Risk factors of Barrett's esophagus and esophageal adenocarcinoma
Nocturnal reflux
Hiatal hernia
Overweight or obese
Tobacco use
Intra-abdominal distribution of fat

Ambulatory 24-h pH monitoring is typically used in the setting of normal or equivocal endoscopic findings with refractory reflux symptoms to confirm diagnosis. A barium swallow and a manometry study will often be requested prior to a surgical procedure and are useful to assess anatomy and/or contraindications to anti-reflux surgery.

Since the development of acid suppression therapy, the number of operations performed for GERD has decreased dramatically. Nonetheless, anti-reflux operations can be a very effective treatment, particularly for medically refractory GERD. Other indications for anti-reflux surgery are listed in Table 5.2. Endoscopic therapies and minimally invasive surgical therapies offer a good alternative for patients who fail to respond to PPI therapy. Laparoscopic fundoplication surgery remains the gold standard of these therapies. In this operation, the stomach is mobilized and wrapped around the esophagus to reinforce the lower esophageal sphincter (Fig. 5.1) [8]. It provides long-standing symptom relief with very low complication rates and short hospital stays (typically 1–3 days). Surgery can often be very durable up to 20 years after the initial operation, though a small subset of patients will still require acid suppression therapy or surgical revision [9]. Because of the association between obesity and reflux, morbidly obese patients will often suffer from GERD. These patients should be referred to a bariatric surgeon as laparoscopic Roux-en-Y gastric bypass is very effective in reducing GERD symptoms in conjunction with significant and long-lasting weight loss [10–12].

Table 5.2 Indications for anti-reflux surgery [7]

• Failed medical management
– Inadequate symptom control
– Severe regurgitation not controlled with acid suppression
– Medication side effects
• Opt for surgery despite successful medical management
– Quality of life
– Lifelong need for medication intake
– Expense of medications
• Complications of GERD
– Severe esophagitis
– Barrett's esophagus[a]
• Extra-esophageal manifestations
– Asthma
– Hoarseness
– Cough
– Chest pain
– Aspiration

[a]Strong indication when symptomatic. However, while patients with asymptomatic Barrett's reportedly regress to a greater degree after surgery, there is no reduction in esophageal adenocarcinoma rates

5.3   Upper Abdominal Pain or Discomfort

Chronic or recurrent upper abdominal (epigastric) pain or discomfort is referred to as dyspepsia. It is often accompanied by other symptoms such as heartburn, reflux, early satiety, a sensation of fullness, bloating, belching, and nausea [13]. The most common organic causes of dyspepsia are peptic ulcer disease, GERD, gastric malignancy, and nonsteroidal anti-inflammatory drug (NSAID)-induced dyspepsia. However, the diagnostic workup for dyspepsia is often negative for any identifiable diseases leading to functional or idiopathic dyspepsia as a diagnosis of exclusion.

In patients younger than 55 years old without alarm symptoms or other risk factors (Table 5.1), it is reasonable to begin with either empiric PPI treatment or *Helicobacter pylori* testing. The latter is preferred in areas where the prevalence of *H. pylori* is greater than 10 % [13]. Starting with either of these approaches appears to be equally cost effective [14]. Treatment failure, age > 55, or alarm symptoms all warrant an upper endoscopy.

5.3.1   Peptic Ulcer Disease

Peptic ulcer disease (PUD) encompasses ulcers occurring in either the stomach or the duodenum. Pain from these ulcers is often described as burning or gnawing hunger. Classical teaching describes gastric ulcer pain occurring shortly after

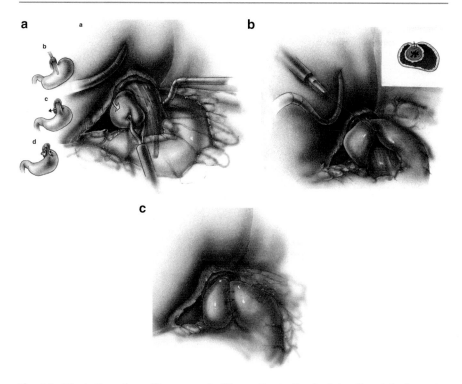

Fig. 5.1 Illustrations from "Laparoscopic Nissen Fundoplication" in *Chassin's Operative Strategy in General Surgery*, 2013, pp. 203–213, Ed. Carol E.H. Scott-Conner. With permission of Springer Science + Business Media. (**a**) In a Nissen fundoplication, the mobilized stomach is brought behind the esophagus. (**b**) Sutures are then used to bring the fundus over the esophagus. The fundoplication should come together without any tension. At least one of the sutures will also incorporate the muscular layer of the esophagus to fix the fundoplication in place. (**c**) The completed fundoplication should be loose enough to allow an instrument to be passed between the wrap and the esophagus. Overly tight wraps can lead to dysphagia

meals, whereas duodenal ulcer pain occurs several hours afterward due to acid secretion in the absence of food. Practically speaking however, once PUD is suspected, then upper endoscopy will confirm or rule out the diagnosis and allow biopsies to be taken for *H. pylori* and malignancy testing. Examples of normal endoscopic anatomy are shown in Fig. 5.2 [15], while benign and malignant ulcers are shown in Fig. 5.3 [16, 17].

The goal of medical management is to heal the ulcer and to treat *H. pylori* if present. Eradication of *H. pylori* reduces ulcer recurrence and complications, although up to 20 % of patients will develop recurrent ulcers [18]. Traditional "triple" therapy with a PPI (twice-daily dosing except for esomeprazole which is once daily), amoxicillin (1 g twice daily), and clarithromycin (500 mg twice daily) for 10–14 days is the recommended first-line treatment for most patients [19, 20]. Metronidazole (500 mg twice daily) can be substituted for amoxicillin in patients with penicillin allergies. However, resistance levels to clarithromycin appear to be rising in many

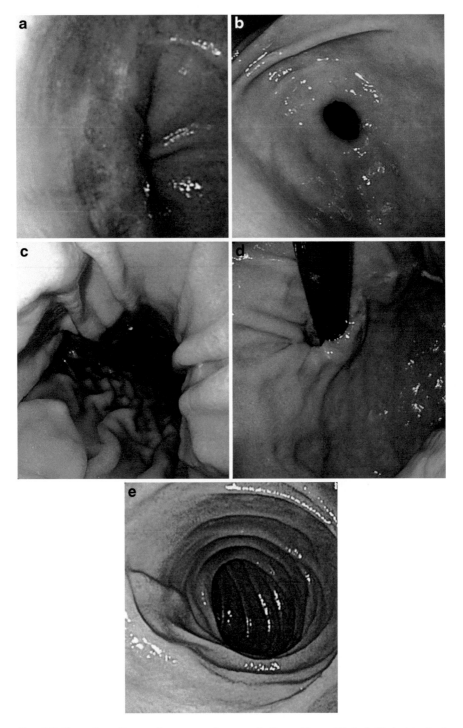

Fig. 5.2 Examples of normal upper endoscopy findings. From Clinical Gastrointestinal Endoscopy: A Comprehensive Atlas, 2014, ed. Hoon Jai Chun, Suk-Kyun Yang, Myung-Gyu Choi. With permission of Springer Science + Business Media. (**a**) Normal gastroesophageal junction. (**b**) Antrum and pylorus. (**c**) Body of the stomach. (**d**) Retroflex view of the cardia. (**e**) Second portion of the duodenum

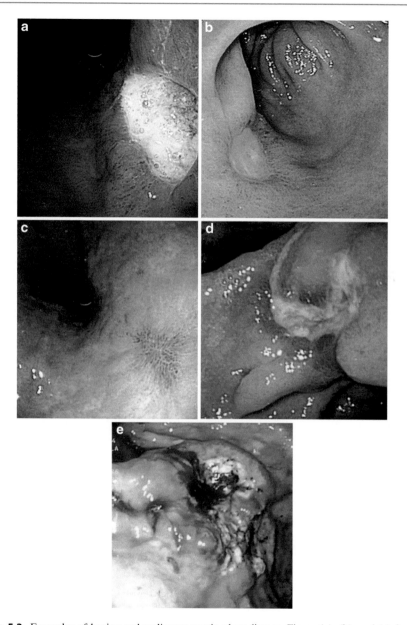

Fig. 5.3 Examples of benign and malignant peptic ulcer disease. Figure (**a**), (**b**), and (**c**) from Clinical Gastrointestinal Endoscopy: A Comprehensive Atlas, 2014, ed. Hoon Jai Chun, Suk-Kyun Yang, Myung-Gyu Choi. With Permission of Springer Science + Business Media. Figure (**d**) and (**e**) from Gastric Cancer, Follow-up endoscopy for benign-appearing gastric ulcers has no additive value in detecting malignancy, 2014, Gielisse EAR, Kuyvenhoven JP, Fig. 1c, d. With permission from the Japanese Gastric Cancer Association, Dr. Eric Gielisse, and Springer Science + Business Media. (**a**) Benign well-circumscribed and deep penetrating ulcer. (**b**) Benign ulcer with a clean base and a regular shape without exudate. (**c**) Well-healed ulcer. (**d**) A 15-mm malignant ulcer with a clean base but an irregular border. (**e**) A 3-cm malignant ulcer with a dirty base as well as an elevated and irregular border

countries leading to treatment failure. In these high-resistance areas or with patients who have failed previous therapy, "quadruple" therapy with a PPI, metronidazole 250 mg and tetracycline 500 mg four times daily, and bismuth (525 mg four times daily) is the recommended regimen. Alternatively, a levofloxacin-based "triple" therapy consisting of a PPI, amoxicillin (1 g twice daily), and levofloxacin (500 mg once daily) can be used.

H. pylori eradication should be confirmed using urea breath testing or stool antigen testing [20]. Patients should also stop NSAID use, alcohol intake, and smoking if possible. For uncomplicated duodenal ulcers, PPI treatment for 4 weeks is usually sufficient and no further testing is necessary [21]. Gastric ulcers should be treated with 8 weeks of PPIs; refractory ulcers should generally receive a twice-daily regimen for another 6–8 weeks. Long-term maintenance therapy with PPIs is generally reserved for high-risk patients with a history of complications (e.g., bleeding, perforation, gastric outlet obstruction) and recurrent or refractory ulcers and those with giant or fibrosed ulcers [20].

The role of follow-up endoscopy in documenting ulcer resolution and allowing for repeat biopsies of concerning lesions remains under some debate. For lesions with equivocal or concerning histology, repeat endoscopy is indicated. However, for patients with initially benign-appearing ulcers (both in endoscopic appearance and histological examination), the rate of malignancy found on follow-up endoscopy is 0–4 % [17, 22, 23]. While earlier detection of cancer may confer some survival benefit, the magnitude of that benefit is not yet well known and follow-up endoscopy is probably not cost effective [23, 24]. Nonetheless, overutilization of follow-up endoscopy, particularly in low-risk patients, appears to be common [25].

Refractory or recurrent ulcers can occur for a wide variety of reasons including persistent *H. pylori* infection, NSAID use, underlying malignancy, or acid hypersecretion (e.g., Zollinger-Ellison syndrome). Identifying and treating the underlying etiology is important to prevent life-threatening complications such as bleeding, perforation, and obstruction [26]. The overall mortality from PUD complications has decreased over time, but is still 3 % for those requiring hospitalization and 11 % for patients undergoing surgery.

If medical therapy is not effective or there is concern about malignancy or the development of complications such as gastric outlet obstruction, then referral to a surgeon is warranted. Surgical options include decreasing acid secretion through vagotomies, removal of the acid-secretion portion of the stomach, excision of ulcers, and gastric drainage procedures to improve emptying.

5.3.2 Biliary Tract Disease

Gallstones are found in approximately 8–10 % of men in the United States and Europe, although that number can be as high as 30 % in certain communities [27]. Most patients are asymptomatic and will not require treatment. The most common symptom is epigastric pain lasting for at least 30 min [28]. Contrary to the classic description of biliary colic, the pain is often steady and constant. Atypical symptoms such as chest pain, belching, early satiety, bloating, burning epigastric or chest pain, and nausea and vomiting may also be seen in patients with gallstones [28].

Patients with symptomatic cholelithiasis will often have an unremarkable physical examination and laboratory tests. The presence of a Murphy's sign (pain on deep inspiration while palpating just below the liver edge) is concerning for cholecystitis. In the presence of fevers, chills, and/or leukocytosis, acute cholecystitis should be considered, and the patient should be referred urgently to the emergency department and a surgeon.

Other diagnoses that should be considered include choledocholithiasis, sphincter of Oddi dysfunction, functional gallbladder disorders (biliary pain in the absence of stones or sludge), GERD, PUD, hepatitis, esophageal disorders, ischemic heart disease, pancreatitis, irritable bowel syndrome, and urinary tract infections or stones. In general, abnormal liver or pancreatic tests in the presence of gallstones should prompt a rapid referral for further evaluation.

The most sensitive and specific test for biliary tract disease is a right upper quadrant ultrasound. If the study is negative but gallstones are still suspected, then a repeat ultrasound after several weeks is reasonable. If both ultrasound studies are negative, then referral to specialists is advisable. Further tests may include upper endoscopy, endoscopic ultrasound, endoscopic retrograde cholangiopancreatography (ERCP), cholescintigraphy (99mTc-hepato-iminodiacetic acid or "HIDA" scans), and esophageal manometry.

Asymptomatic patients with gallstones do not need a prophylactic cholecystectomy as most will not develop symptoms [29]. However, those with symptoms should undergo cholecystectomy because the risk of recurrent symptoms is 30–50 %. Outpatient laparoscopic cholecystectomy is well tolerated by most patients with low rates of serious complications. Cost-effectiveness studies suggest that medical management is actually associated with increased cost and patient disability, added ERCP procedures, and the possible development of gallbladder cancer [30].

Medical management with ursodiol (ursodeoxycholic acid) remains an uncommon treatment for gallstones. It can be an option in select patients with mild or infrequent episodes of biliary pain, biliary sludge or cholesterol gallstones <20 mm in diameter, and a patent cystic duct [31]. In this population, 90 % will have complete dissolution of small stones after 6 months of treatment [32]. The recommended treatment dose is 8–10 mg/kg/day taken at bedtime [31]. Patients should undergo a follow-up ultrasound after 6–12 months of treatment. Patients who have minimal to no decrease in stone size will most likely never dissolve their stones. Once the stones or sludge disappear on ultrasound, patients can transition to low-dose maintenance therapy of 300 mg/day. Maintenance therapy decreases the recurrence of gallstones and future complications such as gallstone pancreatitis [33, 34]. However, medical treatment requires significant patient compliance and is burdened by an extremely high recurrence rate: nearly half of these patients will develop gallstones again after 5 years and up to three-quarters at 12 years [35].

5.4   Esophageal Dysphagia

Esophageal dysphagia (difficulty swallowing) is an alarm symptom which should prompt a careful workup. Unlike oropharyngeal disorders which typically result in symptoms immediately upon food intake, esophageal disorders generally occur a few seconds after swallowing. Patients will often describe a sensation of having food stuck in their chest behind the sternum. The types of foods that cause the dysphagia can help narrow the list of possible diagnoses. Patients reporting problems with both liquids and solids initially are more likely to have an esophageal dysmotility disorder, whereas progressive dysphagia starting with solids and then later with liquids is consistent with mechanical obstruction. Other important questions to ask include whether the patient has a history of radiation therapy to the head and/or neck, smoking or alcohol use, dry mouth or eyes, referred pain, changes in speech, halitosis, food regurgitation, or pain with swallowing.

The workup for esophageal dysphagia generally begins with upper endoscopy [36]. However, if there is a suspicion for a proximal disorder (e.g., Zenker's diverticulum or previous radiation therapy to the neck), a barium swallow can help map out the anatomy. Treatment will vary with the diagnosis, but generally requires consultation with specialists.

5.4.1   Mechanical Obstruction

Mechanical obstruction of the esophagus can be caused by problems within the esophagus or by external compression. The most common disorder is food bolus impaction which is typically seen in the elderly or those with peptic strictures. However, there is an increasing association over time between food bolus impaction and eosinophilic esophagitis (EoE) [37]. EoE is an allergic inflammatory disorder which most commonly presents as dysphagia in adults [38]. First-line treatment starts with dietary modification to identify and avoid inciting allergens and topical corticosteroids.

Benign esophageal strictures can also obstruct the passage of food. They are most commonly associated with GERD, and in these patients, PPI treatment can improve the dysphagia symptoms and decreases the need for repeat balloon dilation [39]. Strictures can also be due to pills, radiation, infection, or lymphocytic esophagitis.

Another source of obstructions is esophageal rings and webs [36]. Esophageal rings are either mucosal (most common) or muscular rings located in the distal esophagus. Esophageal webs are thin mucosal webs commonly found in the cervical esophagus. Barium esophagrams are more sensitive than endoscopy in diagnosing both and treatment is typically esophageal balloon dilation.

Finally, both benign and malignant masses of the esophagus and stomach can obstruct the passage of food. In North America and Europe, the most common esophageal malignancy is adenocarcinoma, whereas squamous cell carcinoma is the predominant malignancy in the rest of the world [40]. The major risk factors for adenocarcinoma are GERD, smoking, and obesity. Alcohol, especially in conjunction with smoking, is the major risk factor for squamous cell carcinoma.

5.4.2 Esophageal Dysmotility

When a dysmotility disorder is suspected or if the upper endoscopy and barium fluoroscopy are unrevealing, the test of choice is esophageal manometry. Some disorders such as achalasia or diffuse esophageal spasm have associated radiological findings ("bird's beak" and "corkscrew," respectively). However, not all patients have the typical radiological findings, and manometry is still needed to establish the diagnosis. Novel therapies such as peroral endoscopic myotomy (POEM) for achalasia can now be performed completely endoscopically with extremely effective functional results [41].

Esophageal dysmotility can also be due to systemic diseases such as scleroderma, systemic lupus erythematosus, rheumatoid arthritis, or mixed connective-tissue disorders [42]. Other disorders to consider include Chagas' disease, chronic idiopathic intestinal pseudo-obstruction, diabetes mellitus, amyloidosis, alcoholism, and multiple sclerosis.

5.4.3 Functional Dysphagia

In order for a patient to be diagnosed with a functional dysphagia, symptoms must persist for at least 3 months, and the symptoms should be present at least 6 months before the diagnosis is made [43]. In addition, GERD, esophageal dysmotility, and structural and metabolic disorders must be excluded.

5.5 Chronic Nausea and Vomiting

Nausea (the feeling of sickness marked by an urge to vomit) and vomiting (the expulsion of stomach contents through the mouth) are caused by a variety of disorders. This section will focus on chronic nausea and vomiting as most acute episodes are self-limiting (e.g., gastroenteritis), easily treated by stopping the inciting cause (e.g., medications), or controllable with anti-nausea medications. The diagnostic workup for chronic disorders should take place in parallel with treatment of the complications and sequela of nausea and vomiting [44]. Patients with chronic vomiting may be dehydrated or have electrolyte imbalances and acid-base disturbances. While there are a wide variety of disorders which cause nausea and vomiting, questions regarding the onset and timing of symptoms, the characteristics of the vomitus, the presence or absence of associated abdominal pain, and other associated symptoms and findings can help elucidate the diagnosis (see Table 5.3) [45].

Upper endoscopy is generally the first step in diagnosing chronic nausea and vomiting. Other tests to consider include CT scans or upper GI fluoroscopy, endocrine workup, gastric motility studies, and a psychological evaluation. A negative workup after these studies suggests a functional disorder.

Table 5.3 A partial list of etiologies causing chronic nausea and vomiting

Type	Diagnoses
Gastrointestinal	GERD
	PUD
	Biliary tract disease
	Irritable bowel syndrome
	Hepatitis
	Pancreatic disease
	Irritable bowel syndrome
	Inflammatory bowel disease
	Chronic intestinal pseudo-obstruction
Obstructive	Esophageal disorders
	Malignancy
	Volvulus
Decreased gastric emptying	Gastroparesis
	Gastric outlet obstruction
	Malignancy
Medications	Antibiotics
	Opioids
	Chemotherapy
	Antiarrhythmics
	Anticonvulsants
Neurogenic	Intracranial neoplasm
	Head injury
	Stroke
	Infection
	Migraines
	Seizures
	Vestibular disease
Psychiatric	Anxiety
	Depression
	Conversion disorder

Adapted from Scorza et al. [45]

5.5.1 Gastroparesis

Gastroparesis is delayed gastric emptying in the absence of mechanical obstruction. The most common causes of gastroparesis are idiopathic, diabetic, and postsurgical, but a variety of other diseases such as Parkinson's, scleroderma, and mesenteric ischemia can be responsible [46]. In addition to nausea and vomiting, patients may also complain of bloating, early satiety, and abdominal pain. Many patients with idiopathic gastroparesis will have functional disorders such as functional dyspepsia (86 %) and irritable bowel syndrome (65 %) [47]. Idiopathic gastroparesis can also occur after a systemic viral illness. Postsurgical gastroparesis is rare but may occur after abdominal surgery (usually in the upper abdomen) [48]. Diabetic gastroparesis is found in 5 % of type 1 diabetics and 1 % of type 2 diabetics [49].

A scintigraphic gastric emptying study where patients eat a radiolabeled egg-white meal is the gold-standard diagnostic test [50]. Patients retaining >90 % at 1 h, >60 % at 2 h, and >10 % of the meal at 4 h are generally considered to have delayed gastric emptying. Alternative forms of testing include wireless capsule motility testing and breath testing.

The first-line management of gastroparesis is dietary modification, nutritional support, and glycemic control [46]. Patients should try eating small and frequent meals and avoid fat and nondigestible fibers (e.g., fruits, vegetables). Those unable to tolerate solids can try pureed foods. Patients should avoid alcohol, smoking, and carbonated beverages. Any caloric, vitamin, or mineral deficiencies should be corrected. Good glycemic control can also improve symptoms. If these interventions are not enough, then a prokinetic drug (typically metoclopramide) is the next step. However, caution should be exercised and patients starting metoclopramide need to discontinue therapy if they develop extrapyramidal side effects such as tardive dyskinesia and dystonia and be counseled on these symptoms. Alternatives include domperidone and erythromycin. Finally, those with refractory or severe disease may consider gastric electrical stimulation using an implanted pacemaker [46]. A recent meta-analysis suggests that gastric electrical stimulation can improve both symptoms and gastric emptying, but further studies are still needed [51].

5.6 Bleeding

When patients present with upper GI bleeding, the most important step is to determine the acuity and severity. The most common symptom prompting a workup is melena (tarry black stools) [52]. Melena or coffee-ground emesis is more consistent with chronic or resolved bleeding, whereas frankly bloody emesis is associated with ongoing moderate to severe bleeding. Frankly bloody stool is more consistent with lower GI bleeding but can be seen in patients with massive upper GI bleeding.

For patients who are hemodynamically stable, the history and physical may suggest a cause for the bleeding. A history of liver disease may suggest variceal bleeding, while a history of smoking, alcohol abuse, or peptic ulcer disease raises concerns about malignancy. Laboratory studies are reasonable but often inconclusive, as patients with acute bleeding will still have a hemoglobin level that is unchanged because the overall concentration in the blood is unchanged. However, microcytic anemia may suggest a chronicity to the disease. A blood urea nitrogen to serum creatinine ratio ≥36 suggests that the bleeding is occurring in the upper rather than lower GI tract [53].

For most patients, the diagnostic workup begins with upper endoscopy followed by a colonoscopy if needed. In patients without variceal bleeding, the most common finding is an ulcer (33 %) followed by mucosal erosion (19 %), although as many as 17 % of patients will have normal study results [52]. Other causes include esophagitis, Mallory–Weiss syndrome, angiodysplasia, neoplasms, Cameron's erosions, and Dieulafoy's lesions. Repeat endoscopy may be necessary to make the diagnosis.

In the past, nasogastric lavage has been used as a diagnostic tool prior to upper endoscopy for determining whether there was ongoing bleeding. However, a recent study suggests that the use of nasogastric lavage does not change mortality, length of hospitalization, or the units of blood transfused [54].

If upper endoscopy and colonoscopy are not diagnostic, the next step is wireless capsule endoscopy [55]. Capsule endoscopy is more likely to identify a source of bleeding than push enteroscopy, small bowel radiographic series, and colonoscopy with ileoscopy [56]. In patients under the age of 40 years, small bowel bleeding is typically from neoplasms (e.g., lymphoma, carcinoids, and adenocarcinoma), Meckel's diverticulum, Dieulafoy's lesion, and Crohn's disease [55]. Patients older than 40 years typically bleed from vascular lesions (e.g., angiectasis) or NSAID-related disease. Celiac disease can present at any age.

5.7   Conclusion

Many men will develop upper GI tract symptoms over the course of their lifetime. A careful history and physical examination can narrow the range of possible etiologies. Watch out for alarm symptoms which should prompt further workup. Medical management will be successful for most disorders but patients with refractory or recurrent symptoms should be referred to specialists.

References

1. Camilleri M, Dubois D, Coulie B, Jones M, Kahrilas PJ, Rentz AM, et al. Prevalence and socioeconomic impact of upper gastrointestinal disorders in the United States: results of the US Upper Gastrointestinal Study. Clin Gastroenterol Hepatol. 2005;3(6):543–52.
2. Drossman DA, Li Z, Andruzzi E, Temple RD, Talley NJ, Thompson WG, et al. U.S. house-holder survey of functional gastrointestinal disorders. Prevalence, sociodemography, and health impact. Dig Dis Sci. 1993;38(9):1569–80.
3. Vakil N, van Zanten SV, Kahrilas P, Dent J, Jones R, The Global Consensus Group. The Montreal definition and classification of gastroesophageal reflux disease: a global evidence-based consensus. Am J Gastroenterol. 2006;101(8):1900–20.
4. Dent J, El-Serag HB, Wallander M-A, Johansson S. Epidemiology of gastro-oesophageal reflux disease: a systematic review. Gut. 2005;54(5):710–7.
5. Bytzer P, Jones R, Vakil N, Junghard O, Lind T, Wernersson B, et al. Limited ability of the proton-pump inhibitor test to identify patients with gastroesophageal reflux disease. Clin Gastroenterol Hepatol. 2012;10(12):1360–6.
6. Katz PO, Gerson LB, Vela MF. Guidelines for the diagnosis and management of gastroesopha-geal reflux disease. Am J Gastroenterol. 2013;108(3):308–29.
7. Stefanidis D, Hope WW, Kohn GP, Reardon PR, Richardson WS, Fanelli RD, et al. Guidelines for surgical treatment of gastroesophageal reflux disease. Surg Endosc. 2010;24(11): 2647–69.

8. Scott-Conner CE. Laparoscopic Nissen Fundoplication. In: Scott-Conner CE, editor. Chassin's operative strategy in general surgery. 4th ed. New York: Springer; 2014.
9. Robinson B, Dunst CM, Cassera MA, Reavis KM, Sharata A, Swanstrom LL. 20 years later: laparoscopic fundoplication durability. Surg Endosc. 2014.
10. Frezza EE, Ikramuddin S, Gourash W, Rakitt T, Kingston A, Luketich J, et al. Symptomatic improvement in gastroesophageal reflux disease (GERD) following laparoscopic Roux-en-Y gastric bypass. Surg Endosc. 2002;16(7):1027–31.
11. Perry Y, Courcoulas AP, Fernando HC, Buenaventura PO, McCaughan JS, Luketich JD. Laparoscopic Roux-en-Y gastric bypass for recalcitrant gastroesophageal reflux disease in morbidly obese patients. JSLS. 2004;8(1):19–23.
12. Varela JE, Hinojosa MW, Nguyen NT. Laparoscopic fundoplication compared with laparoscopic gastric bypass in morbidly obese patients with gastroesophageal reflux disease. Surg Obes Relat Dis. 2009;5(2):139–43.
13. Talley NJ, Vakil N. The Practice Parameters Committee of the American College of Gastroenterology. Guidelines for the management of dyspepsia. Am J Gastroenterol. 2005;100(10):2324–37.
14. Delaney BC, Qume M, Moayyedi P, Logan RFA, Ford AC, Elliott C, et al. Helicobacter pylori test and treat versus proton pump inhibitor in initial management of dyspepsia in primary care: multicentre randomised controlled trial (MRC-CUBE trial). BMJ. 2008;336(7645):651–4.
15. Kim KO. Normal upper GI findings and normal variants. In: Chun HJ, Yang S-K, Choi M-G, editors. Clinical gastrointestinal endoscopy. Berlin: Springer; 2014.
16. Kim SG. Early gastric cancers. In: Chun HJ, Yang S-K, Choi M-G, editors. Clinical gastrointestinal endoscopy. Berlin: Springer; 2014.
17. Gielisse EAR, Kuyvenhoven JP. Follow-up endoscopy for benign-appearing gastric ulcers has no additive value in detecting malignancy. Gastric Cancer. 2014:1–7.
18. Laine L, Hopkins R, Girardi L. Has the impact of Helicobacter pylori therapy on ulcer recurrence in the United States been overstated? A meta-analysis of rigorously designed trials. Am J Gastroenterol. 1998;93(9):1409–15.
19. Chey WD, Wong BCY. Practice parameters committee of the American College of Gastroenterology. American College of Gastroenterology guideline on the management of helicobacter pylori infection. Am J Gastroenterol. 2007;102(8):1808–25.
20. Malfertheiner P, Megraud F, O'Morain CA, Atherton J, Axon ATR, Bazzoli F, et al. Management of helicobacter pylori infection--the Maastricht IV/Florence consensus report. Gut. 2012;61(5):646–64.
21. Yuan Y, Padol IT, Hunt RH. Peptic ulcer disease today. Nat Clin Pract Gastroenterol Hepatol. 2006;3(2):80–9.
22. Thomopoulos KC, Melachrinou MP, Mimidis KP, Katsakoulis EC, Margaritis VG, Vagianos CE, et al. Gastric ulcers and risk for cancer. Is follow-up necessary for all gastric ulcers? Int J Clin Pract. 2004;58(7):675–7.
23. Hopper AN, Stephens MR, Lewis WG, Blackshaw GRJC, Morgan MA, Thompson I, et al. Relative value of repeat gastric ulcer surveillance gastroscopy in diagnosing gastric cancer. Gastric Cancer. 2006;9(3):217–22.
24. Yeh JM, Ho W, Hur C. Cost-effectiveness of endoscopic surveillance of gastric ulcers to improve survival. Gastrointest Endosc. 2010;72(1):33–43.
25. Saini SD, Eisen G, Mattek N, Schoenfeld P. Utilization of upper endoscopy for surveillance of gastric ulcers in the united states. Am J Gastroenterol. 2008;103(8):1920–5.
26. Wang YR, Richter JE, Dempsey DT. Trends and outcomes of hospitalizations for peptic ulcer disease in the United States, 1993 to 2006. Ann Surg. 2010;251(1):51–8.
27. Shaffer EA. Epidemiology of gallbladder stone disease. Best Pract Res Clin Gastroenterol. 2006;20(6):981–96.
28. Diehl AK, Sugarek NJ, Todd KH. Clinical evaluation for gallstone disease: usefulness of symptoms and signs in diagnosis. Am J Med. 1990;89(1):29–33.
29. Ransohoff DF, Gracie WA. Treatment of gallstones. Ann Intern Med. 1993;119(7 Pt 1):606–19.

30. Internal Clinical Guidelines Team (UK). Gallstone Disease: Diagnosis and management of cholelithiasis, cholecystitis and choledocholithiasis. London: National Institute for Health and Care Excellence (UK); 2014.
31. Rubin RA, Kowalski TE, Khandelwal M, Malet PF. Ursodiol for hepatobiliary disorders. Ann Intern Med. 1994;121(3):207–18.
32. Jazrawi RP, Pigozzi MG, Galatola G, Lanzini A, Northfield TC. Optimum bile acid treatment for rapid gall stone dissolution. Gut. 1992;33(3):381–6.
33. Villanova N, Bazzoli F, Taroni F, Frabboni R, Mazzella G, Festi D, et al. Gallstone recurrence after successful oral bile acid treatment. A 12-year follow-up study and evaluation of long-term postdissolution treatment. Gastroenterology. 1989;97(3):726–31.
34. Ros E, Navarro S, Bru C, Garcia-Puges A, Valderrama R. Occult microlithiasis in "idiopathic" acute pancreatitis: prevention of relapses by cholecystectomy or ursodeoxycholic acid therapy. Gastroenterology. 1991;101(6):1701–9.
35. Petroni ML, Jazrawi RP, Pazzi P, Zuin M, Lanzini A, Fracchia M, et al. Risk factors for the development of gallstone recurrence following medical dissolution. The British-Italian Gallstone Study Group. Eur J Gastroenterol Hepatol. 2000;12(6):695–700.
36. Spechler SJ. AGA technical review on treatment of patients with dysphagia caused by benign disorders of the distal esophagus. Gastroenterology. 1999;117(1):233–54.
37. Mahesh VN, Holloway RH, Nguyen NQ. Changing epidemiology of food bolus impaction: Is eosinophilic esophagitis to blame? J Gastroenterol Hepatol. 2013;28(6):963–6.
38. Dellon ES, Liacouras CA. Advances in clinical management of eosinophilic esophagitis. Gastroenterology. 2014;147(6):1238–54.
39. Smith PM, Kerr GD, Cockel R, Ross BA, Bate CM, Brown P, et al. A comparison of omeprazole and ranitidine in the prevention of recurrence of benign esophageal stricture. Restore Investigator Group. Gastroenterology. 1994;107(5):1312–8.
40. Rustgi AK, El-Serag HB. Esophageal carcinoma. N Engl J Med. 2014;371(26):2499–509.
41. Talukdar R, Inoue H, Reddy DN. Efficacy of peroral endoscopic myotomy (POEM) in the treatment of achalasia: a systematic review and meta-analysis. Surg Endosc. 2014:1–17.
42. Richter JE. Oesophageal motility disorders. Lancet. 2001;358(9284):823–8.
43. Galmiche JP, Clouse RE, Bálint A, Cook IJ, Kahrilas PJ, Paterson WG, et al. Functional esophageal disorders. Gastroenterology. 2006;130(5):1459–65.
44. American Gastroenterological Association medical position statement. Nausea and vomiting. Gastroenterology. 2001;120(1):261–2.
45. Scorza K, Williams A, Phillips JD, Shaw J. Evaluation of nausea and vomiting. Am Fam Physician. 2007;76(1):76–84.
46. Camilleri M, Parkman HP, Shafi MA, Abell TL, Gerson L. American College of Gastroenterology. Clinical guideline: management of gastroparesis. Am J Gastroenterol. 2013;108(1):18–37.
47. Parkman HP, Yates K, Hasler WL, Nguyen L, Pasricha PJ, Snape WJ, et al. Clinical features of idiopathic gastroparesis vary with sex, body mass, symptom onset, delay in gastric emptying, and gastroparesis severity. Gastroenterology. 2011;140(1):101–15.
48. Quigley EM. Other forms of gastroparesis: postsurgical, Parkinson, other neurologic diseases, connective tissue disorders. Gastroenterol Clin North Am. 2015;44(1):69–81.
49. Choung RS, Locke GR, Schleck CD, Zinsmeister AR, Melton LJ, Talley NJ. Risk of gastroparesis in subjects with type 1 and 2 diabetes in the general population. Am J Gastroenterol. 2012;107(1):82–8.
50. Abell TL, Camilleri M, Donohoe K, Hasler WL, Lin HC, Maurer AH, et al. Consensus recommendations for gastric emptying scintigraphy: a joint report of the American Neurogastroenterology and Motility Society and the Society of Nuclear Medicine. Am J Gastroenterol. 2008;103(3):753–63.
51. Chu H, Lin Z, Zhong L, McCallum RW, Hou X. Treatment of high-frequency gastric electrical stimulation for gastroparesis. J Gastroenterol Hepatol. 2012;27(6):1017–26.

52. Enestvedt BK, Gralnek IM, Mattek N, Lieberman DA, Eisen G. An evaluation of endoscopic indications and findings related to nonvariceal upper-GI hemorrhage in a large multicenter consortium. Gastrointest Endosc. 2008;67(3):422–9.
53. Richards RJ, Donica MB, Grayer D. Can the blood urea nitrogen/creatinine ratio distinguish upper from lower gastrointestinal bleeding? J Clin Gastroenterol. 1990;12(5):500–4.
54. Huang ES, Karsan S, Kanwal F, Singh I, Makhani M, Spiegel BM. Impact of nasogastric lavage on outcomes in acute GI bleeding. Gastrointest Endosc. 2011;74(5):971–80.
55. Raju GS, Gerson L, Das A, Lewis B. American Gastroenterological Association (AGA) Institute technical review on obscure gastrointestinal bleeding. Gastroenterology. 2007; 133(5):1697–717.
56. Lewis BS, Eisen GM, Friedman S. A pooled analysis to evaluate results of capsule endoscopy trials. Endoscopy. 2005;37(10):960–5.

His Lower GI

6

Cindy Kin

6.1 Introduction: Approach to the Patient with a Lower Gastrointestinal Problem

This chapter will provide a broad overview of lower gastrointestinal symptoms and diagnoses, along with practical management and work-up guidelines. One of the most important aspects of managing lower gastrointestinal conditions is one's approach to the patient, with regard to both communication and physical examination. While this volume is focused specifically on men's health, the diagnoses outlined in this chapter are applicable to both men and women. Rectal prolapse and pelvic floor dyssynergia are less commonly seen in men, but levator spasm is more common in men.

Health-care professionals must exercise both sensitivity and candor to effectively diagnose and manage ailments affecting the lower gastrointestinal tract. Many patients find it embarrassing to discuss such issues and thus are likely to have already procrastinated from seeking medical attention for their symptoms. The patients who have finally made their way into a physician's office are likely to not only be rather anxious about what ails them "down there" but also may find it difficult to describe their symptoms. Thus, the responsibility of helping the patient describe the nature of the problem rests on the physician and requires the physician to put the patient at ease and ask those "difficult" questions so that the patient does not face the barrier of having to bring up those sensitive topics himself.

When discussing lower gastrointestinal symptoms, health-care providers must be willing to ask detailed questions to help patients describe exactly what they are experiencing. For example, a patient who states that he has constipation may mean that he has hard stools, or infrequent stools, or difficulty with defecation, or all of these symptoms—and it is the responsibility of the health-care provider to define

C. Kin, M.D. (✉)
Department of Surgery, Stanford University School of Medicine,
300 Pasteur Drive, H3680K, Stanford, CA 94305, USA
e-mail: cindykin@stanford.edu

© Springer Science+Business Media New York 2016
J.M. Potts (ed.), *Men's Health*, DOI 10.1007/978-1-4939-3237-5_6

explicitly what the patient means. A complete discussion of lower gastrointestinal issues also requires a discussion of genitourinary symptoms as many of these conditions have overlapping symptoms involving urinary function and sexual function.

The physician must also have a low threshold to perform an examination of the anus and perineum. Patients commonly assume symptoms of bleeding, pain, itching, swelling, or drainage are all attributable to hemorrhoids. Physicians must not rely on the patients' self-diagnosis; rather they must look for themselves to avoid delaying diagnosis and treatment of other benign anorectal problems or malignancies. Again, patients who seek medical help regarding a lower gastrointestinal concern will likely be anxious about undergoing such an examination, but it is the job of the medical professional to put the patient at ease and be as efficient and sensitive as possible with this part of the examination. Most patients will expect to undergo an internal exam, but it is important to be explicit about the examination to make sure the patient agrees to it. In many cases, it is wise and helpful to have at least one other medical personnel in the examination room as a chaperone as well as source of support for the patient. Finally, if the patient is accompanied by a family member, it is important to ask if the patient prefers to have the family member in the room for the exam or not. In most cases of lower gastrointestinal concerns, at least a digital exam is warranted if not also anoscopy. Internal examination can be deferred if the pathology is clearly visible on external exam and digital examination or anoscopy would cause undue discomfort to the patient.

Patients undergoing anorectal and perineal examination can be positioned in either left lateral decubitus position or knee-chest position (otherwise known as prone jackknife position) if one has access to an examination table that allows for that mode of positioning. Left lateral decubitus position is generally more comfortable for the patient; examiners who prefer the knee-chest position should also be facile with the left lateral decubitus position as patients with knee problems may not be able to kneel.

Examination of the anal canal can be accomplished with a variety of anoscopes—some equipped with lights which can facilitate vision of anal canal and distal rectal mucosa. It is helpful to have a variety of lengths and diameters available, as some patients cannot tolerate examination with a large anoscope, some patients have deeper buttocks with longer anal canals that require longer anoscopes, and procedures like hemorrhoid ligation require a larger caliber anoscope which will accommodate the banding device.

Rigid proctoscopes are necessary for examination of the more proximal rectal mucosa and, compared to flexible sigmoidoscopes, are less expensive and easier to maintain. They are also important for obtaining accurate measurements of distance of a lesion from the anal canal.

A bright light source is also very helpful for examination of the buttock and perianal skin and should be either freestanding or a headlight to allow the examiner to use both hands for retraction and examination.

A suction machine is necessary if one wishes to use the suction banders for hemorrhoid ligation and can also come in handy during proctologic examinations to clear stool or liquid. Other handy supplies are listed in Table 6.1.

Table 6.1 Equipment and supplies for proctologic examinations and procedures

Equipment	Supplies
Proctologic examination table which raises and tilts in Trendelenburg	Lubricant
Anoscopes—variety of diameters and lengths, prefer with a light source	Scalpels
Proctoscopes	Cotton-tip applicators
Light source: freestanding or headlamp	Silver nitrate
Suction machine	Lidocaine: prefer 2 % with epinephrine
Hemorrhoid banders: suction or manual	Betadine swabs
Allis clamps	Suture removal kits (forceps and scissors)
	Gauze

6.2   Symptoms

6.2.1   Blood per Rectum

Patients who present with symptoms of rectal or anal bleeding, or blood in the stool, may have essentially any diagnosis covered in this chapter. A complete list is provided in Table 6.2. Eliciting the details of the exact nature of the bleeding is key to developing a complete differential diagnosis and will help reduce the risk of missing an important diagnosis. The bleeding should be characterized as bright red, dark red, or black. One should also determine if the blood is separate from the stool—dripping into the toilet bowl or evident on the toilet paper after wiping—as opposed to mixed into the stool. It is also important to ask whether the bleeding is associated with bowel movements and, if so, if the bowel movements are associated with pain. All of these details can help the health-care provider develop a list of the most likely diagnoses and direct the examination.

In the office, examination of the external skin with effacement of the buttocks should be performed to look for perianal lesions such as external fistula openings, perianal skin excoriation, and masses. Next, one should look for a fissure by gently everting the anus a bit more; they are usually located in the posterior midline but could occur at any location. The next step is a digital examination and anoscopy to look for masses or hemorrhoids. If still no source of bleeding is found, then proctoscopy is warranted to look for lesions in the rectum.

Young patients with no other cancer risk factors presenting with bright red bleeding per rectum and who are found on examination to have an obvious source of bleeding such as hemorrhoids or fissure may not require colonoscopy, as long as they do not meet standard screening criteria. However, lower endoscopy (at least flexible sigmoidoscopy) is warranted if no source of bright red bleeding is found, even in a young patient of average cancer risk. Bloody stools and melena in any

Table 6.2 Differential diagnosis of rectal bleeding

Symptom	Benign etiologies	Neoplastic etiologies
Bright red blood per rectum (described as dripping into the toilet bowl, staining the underwear, or noticed on the toilet paper after wiping)	Fistula Abscess Internal hemorrhoids Proctitis or colitis (inflammatory, infectious, ischemic, radiation induced) Diverticulosis Fissure Perianal skin breakdown Arteriovenous malformation Sexually transmitted diseases: gonorrhea, herpes, chlamydia	Anal cancer Anal warts Anal dysplasia Perianal cancer Rectal cancer
Bloody stools (streaks of blood in the stool, reddish stool)	Colitis (inflammatory, infectious, ischemic, radiation induced) Diverticulosis Arteriovenous malformation	Colorectal polyps Colon cancer Rectal cancer Anal cancer
Melena (black stool)	Diverticulosis Colitis (inflammatory, infectious, ischemic, radiation induced) Peptic ulcer Arteriovenous malformation	Colon cancer (likely more proximal, like right colon) Small bowel tumor Gastric cancer

patient are indications for endoscopic examination; for the latter, upper endoscopy is also recommended to rule out a gastric or duodenal bleeding source. Of course, any patient who meets standard criteria for colorectal cancer screening and presents with rectal bleeding should undergo lower endoscopic examination. Screening and surveillance guidelines are detailed in Tables 6.3 and 6.4. It is important to maintain a high index of suspicion for colorectal malignancy even in young people, as the rates of colorectal cancer in patients under 50 years old are on the rise, while the incidence of colorectal cancer in patients over 50 years old is decreasing [1].

6.2.2 Constipation

As with rectal bleeding, constipation is a symptom that must be explored in greater detail, as it can mean a variety of different things to different people, ranging from hard stools to small-caliber stools to difficulty with evacuation to infrequent defecation. These can all be attributed to different etiologies. Elucidating the cause of constipation is akin to understanding the reasons for why one is sitting in a traffic jam on the highway: it may be due to slow drivers or slow cars (suboptimal stool consistency), a slow bumpy road (colonic inertia), a merging of multiple lanes into fewer lanes (stricture), a roadblock due to a collision (obstruction), or a back-up on one of the exits (functional outlet obstruction). Similarly, constipation can be

Table 6.3 Screening recommendations for colorectal cancer

Asymptomatic patients with no prior history of CRC or adenomas	Recommended screening
Average risk (age > 50 years, without other risk factors)	Starting at age 50[a]: Annual fecal occult blood test (FOBT) Flexible sigmoidoscopy every 5 years Annual FOBT plus flex sig every 5 years Colonoscopy every 10 years Barium enema every 5 years
First-degree relative (parent, sibling, child) with CRC or adenomas diagnosed at age ≤ 60 years or two first-degree relatives of any age	Colonoscopy every 5 years, starting at age 40 or 10 years before age at diagnosis of youngest affected relative whichever is first
First-degree relative with CRC or adenoma at age > 60 years, or two second degree with CRC	Same as average risk but start at age 40
Familial adenomatous polyposis	Refer for genetic testing Annual screening by sigmoidoscopy starting at age 10–12
Hereditary nonpolyposis colorectal cancer	Refer for genetic testing Colonoscopy every 1–2 years beginning at age 20–25 or 10 years younger than youngest age at cancer diagnosis in family
Ulcerative colitis or Crohn's colitis	Start annual colonoscopy 10 years after diagnosis with systematic biopsies

Source: Levin et al. [4]
[a]Start at 45 years for African American patients

Table 6.4 Surveillance recommendations for colorectal cancer (patients with a personal history of colorectal cancer or adenomas)

History	Recommended surveillance
Personal hx of adenomas	
1–2 tubular adenomas <1 cm in size	5 years
3 or more adenomas	3 years
Advanced adenomas (>1 cm, high-grade dysplasia or villous elements)	3 years
Numerous adenomas or lg sessile adenoma removed piecemeal	Short interval based on clinical judgment
Follow-up exam normal (patients with only hyperplastic polyps are generally considered to have a normal examination)	5 years
Personal history of colorectal cancer	
At diagnosis	Colonoscopy pre-operatively or within 6 months post-op if pre-operative obstruction precluded complete colonoscopy
After resection	One year after diagnosis. Subsequent intervals depend on findings

Source: Levin et al. [4]

attributed to poor diet with inadequate fiber and water intake, colonic inertia due to an intrinsic motility disorder, stricture or obstruction due to inflammation or mass, and functional outlet obstruction due to pelvic floor dysfunction. Thus, it is important to ask the patient about his fiber and water intake, stool consistency and caliber, frequency of bowel movements, abdominal or anal pain with bowel movements, recent changes in bowel movement frequency or stool caliber, blood in the stool, amount of time that he sits on the toilet, the degree to which he strains to have a bowel movement, whether he needs to change positions in order to defecate, and whether there are symptoms of urgency or tenesmus.

Focused examination in the office should include an abdominal and digital rectal exam. Proctoscopy or flexible sigmoidoscopy can also be performed to assess for a distal obstruction.

Most cases of constipation in the USA can be attributed to the low fiber content of the typical Western diet and can be successfully managed with increased water intake and fiber supplementation. Stool softeners and other laxatives can be used as adjunct therapy as needed. However, if the symptoms of constipation are suspected to be due to other etiologies, then further diagnostic testing is warranted.

Additional studies to help determine the etiology for the symptoms include endoscopic examination with colonoscopy or flexible sigmoidoscopy to assess for a partially obstructing mass, contrast enema to assess for stricture, and intestinal transit studies to assess for motility disorders (Fig. 6.1). Colonoscopy should be performed in all patients who meet standard screening criteria and also in the presence of other worrisome symptoms and signs such as a change in bowel habits, narrower caliber stools, blood in the stool, weight loss, anemia, abdominal discomfort, or tenderness. Colonic transit can be measured by radiopaque markers, which are swallowed by the patient in pill form and then disperse throughout the intestine. Abdominal radiograph taken at 5 days demonstrating less than 20 % residual markers remaining signifies normal colonic motility; more than 20 % residual markers scattered throughout the colon is suspicious for colonic inertia (Fig. 6.2). If the remaining markers are clustered in the rectosigmoid colon, then functional outlet obstruction such as pelvic floor dysfunction should be suspected (Fig. 6.3). The wireless motility capsule (SmartPill—SmartPill Corporation, Buffalo, NY) offers comparable results and also offers information on small bowel motility [2].

6.2.3 Anal Pain

The majority of patients presenting with anal pain assume that it is due to hemorrhoids and have already tried a variety of over-the-counter remedies for hemorrhoids by the time they present to a physician. However, hemorrhoids are often not the cause of anal pain. Rather, the most common etiology of anal pain is a fissure in ano, and symptoms usually consist of sharp anal pain exacerbated by bowel movements and often associated with bright red blood. These symptoms may be acute or chronic. Thrombosed external hemorrhoids and perianal abscesses are common causes of acute anal pain. Levator ani syndrome is another cause of anal pain that is

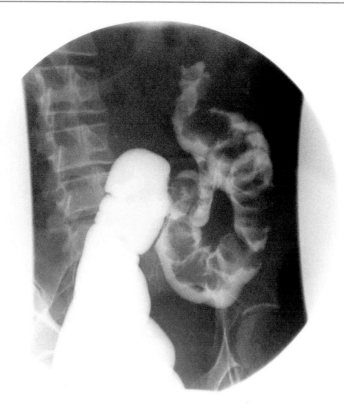

Fig. 6.1 Patient presented with constipation and abdominal pain. Colonoscopy could not be completed due to a narrowing of the sigmoid colon. Contrast enema demonstrated a fixed stricture concerning for a near-obstructing tumor

usually described as spasmodic and sharp, occurring at random times and rarely exacerbated by bowel movements. Malignancies such as anal cancer or distal rectal cancers can also cause anal pain due to invasion of the sphincter complex; rectal tumors can also cause pelvic pressure and tenesmus even without invasion of the sphincter muscle. Presacral tumors may also be a case of anal pain or tailbone pain.

Examination in the office should consist of buttock effacement and palpation of the buttock and perianal tissue externally to assess for areas of fluctuance or tenderness. An external thrombosed hemorrhoid or abscess would be visible by external exam, and digital exam should be deferred until a later time due to discomfort. Special notice should be taken of the tension of the gluteal muscles, pelvic floor, and anal sphincter. The anus should be effaced a bit more to examine for a fissure, usually located in the posterior midline. Often, patients with a fissure in ano will have considerable discomfort with just the external exam and may not be able to tolerate a digital exam or anoscopy. These examinations can be deferred until after the patient has some improvement with treatment and is able to tolerate an exam.

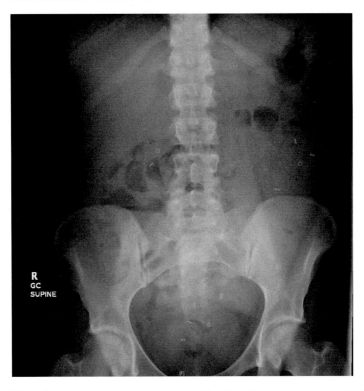

Fig. 6.2 This radiopaque marker test is consistent with colonic inertia, as more than 20 % of the markers are still present throughout the colon after 7 days

Digital exam and anoscopy should be performed to rule out an anal canal or distal rectal mass. Fluctuance within the anal canal is indicative of an intersphincteric abscess which can cause considerable pain in the absence of the typical fluctuance or erythema visible on external examination with other perianal abscesses. Reproduction of the pain specifically with palpation of the levators raises the suspicion for levator ani syndrome. Any mucosal lesions should be examined with anoscopy and biopsied. Masses of the anal canal and distal rectum should be characterized based on location, size, distance from the top of the anorectal ring, and whether it is mobile, tethered, or fixed. Submucosal or presacral masses may also be palpated.

If no etiology of the pain is found on physical exam, colonoscopy or flexible sigmoidoscopy should be performed to rule out an intra- or extra-luminal mass that is the cause of the pain. If still nothing is found on endoscopy, then cross-sectional imaging of the pelvis and lower spine is indicated to rule out a presacral or sacrococcygeal mass, which can cause pelvic, anal, or tailbone pain.

Idiopathic pelvic pain is a diagnosis of exclusion and should be referred for treatment with a pain specialist.

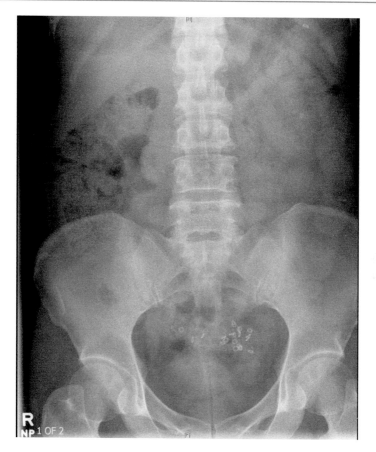

Fig. 6.3 This radiopaque marker test is consistent with pelvic floor dysfunction, as the remaining markers are clustered in the rectosigmoid region, indicating normal transit through the colon but a functional outlet obstruction

6.2.4   Pruritus Ani

A number of diagnoses may cause itchiness of the anus and perianal skin. In addition to determining the timing and severity of the symptoms, it is also important to determine what sort of skin cleansers and lotions the patient is using, as many of these products can exacerbate the symptoms.

Examination of the perianal skin may reveal superficial fissuring, excoriation, maceration, or other signs of dermatitis. Moisture of the perianal skin or fecal seepage should be noted, as chronic moisture of the skin can cause pruritus. Prolapsed internal hemorrhoids or mixed external and internal hemorrhoids can allow tracking of mucus and fecal matter onto the perianal skin which can in turn cause pruritus. Finally, digital exam and anoscopy should be performed to rule out an anal or distal rectal lesion and to look for prominent internal hemorrhoids that may prolapse intermittently.

Special attention should be given to any well-demarcated areas of erythema; a skin biopsy should be taken to rule out Paget's disease, a rare but potentially malignant cause of pruritus and/or perianal bleeding. As Paget's disease of the perianal skin is frequently misdiagnosed as dermatitis, often leading to long delays in proper treatment, a high index of suspicion must be maintained to make the correct diagnosis. Other uncommon causes of pruritic lesions include anal intraepithelial neoplasia of the perianal skin and anal canal. Any abnormal biopsy finding should be referred to a surgeon experienced in treating these conditions. The management of perianal Paget's disease includes full colonoscopy to rule out a synchronous colorectal cancer, followed by wide local excision of Paget's disease, or even abdomino-perineal resection if it is invasive. As local recurrence of perianal Paget's disease is common, follow-up includes proctoscopy and digital rectal examination at regular intervals. Invasive perianal disease can metastasize to inguinal lymph nodes as well as the liver and lungs [3].

6.2.5 Anal Mass

Patients presenting with an anal mass are commonly assumed to have hemorrhoids, but a host of other diagnoses are in the differential. Physical examination may reveal external or internal hemorrhoids, sentinel tag, or hypertrophic anal papilla from a chronic anal fissure, perianal abscess, anal condyloma, anal cancer or prolapsing rectal polyp or cancer, or rectal prolapse.

6.2.6 Fecal Incontinence

Patients are often embarrassed to bring up symptoms of fecal incontinence, and health-care providers must be candid and explicit in their discussion with patients in order to elicit this history. Symptoms may range from fecal seepage to compromised control over flatus, liquid stool, and/or solid stool. The patient's anorectal sensation may be altered such that they are not aware of stool in the rectum, or the passage of stool, so it is important to ask whether patients notice the urge to defecate or not. Finally, the consistency of the stool can affect continence, as looser stools are much more difficult to control than solid stool.

When examining the perianal skin, one should look for evidence of chronic fecal soiling such as skin maceration or signs of dermatitis. On effacement of the buttocks, one should notice whether the anus is patulous. When asking the patient to squeeze the sphincter, as if to hold in a bowel movement, one should note whether the anus actually tightens or if the patient is squeezing the gluteal muscles together instead. When asking the patient to push as if to have a bowel movement, one should note whether the perineum descends and whether there is any mucosal or full-thickness prolapse. The same squeeze and push maneuvers should be performed during the digital exam, and the tone of the anal sphincter noted. Anoscopy should also be performed to examine for hemorrhoids or lesions.

6.3   Neoplastic Diagnoses

6.3.1   Colorectal Polyps and Cancer

Colorectal cancer is the second most common cause of cancer and third most common cause of cancer death in the USA. Screening for colorectal cancer starts at the age of 50 for people with no family history or other risk factors for colorectal cancer and should continue at regular intervals depending on symptoms and risk level [4] (Tables 6.3 and 6.4). According to the US Preventive Services Task Force, screening for colorectal cancer is not generally recommended for people over the age of 85, although elderly patients with worrisome symptoms who are otherwise healthy should be considered for diagnostic testing. Fecal occult blood test (FOBT) can be performed with either guaiac testing or immunochemistry and requires three separate patient-collected stool samples collected at least one day apart. The immunochemical FOBT has been shown in a few studies to have increased sensitivity without a loss of specificity compared to traditional guaiac [5]. CT colonography or "virtual colonoscopy" is an alternative way to detect polyps and masses but has not been widely adopted for screening. Patients still must undergo bowel preparation, but do not undergo sedation for the procedure which involves air insufflation of the colon. The downside of CT colonography is that patients will require colonoscopy for removal of polyps or biopsy of lesions that are detected, whereas patients undergoing colonoscopy as the screening test will undergo polypectomy and/or biopsy at the same time.

While most polyps can be removed easily with biopsy forceps or snare techniques at the time of colonoscopy, some polyps are larger or sessile and are associated with a higher risk of perforation with polypectomy (Fig. 6.4). More advanced

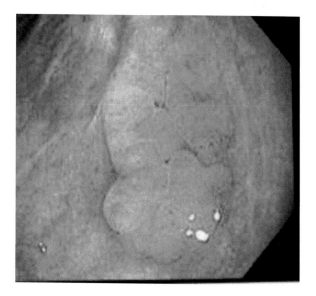

Fig. 6.4 Rectal polyp requiring transanal excision due to size and location

endoscopic techniques, including endoscopic mucosal resection (EMR) and endoscopic submucosal dissection (ESD), have been developed for this indication and are often successful in complete polyp removal and thus avoidance of segmental colectomy. Patients with these large or sessile polyps should be referred to an experienced interventional gastroenterologist or surgeon who can discuss the option of EMR or ESD, before committing the patient to surgical resection.

Patients found to have colon or rectal cancer should undergo CT scan of the chest, abdomen, and pelvis to rule out the presence of metastatic disease and should be referred expeditiously to a surgeon experienced in intestinal surgery, as well as a medical oncologist for consideration of neoadjuvant or adjuvant chemotherapy. Patients with rectal cancer should also undergo either MRI of the pelvis or transrectal ultrasound to determine tumor depth and lymph node status, which will determine whether the patient should undergo neoadjuvant chemoradiation prior to surgical resection. A multidisciplinary approach is crucial for the successful treatment of colorectal cancers.

6.3.2   Anal Dysplasia and Anal Cancer

Screening for anal dysplasia and anal cancer is under considerable debate, and there are no universally accepted guidelines. Digital rectal exam, an inexpensive and benign screening tool, should be performed at least for high-risk or at-risk populations including men with HIV infection or a history of anogenital condyloma, men who have sex with men, and men with prior history of dysplasia. Some recommend annual anal Pap smear for high-risk populations. A Dacron cotton swab is inserted into the anus to 5 cm, placing firm lateral pressure to the handle while rotating it and withdrawing it from the anal canal. Liquid cytology is preferred, but air-drying and fixation can also be used if the former is unavailable [6]. Anal Pap smears can be collected by the patient or a health-care provider, although specimens collected by providers are more sensitive [7].

Suspicious lesions in the anal canal should be biopsied and/or referred to a surgeon with experience in treating anorectal disorders. Any finding of dysplasia (anal intraepithelial neoplasia, squamous carcinoma in situ) in the anal canal should be referred to a colorectal surgeon, as further evaluation and biopsy may be warranted. High-resolution anoscopy with targeted destruction or excision of dysplastic lesions may be considered, but this is also controversial as the risk of progression to anal cancer is low in the general population, albeit higher in immunosuppressed patients [8]. The use of the quadrivalent HPV vaccine was found to reduce the rates of dysplasia in the anal canal among men who have sex with men, but there is no definitive evidence demonstrating the benefit of administering the vaccine to high-risk people over the age of 26 to prevent dysplasia, warts, or cancer [9]. Certainly, all patients 26 years and under should routinely undergo vaccination to prevent HPV infection.

Finally, any finding of malignancy in the anal canal, most commonly squamous cell carcinoma but rarely anal adenocarcinoma or anorectal melanoma, should be

Fig. 6.5 Perianal
condyloma

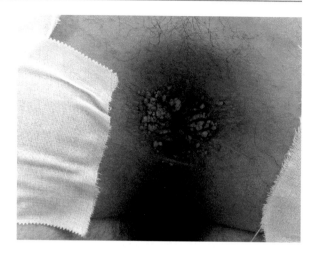

referred expeditiously for consultation at a cancer center, as these malignancies require a cohesive multidisciplinary approach including radiation oncology, medical oncology, and surgery.

6.3.3   Condyloma Acuminatum

Anal condyloma is due to infection with HPV. Patients often present with a bump inside the anus or on the perianal skin (Fig. 6.5). They may note symptoms of itching or bleeding, but rarely have pain. The diagnosis is confirmed with examination of the perianal skin and anoscopy. A variety of patient-administered and provider-administered therapies can successfully treat condyloma. For limited disease, topical therapies including imiquimod and podophyllotoxin can be prescribed for the patient to apply at home. Bi- or trichloroacetic acid can be applied in the office as well. For more extensive disease, ablation with cryotherapy or the CO_2 laser can be performed. Excision and fulguration with electrocautery are very effective for removal of these lesions as well. Referral to a surgeon for ablation or excision is indicated for more advanced disease and certainly in cases of suspected malignancy.

6.4   Benign Diagnoses

6.4.1   Diverticular Disease

Diverticulosis and diverticulitis are very common in the Western world, presumably due to a lack of fiber in the diet leading to small-caliber stools that generate greater intraluminal forces within the colon. Diverticula are often seen incidentally on screening colonoscopy, and the majority of patients with diverticula will never have associated symptoms. Some patients may develop a lower gastrointestinal bleed from the diverticula, usually in the absence of inflammation—the vast majority of these bleeds are self-limited and require no intervention. Diverticulitis can range widely in severity from mild localized inflammation causing pain in the left lower quadrant and treated successfully on an outpatient basis with oral antibiotics to a large perforation in the colon causing peritonitis and sepsis requiring emergency surgery.

Even in mild cases of diverticulitis, it is important that the patient undergo colonoscopy after he has recovered from the acute bout of inflammation to rule out an underlying malignancy. Patients with one or two bouts of mild uncomplicated diverticulitis can be managed nonoperatively with antibiotics for the acute inflammatory phase and improvement of bowel function with increased fiber intake and water after the inflammation subsides. Patients with diverticular disease have been traditionally advised to avoid all nuts and seeds in the diet, but this has not been shown to decrease future bouts of inflammation.

Referral to a colorectal surgeon to discuss possible resection is reasonable for patients with multiple recurrent bouts of diverticulitis, especially for those whose symptoms are worsening or increasing in frequency or who have required inpatient hospitalization for intravenous antibiotic therapy [10]. In such cases, even if mild and treated successfully with outpatient oral antibiotics, at least one CT scan of the abdomen and pelvis during an acute attack is helpful to confirm the presence of inflammation in the event that surgical resection is considered. Another strong indication for referral to a colorectal surgeon to discuss surgical resection include patients with diverticulitis complicated by abscess formation, as these cases have a higher risk of recurrence and poor outcomes especially in younger patients [11]. Finally, patients with a history of diverticulitis and symptoms suspicious for fistula formation such as pneumaturia, fecaluria, or recurrent urinary tract infections should be referred to a colorectal surgeon as this is an important indication for surgical resection.

6.4.2 Hemorrhoids

Hemorrhoids are the scapegoat of all anorectal complaints and must be distinguished from other common benign anorectal disorders such as fissure, abscess, or fistula, as well as more serious diagnoses such as anal cancer or rectal cancer. Most symptoms of hemorrhoids can and should be treated without surgical intervention. It is important to appreciate that hemorrhoids are a normal part of anal anatomy and play an important role in maintaining continence to flatus and stool. Additionally, while rubber band ligation is not painful, recovery from excisional hemorrhoidectomy is usually characterized by significant pain for a week or more, so hemorrhoidectomy should be reserved for only the most severely symptomatic cases that are refractory to maximal medical measures.

In addition to improving stool consistency with fiber supplementation and increased water intake, patients must also be advised to reduce straining and reduce the time they spend sitting on the toilet to several minutes. Sitting on a "donut" pillow should also be discouraged as this can also increase the blood flow to the hemorrhoidal cushions and exacerbate the symptoms. Topical preparations may also be helpful for their anti-inflammatory effects.

Grade 1 bleeding internal hemorrhoids usually cause painless bright red bleeding occurring with bowel movements. Grade 2 internal hemorrhoids may prolapse with bowel movements but reduce spontaneously. Grade 1 and grade 2 internal hemorrhoids can be successfully treated with medical therapy and optimization of bowel habits and rarely require any surgical intervention. Grade 3 prolapsed internal hemorrhoids which require manual reduction may also improve with medical therapy and optimization of bowel habits; persistent symptoms may be treated with rubber band ligation or excisional hemorrhoidectomy. Grade 4 prolapsed internal hemorrhoids, which cannot be manually reduced, must be evaluated for strangulation, necrosis, and gangrene, which are clear indications for emergent operative excisional hemorrhoidectomy (Table 6.5).

External thrombosed hemorrhoids present acutely with severe anal pain and swelling, and there are two methods of managing them depending on the timing and severity of the symptoms. If the patient presents within the first 2 days of symptoms and the pain has not started to abate, then evacuation of the thrombus with excision of the external hemorrhoid is the recommended treatment to speed the resolution of symptoms and reduce the risk of recurrence [12]. Excision of a thrombosed external hemorrhoid should not be performed in the emergency room or office setting if there is an associated grade 4 internal hemorrhoid, coagulopathy or current treatment with anticoagulants, concern for a perianal infection, or portal hypertension or liver disease. If the excision of the thrombosed external hemorrhoid cannot be performed safely in this setting, it is best to refer the case to a surgeon who will be able to perform the operation in the controlled setting of the operating room.

If the patient presents more than 2 days after the onset of symptoms, and the pain has started to abate, then the recommendation is symptom management with warm water soaks and pain control, because excision of the hemorrhoid at this point will not speed the resolution of symptoms. The exception to this is if there is evidence of necrosis or gangrene of the overlying skin, in which case surgical excision in the operating room is appropriate.

6.4.3   Fissure-in-Ano

Anal fissures are very common and present with severe anal pain and bright red bleeding per anus, exacerbated by bowel movements. Patients often describe the sensation of "passing shards of glass" or a "tearing" sensation and may even avoid having bowel movements due to the pain. These patients often attribute these symptoms to hemorrhoids and have already tried over-the-counter hemorrhoid topical preparations without any success. Diagnosis of a fissure-in-ano is made on the grounds of history of painful bleeding from the anus, and physical examination, which may be difficult given the level of pain and sphincter hypertonicity. Gentle effacement of the buttocks to expose the anus may reveal a sentinel tag at the anal

Table 6.5 Hemorrhoidal symptoms and recommended management

Type of hemorrhoid	Symptoms/signs	Recommended treatment
Internal hemorrhoids		
Grade 1	Bleeding with BMs	Increase fiber/water Reduce straining and time sitting on toilet Topical medications
Grade 2	Prolapse with spontaneous reduction ± Bleeding with BMs	Increase fiber/water Reduce straining and time sitting on toilet Topical medications Consider rubber band ligation if still symptomatic despite above measures
Grade 3	Prolapse with manual reduction ± Bleeding with BMs	Increase fiber/water Reduce straining and time sitting on toilet Topical medications Consider rubber band ligation if still symptomatic despite above measures Consider excisional hemorrhoidectomy if still symptomatic despite above measures
Grade 4	Incarcerated prolapse	Excisional hemorrhoidectomy if symptomatic
External hemorrhoids		
Acutely thrombosed (<48 h)	Severe acute anal pain, with swelling at the anus Swollen and extremely tender external hemorrhoid with thrombus	Evacuation of thrombosis and excision of hemorrhoid
Thrombosed >48 h ago	Anal pain starting >48 h ago, with at least some improvement Swollen and tender external hemorrhoid with thrombus	Warm water soaks Topical medications Pain control If strangulation, necrosis or gangrene → excisional hemorrhoidectomy
Non-thrombosed	Skin tags at anal verge, nontender	No intervention indicated

verge, which is a marker of a chronic fissure. Further eversion of the anus can be done with the aid of cotton-tip applicators to expose the fissure, which is usually in the posterior midline. Fissures in other locations raise the suspicion for Crohn's disease. The white fibers of the internal sphincter muscle are often exposed, and chronic fissures may have rolled edges with a hypertrophic anal papilla at the proximal end of the fissure (Fig. 6.6). One might also observe that the sphincter muscles are activated and even contracting during the external exam, a testament to the level of pain caused by the fissure. Digital rectal exam and anoscopy are often not possible due to the patient's discomfort and should be deferred until a later date when the patient is feeling better.

Fig. 6.6 Chronic
fissure-in-ano with a large
sentinel tag in the posterior
midline

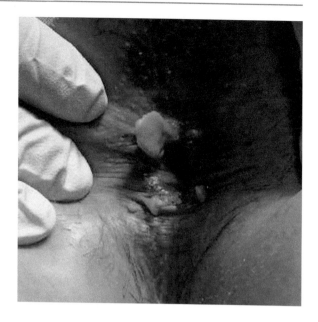

The pathophysiology of anal fissures is that a hard bowel movement causes a tear in the anoderm, exposing the underlying internal sphincter muscle, which promptly goes into spasm and not only causes the large majority of the pain but also causes relative ischemia of the posterior midline, thus preventing healing of the fissure. First-line management of an anal fissure consists of fiber supplementation, increased water intake, and stool softeners to prevent hard stools and exacerbation of the fissure, as well as warm water soaks to help relax the sphincter muscles. Topical therapies are the next line of treatment and are targeted toward decreasing the hypertonicity of the internal sphincter. Nitroglycerine ointment is widely used in various concentrations from 0.05 % to 0.4 %, but is poorly tolerated due to severe headache in 30% of patients. Calcium channel blockers such as diltiazem and nifedipine are as effective as nitroglycerine, but have fewer adverse side effects. These are commonly compounded with lidocaine ointment to aid with pain control [13]. Chemodenervation of the internal anal sphincter using botulinum toxin has equivalent results to the topical treatments. A wide range of doses (10–100 units) has been used in various locations along the internal sphincter; it appears that injecting the equal amounts on either side of the anterior midline is most effective. All of these nonsurgical treatments have success rates ranging between 60 and 80 %, with a 50 % risk of recurrent fissure.

If the patient experiences no relief from these therapies, then lateral internal sphincterotomy is indicated, with a success rate over 90 % and a lower risk of recurrence. Contrary to popular belief, there is a very low risk of a change in continence to flatus or stool because patients with such severe fissures tend to have very high baseline internal sphincter tone, and targeted partial lateral internal sphincterotomy is unlikely to bring the tone even below a normal level.

6.4.4   Perianal Abscess and Fistula-in-Ano

Perianal abscesses present with a feeling of painful pressure at the anus, often associated with a tender swelling on the perianal skin. Patients may notice purulent or bloody drainage from the perianal skin or from the anus. Severe pain exacerbated by bowel movements without a perianal swelling may also occur and may be confused with a fissure in ano. Patients may also present with pelvic pain, tailbone pain, or urinary retention. Ischioanal or ischiorectal abscesses are usually evident on external exam as a tender erythematous swelling (Fig. 6.7). Intersphincteric abscesses are often not evident on external exam as they may not cause a swelling, but they cause significant pain and anal spasm due to their location between the internal and external sphincter.

The initial management of a perianal abscess is incision and drainage. Simple abscesses are amenable to drainage in the office with local anesthetic. Either a cruciate or a radial elliptical incision over the most fluctuant part of the swelling is effective for drainage; the cavity can be packed with a gauze strip for hemostasis for a few hours. After removal of the dressing, the wound does not require further packing but rather several warm water soaks per day. Antibiotics should only be given in case of extensive induration of the surrounding soft tissue.

Complicated abscesses include larger or recurrent abscesses, abscesses causing sepsis, and abscesses occurring in immunocompromised patients. These abscesses should be expeditiously drained and are likely to require operative management.

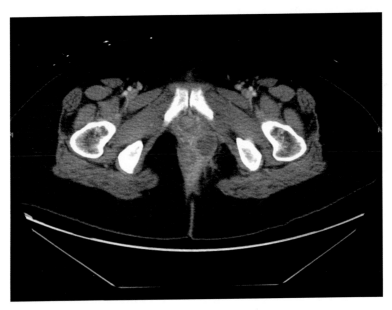

Fig. 6.7 While CT scan is usually not a necessary part of the work-up for perianal abscess, this patient presented with severe anal pain but without any external signs of swelling or erythema. Abscess drainage was performed

Health-care providers must maintain a high level of suspicion for a necrotizing soft tissue infection in this location, as these potentially infections progress rapidly to cause septic shock and death, with a median mortality rate over 30 %. Classic symptoms and signs of necrotizing fasciitis include pain out of proportion to examination, vital sign abnormalities consistent with sepsis, dishwater drainage from open wounds, and a black spot on the scrotum, which is indicative of underlying necrosis. Such patients must be emergently resuscitated, treated with broad-spectrum antibiotics, and undergo emergent aggressive operative debridement.

If the incision site fails to close completely, or if an abscess recurs, then an underlying fistula in ano is likely and requires referral to a surgeon specialized in treating anorectal conditions. Often, physical exam will reveal the fistula tract as a palpable cord under the skin between the opening on the skin and the anus. Generally, radiological studies are not a necessary part of the work-up as an experienced surgeon will be able to find the fistula tract during anal exam under anesthesia.

6.4.5   Pelvic Floor Disorders

Pelvic floor disorders include levator ani syndrome, proctalgia fugax, and pelvic floor dyssynergia. Patients who present with pelvic or anal pain should be evaluated for other etiologies such as fissure, anal or distal rectal mass or lesion, abscess or fistula, presacral mass, or sacrococcygeal masses [14]. If these diagnoses are ruled out by physical exam and cross-sectional imaging, then levator ani syndrome or proctalgia fugax should be considered. Differentiating characteristic of these diagnoses includes episodic pain that is unrelated to bowel movements and may even wake the patient up from sleep. Treatment options include biofeedback, tricyclic antidepressants, botulinum toxin injection, massage or physical therapy, and sacral nerve stimulation [15, 16]. Referral to pain specialists is appropriate for these conditions.

Pelvic floor dyssynergia, or pelvic floor dysfunction, should be suspected in patients with difficulty with defecation, which is often diagnosed as constipation. Anorectal manometry and electromyography confirm the diagnosis. Defecography can also be helpful in making the diagnosis. Biofeedback therapy is the mainstay of treatment for pelvic floor dysfunction.

Relevant Financial Disclosures None.

References

1. Ahnen DJ, Wade SW, Jones WF, Sifri R, Mendoza Silveiras J, Greenamyer J, et al. The increasing incidence of young-onset colorectal cancer: a call to action. Mayo Clin Proc. 2014;89(2):216–24.
2. Rao SS, Kuo B, McCallum RW, Chey WD, DiBaise JK, Hasler WL, et al. Investigation of colonic and whole-gut transit with wireless motility capsule and radiopaque markers in constipation. Clin Gastroenterol Hepatol. 2009;7(5):537–44.

3. Perez DR, Trakarnsanga A, Shia J, Nash GM, Temple LK, Paty PB, et al. Management and outcome of perianal Paget's disease: a 6-decade institutional experience. Dis Colon Rectum. 2014;57(6):747–51.
4. Levin B, Lieberman DA, McFarland B, Smith RA, Brooks D, Andrews KS, et al. Screening and surveillance for the early detection of colorectal cancer and adenomatous polyps, 2008: a joint guideline from the American Cancer Society, the US Multi-Society Task Force on Colorectal Cancer, and the American College of Radiology. CA Cancer J Clin. 2008;58(3): 130–60.
5. Parra-Blanco A, Gimeno-García AZ, Quintero E, Nicolás D, Moreno SG, Jiménez A, et al. Diagnostic accuracy of immunochemical versus guaiac faecal occult blood tests for colorectal cancer screening. J Gastroenterol. 2010;45(7):703–12.
6. Bean SM, Chhieng DC. Anal-rectal cytology: a review. Diagn Cytopathol. 2010;38(7): 538–46.
7. Chin-Hong PV, Berry JM, Cheng SC, Catania JA, Da Costa M, Darragh TM, et al. Comparison of patient- and clinician-collected anal cytology samples to screen for human papillomavirus-associated anal intraepithelial neoplasia in men who have sex with men. Ann Intern Med. 2008;149(5):300–6.
8. Goldstone SE, Johnstone AA, Moshier EL. Long-term outcome of ablation of anal high-grade squamous intraepithelial lesions: recurrence and incidence of cancer. Dis Colon Rectum. 2014;57(3):316–23.
9. Palefsky JM, Giuliano AR, Goldstone S, Moreira ED, Aranda C, Jessen H, et al. HPV vaccine against anal HPV infection and anal intraepithelial neoplasia. N Engl J Med. 2011;365(17): 1576–85.
10. Binda GA, Arezzo A, Serventi A, Bonelli L, Facchini M, Prandi M, et al. Multicentre observational study of the natural history of left-sided acute diverticulitis. Br J Surg. 2012;99(2): 276–85.
11. Ho VP, Nash GM, Milsom JW, Lee SW. Identification of diverticulitis patients at high risk for recurrence and poor outcomes. J Trauma Acute Care Surg. 2015;78(1):112–9.
12. Greenspon J, Williams SB, Young HA, Orkin BA. Thrombosed external hemorrhoids: outcome after conservative or surgical management. Dis Colon Rectum. 2004;47(9):1493–8.
13. Nelson RL, Thomas K, Morgan J, Jones A. Non surgical therapy for anal fissure. Cochrane Database Syst Rev. 2012;2, CD003431.
14. Singer MA, Cintron JR, Martz JE, Schoetz DJ, Abcarian H. Retrorectal cyst: a rare tumor frequently misdiagnosed. J Am Coll Surg. 2003;196(6):880–6.
15. Atkin GK, Suliman A, Vaizey CJ. Patient characteristics and treatment outcome in functional anorectal pain. Dis Colon Rectum. 2011;54(7):870–5.
16. Chiarioni G, Nardo A, Vantini I, Romito A, Whitehead WE. Biofeedback is superior to electrogalvanic stimulation and massage for treatment of levator ani syndrome. Gastroenterology. 2010;138(4):1321–9.

Cardiovascular Prevention in Men

7

Rony Lahoud and Irving Franco

7.1 Introduction

Cardiovascular disease (CVD) which encompasses coronary heart disease, stroke, and peripheral artery disease remains the leading cause of mortality in the developed world, notwithstanding significant advances in the prevention and acute management of these syndromes [1]. Despite a remarkable decline in mortality due to therapeutic and preventive measures, CVD still accounts for 33.6 % of all deaths in the USA and is the cause of 1 death every 36 s in the USA alone. Notably, males continue to experience far higher mortality rates at earlier ages than their female counterparts.

The economic burden of CVD was estimated at $444 billion in 2010, with the treatment of these diseases accounting for $1 of every $6 spent on healthcare in the USA. CVD remains the leading cause of hospitalization in the USA.

Most known risk factors for developing CVD are modifiable by preventive measures. These risk factors include cigarette smoking, sedentary lifestyle, dyslipidemia, hypertension, diabetes, metabolic syndrome, abdominal obesity, lack of regular exercise, and poor diet. According to the CDC, an estimated 68 million adults have hypertension (with only one half having their blood pressure controlled adequately) and 71 million have hyperlipidemia (with only one third having adequate treatment for this condition).

Simply stated, prevention saves lives. This chapter will address primary prevention strategies in males, divided by the major known contributors to CVD.

R. Lahoud, M.D.
Department of Cardiology, Cleveland Clinic Foundation, Cleveland, OH, USA

I. Franco, M.D. (✉)
Heart and Vascular Institute, Cleveland Clinic, 9500 Euclid Avenue, J2-3,
Cleveland, OH 44195, USA
e-mail: francoi@ccf.org

© Springer Science+Business Media New York 2016
J.M. Potts (ed.), *Men's Health*, DOI 10.1007/978-1-4939-3237-5_7

7.2   Major Components of Primary Prevention

7.2.1   Physical Activity

Sedentary persons have almost double the risk for CAD death as that of active persons. Even moderate physical activity provides a reduction in risk. Numerous studies have shown a strong graded response between levels of physical activities and decreased CV events. In addition, regular exercise is associated with improvement in the BP (mean reduction by 5 mmHg in those with hypertension), improves HDL, reduces triglyceride levels, and increases LDL particle size (without an effect on lowering LDL levels). Interestingly, these favorable effects are independent of weight loss associated with exercise and have a somewhat linear relationship with the intensity of exercise. Only 22 % of US adults engage in 30 min (or more) of exercise five times weekly. The American Heart Association recommends that adults perform at least 30 min of moderate intensity physical activity on most (and preferably all) days of the week. The rate of death decreased by 50 % by men 60 years and older whose status changed from unfit to fit over an 18-year follow-up period.

The mechanisms by which exercise exerts its beneficial effects are several and include improvement in CV risk factors (namely, hypertension, hyperlipidemia, and potential weight loss), as well as improve insulin sensitivity in diabetic patients. In fact, moderate intensity exercise has been associated with a reduced incidence of diabetes.

7.2.2   Tobacco

Despite the decline in the number of smokers in the Unites States in the past decade, nearly 20 % of adult Americans remain current smokers (with an increased rate of use in some populations including adolescents and young adults). There are more men than women who continue to smoke (21.5 % vs. 17.3 %), notwithstanding the recent rise in the rates of tobacco use among women [2].

Tobacco use is the single most important modifiable cardiovascular disease risk factor. In fact, cigarette use remains the leading cause of death in the USA, accounting for >400,000 deaths annually from CV and non-CV causes. There is a two- to threefold increase in the rates for coronary heart disease among those who consume >20 cigarettes daily. It is also important to remember that even passive exposure to tobacco or very low levels of consumption (<4 cigarettes daily) are also associated with increased rate of coronary artery disease. It has been clearly shown that continuation of smoking increases the risk for recurrent MI and need for repeat revascularization after the initial episode. Complete cessation is advocated and has been shown to reduce the risk of recurrent MI to levels equal to that of a nonsmoker within 3 years [3]. If complete cessation is not achievable, even a reduction of consumption by an increment of 5 cigarettes is associated with an 18 % decrease in mortality for each increment in patients who quit after MI [4].

Smoking leads to increased atherosclerosis and subsequent CVD. This occurs via several pathways which include acute unfavorable effects on blood pressure, myocardial oxygen supply, and sympathetic tone and longer-term vasomotor and endothelial dysfunction, increased inflammatory response, adverse lipid profile, platelet dysfunction, and a pro-coagulation state.

The importance of smoking cessation in any preventive clinic can hardly be overstated. The "5As" model for treating tobacco dependence has been shown to be effective and consists of the following components: ask, advise, assess, assist, and arrange. Patients should be asked about tobacco use at every encounter, and then every patient should be advised to quit (if current smoker) or provided with positive reinforcement (if past smoker). After identification, a physician should assess their readiness to quit. A commonly used model includes the following stages: precontemplation (no change intended), contemplation (intention to quit in the next 6 months), preparation (intend to quit within 1 month), action (discontinued smoking within the past 6 months), and maintenance (quit greater than 6 months prior). After assessment, the physician should assist the patient in quitting through counseling, providing resources (such as access to a support line), and pharmacotherapy. Although 70 % of all smokers state their intention to stop smoking, only ~4 % will be successful in doing so unaided, hence the importance of this step in successful smoking cessation. Counseling (as brief as 3 min or less during an office visit) has been shown to increase cessation rates by 30 %. The importance of community education regarding the dangers of smoking (severely lacking in developing countries and still important in developed countries) and physician-based primary prevention in the office remain paramount. Pharmacotherapy approaches are broadly divided into nicotine replacement therapies (via patch, gum, or nasal spray), and non-nicotine therapy (which includes sustained release bupropion, varenicline, clonidine, or nortriptyline) can also significantly increase abstinence rates. Interestingly, social influences can have a tremendous effect, with a ~2/3 increase in the chances of abstinence among smokers whose spouse also quits smoking and ~1/3 among those with a friend or coworker quitting smoking.

7.2.3 Hypertension

Hypertension is defined as a systolic blood pressure (BP) of 140 mmHg or greater and/or a diastolic blood pressures of 90 mmHg or greater among those not taking antihypertensive medications. Patients with a systolic BP of 120–140 mmHg and/or diastolic BP of 80–90 mmHg are classified as prehypertensive. It is thought to be present in~30 % of the US population and is increasingly prevalent with advanced age. Strikingly, a normotensive 55-year-old person might have a 90 % lifetime risk of developing hypertension as suggested by the Framingham Heart Study. In the National Health and Nutrition Examination Survey, only 68 % of participants were aware of their hypertension, and less than half of those aware of having hypertension had their BP adequately controlled. Although there remains a great deal of discussion regarding the relative importance of systolic vs. diastolic

BP, ambulatory vs. office-based measurements, diurnal variations in blood pressures, etc., greater emphasis has been placed on systolic blood pressure as a predictor of cardiovascular risk.

Primary (also called essential or idiopathic) hypertension accounts for 90 % of all cases of hypertension, while secondary hypertension (due to a variety of mostly treatable conditions) accounts for the rest. It is a complex disease with several environmental and genetic determinants. There is long-established graded relationship between blood pressure and cardiovascular risk, which holds even for those in the prehypertensive range. Beginning at 115/75 mmHg, each increase in 20/10 mmHg doubles the risk of cardiovascular disease. Importantly, the gradual rise of blood pressure over most patients' lifetime is not benign, and treatment of hypertension even in the elderly population has been shown to be beneficial.

Sodium reduction (e.g., DASH diet), weight loss, and exercise and discontinuation of tobacco and alcohol use are non-pharmacological approaches to reduce BP that could be successful in compliant patients. Nonetheless, the long-term effects of solely non-pharmacological approaches have generally been disappointing. The initiation of relatively simple mono or combination pharmacotherapies has been shown to be effective in treating hypertension and has a significant reduction in cardiovascular complications. The selection of the specific class of antihypertensive should be based on demographic factors and presence of concomitant comorbidities. For example, alpha-blockers should be considered for patients with benign prostatic hypertrophy, while ACE-inhibitors should be considered for those with diabetic nephropathy.

7.2.4 Hyperlipidemia

There is an estimate of more than 33 million Americans with elevated cholesterol levels [5]. Observational studies have repeatedly showed a strong graded relation between total cholesterol and LDL levels with cardiovascular events.

All patients with elevated total cholesterol or LDL should receive counseling on appropriate lifestyle modifications which include aerobic exercise, weight loss (for overweight patients), and a healthy diet.

Statins (HMG-CoA reductase inhibitors) represent the mainstay of pharmacologic therapy for patients with hyperlipidemia. Other lipid-lowering therapies (fibrates, niacin) have not shown convincing reductions in CV events despite their effect on improving lipid profiles. Newer therapies (such as PCSK-9 inhibitors) have shown great promise in early trials, but much more additional data is needed prior to widespread clinical use. Patients with known cardiovascular disease, CAD risk equivalents, or combination of multiple CV risk factors clearly benefit from initiation of statin therapy. For the remaining of the patients, the decision to initiate statin therapy depends on their baseline risk for CVD events and the potential for absolute risk reduction with addition of statin therapies. Several risk calculators are available and include the Framingham risk score, the recently issued AHA/ACC CV risk calculator in order to guide the clinician in appropriate risk stratification.

Recent guidelines have focused on identifying populations who would benefit from initiation of moderate vs. high-potency statins and have downplayed the importance of achieving specific LDL targets (except when checking for compliance with statin use). Examples of low-to-moderate statin doses include pravastatin 40 mg, lovastatin 20–40 mg, simvastatin 40 mg, and atorvastatin 10–20 mg, while high intensity statin doses include atorvastatin 40–80 mg and rosuvastatin 10–20 mg. Dose of statin should not be intensified for any LDL target. Statin intolerance (most commonly due to myalgia) is unfortunately not uncommon. While this could be resolved in some instances (by dose modification or switching statins), statins might have to be discontinued all together if the benefit of primary prevention does not outweigh the adverse effects. Patients should also undergo monitoring for the serious side effects of transaminitis (periodic monitoring of LFTs is recommended, frequency remains debated) and myopathy (clinicians should check CK for symptomatic patients only).

7.2.5 Diabetes and Metabolic Syndrome

Diabetes mellitus is the seventh leading cause of death in the USA. The prevalence of type 2 diabetes (which accounts for 90 % of cases) has unfortunately been on the rise, following the increase in rates of obesity in the USA and worldwide. The number of diabetics worldwide has increased from 35 million in 1985 to 171 million in 2000. Two million people are newly diagnosed with diabetes each year in the USA alone. The prevalence of diabetes is higher in men compared to women.

Simply stated, diabetes is a metabolic disorder characterized by inadequate insulin secretion necessary to maintain normal plasma glucose levels. Type II diabetes is characterized by increased insulin resistance, requiring ever-increasing levels of insulin production in order to maintain glycemic control. The definition of diabetes (according to the American Diabetes Association in 2011) is a fasting plasma glucose ≥ 126 mg/dl, a random plasma glucose ≥ 200 mg/dl (with hyperglycemic symptoms), 2-h plasma glucose ≥ 200 mg/dl, or a hemoglobin $A_{1C} \geq 6.5$ %.

It is important to note that CAD accounts for 75 % of deaths among diabetics, while CAD accounts for 30 % in nondiabetics. The 10-year risk of coronary heart disease (MI or death) is almost equal to those with a prior history of MI; therefore, DM is recognized as a CHD risk equivalent. Diabetic complications are generally divided into 2 categories: microvascular and macrovascular complications. Notably, hyperglycemia has a linear causal relationship with microvascular complications (such as retinopathy and nephropathy). Tight glucose control has been convincingly shown to lower diabetic retinopathy and nephropathy trials in two large trials: the Diabetes Control and Complications Trial and the UK Prospective Diabetes Study, both completed in the 1990s. On the other hand, insulin resistance promotes atherosclerosis even before frank diabetes occurs. In fact, patients with prediabetes have threefold increase in rate of myocardial infarctions, almost as high patients diagnosed with diabetes. There has been a relative paucity of data supporting intensive glucose control strategies for prevention of macrovascular complications (such as MI) when compared to prevention of microvascular complications. The current recommended target in a hemoglobin A_{1C} is ≤ 7 % and unfortunately has been shown to reach in only 31 % of participants in the NHANES registry.

Diabetes is a preventable disease and can be prevented or delayed by specific interventions such as 5–10 % weight loss, moderate exercise, avoiding tobacco use, and pharmacotherapy when indicated (metformin).

The term "metabolic syndrome" has slightly differing definitions according to different organizations. The joint AHA/IDF criteria for the diagnosis of metabolic syndrome consist of the following: (1) waist circumference in excess of population-/country-specific dimensions, (2) triglycerides ≥ 150 mg/dl (or drug treatment for hypertriglyceridemia), (3) HDL < 40 mg/dL in males (or drug treatment for low HDL), (4) systolic BP ≥ 130 mmHg and/or diastolic BP ≥ 85 mmHg (or drug treatment for hypertension), and (5) fasting glucose ≥ 100 mg/dL (or drug treatment for hyperglycemia). There has been some recent controversy on whether the sum of parts (metabolic syndrome) offers any additional risk prediction when compared to the sum of its parts (individual criteria). Controversies notwithstanding the identification of metabolic syndrome should focus the attention of the clinician on patients who are at a clearly higher risk of cardiovascular events.

7.2.6   Diet

The importance of a healthy eating pattern was emphasized in the 2006 American Heart Association Diet and Lifestyle recommendations for CVD risk reduction. General recommendations consist of (1) balanced calorie intake with physical activity to achieve a healthy weight; (2) consumption of fruits and vegetables; (3) choosing high-fiber, whole grain options; (4) at least twice weekly consumption of fish; (5) minimization of intake of beverages and foods with added sugars; (6) choosing/preparing foods with little or no added salt; and (7) moderate alcohol use if consumed. Specific recommendations include limiting intake of saturated fat to < 7 %, trans fat to < 1 %, total fat to 25–35 % of total energy intake daily, and cholesterol to < 300 mg daily. Some specific dietary patterns, such as the Mediterranean diet, have been the subject of large observational studies and have been associated with beneficial long-term effects on known CV risk factors. Although randomized trials have generally been disappointing, a Mediterranean diet might be associated with decreased cardiovascular events compared to a control group (who only received advice on low fat diet), with an observed absolute reduction in risk of ~3 CV deaths per 1000 person/year [6].

The issue of alcohol use has received significant attention recently. Moderate consumption of alcohol is defined as 2 drinks or less per day for men (1 or less for women). Men who have a moderate intake do not need to be counseled to discontinue, while those who do not consume alcohol do not need to start.

7.2.7 Obesity

Rate of obesity remains on the rise, and recent statistics show that a majority of Americans (66 %) are overweight (defined as BMI > 25 kg/m²), while 32 % are obese (defined as BMI > 30 kg/m²). The percentage of obese Americans has more than doubled in the past decade alone. This is a critical issue, especially in light of the steep rise in rates of obesity among adolescents. Numerous studies have shown that obesity has a linear relationship with the CV risk factors of hypertension, hyperlipidemia, and diabetes. Even after adjusting for known CV risk factors, higher BMI is clearly associated with cardiovascular mortality. Interestingly, obesity is associated with increased vascular events regardless of levels of physical activity. The waist-to-hip ratio, which is a marker of abdominal adiposity, has been shown to be an accurate predictor of coronary artery disease. Moreover, central obesity is a component of the diagnosis of metabolic syndrome, discussed separately in this chapter.

The main approach of therapy remains achieving a desirable balance between calorie restriction and exercise, along with general lifestyle improvement. Every patient presenting at a preventive clinic should receive advice and encouragement for lifestyle changes of proven benefit. Medications could be used for temporary management, but the effects of long-term use are uncertain. Surgical therapy is available in extreme cases and is associated with generally positive outcomes.

7.3 Conclusions

Primary prevention focusing on modification of known risk factors saves lives and is essential in our daily practice. These modifiable risk factors include cigarette smoking, sedentary lifestyle, dyslipidemia, hypertension, diabetes, metabolic syndrome, abdominal obesity, lack of regular exercise, and poor diet. Preventive interventions include both therapeutic lifestyle changes and adjunctive drug therapies when indicated, with additive beneficial effects achieved with the targeting of all relevant risk factors.

References

1. Johnson NB, Hayes LD, Brown K, Hoo EC, Ethier KA. CDC National Health Report: leading causes of morbidity and mortality and associated behavioral risk and protective factors--United States, 2005-2013. MMWR Surveill Summ. 2014;63 Suppl 4:3–27.
2. Gfroerer J, Dube SR, King BA, Garrett BE, Babb S, McAfee T. Vital signs: current cigarette smoking among adults aged ≥ 18 years with mental illness – United States, 2009-2011. MMWR Morb Mortal Wkly Rep. 2013;62:81–7.
3. Rea TD, Heckbert SR, Kaplan RC, Smith NL, Lemaitre RN, Psaty BM. Smoking status and risk for recurrent coronary events after myocardial infarction. Ann Intern Med. 2002;137: 494–500.

4. Gerber Y, Rosen LJ, Goldbourt U, Benyamini Y, Drory Y, Myoca ISGFA. Smoking status and long-term survival after first acute myocardial infarction a population-based cohort study. J Am Coll Cardiol. 2009;54:2382–7.
5. Roger VL, Go AS, Lloyd-Jones DM, et al. Heart disease and stroke statistics--2011 update: a report from the American Heart Association. Circulation. 2011;123:e18–209.
6. Estruch R, Ros E, Salas-Salvado J, et al. Primary prevention of cardiovascular disease with a Mediterranean diet. N Engl J Med. 2013;368:1279–90.

Metabolic Syndrome: The Vicious Cycle

8

Jeannette M. Potts

8.1 Introduction

The metabolic syndrome (MetS) has been defined as a cluster of risk factors for cardiovascular disease and type 2 diabetes mellitus, occurring together more often than could be attributed to chance alone. It is characterized by the co-occurrence of impaired glucose tolerance, central obesity, high levels of triglycerides, low levels of high-density lipoprotein, and hypertension.

The first unified agreement about the definition of the metabolic syndrome was drawn up during a meeting organized by the International Diabetes Federation in 2005. The major contributing factor to MetS, determined by this consensus, is obesity, measured by waist circumference and body mass index (BMI). Generally speaking, the majority of patients are obese, older, and sedentary and have insulin resistance. The determining factors in order are weight, genetics, aging, lifestyle, and excess caloric intake [1]. There are exceptions, however, with rare patients who meet the criteria for MetS diagnosis, but are not obese.

The metabolic syndrome is diagnosed when at least three of five of the following alterations are present: visceral obesity (waist circumference >102 cm in men or >88 cm in women), raised arterial blood pressure (>130/85 mmHg), dysglycemia (fasting plasma glucose >100 mg dL), raised triglyceride concentrations (>150 mg dL), and low HDL cholesterol (<40 mg dL in men or <50 mg dL in women).

J.M. Potts, M.D. (✉)
Vista Urology & Pelvic Pain Partners, 2998 South Bascom Avenue, Suite 100,
San Jose, CA 95124, USA
e-mail: DrPotts@VistaUrology.com

© Springer Science+Business Media New York 2016
J.M. Potts (ed.), *Men's Health*, DOI 10.1007/978-1-4939-3237-5_8

8.2   A Vicious Cycle

The increasing prevalence of MetS correlates to the growing numbers of obese persons. Theories for this phenomenon include genetic predisposition, diet [and a "super size" fast food culture], decrease physical activity, and physiological differences in taste and satiety.

Taken alone, each of the components of the metabolic syndrome confers their own set of risk factors and impairment, some of which initiate a cascade effect of other risk factors and diseases. These individual disorders or imbalances contribute to oxidative stress by causing an overproduction of reactive oxygen species (ROS), decreasing cellular antioxidant capacity (TAC), or both. This results in chronic end organ as well as systemic oxidative stress, which in turn affects other metabolic functions of the body [1]. Together, as the metabolic syndrome, the chronic systemic oxidative stress is even greater leading to more lethal disease and the overall acceleration of the aging process. To make matters worse, the very factors which perpetuate disease also act as obstacles toward reversing or interrupting the cycle. For example, depression and abnormal eating habits make it even more challenging for patients to initiate a program of regular exercise. Sleep disorders perpetuate imbalances of the HPA, negatively impacting motivation and compliance as well as exacerbating depressive symptoms (Fig. 8.1).

Thyroid dysfunction may also be a consequence or a perpetuating factor of MetS. One group found that within a euthyroid population, the incidence of MetS increased along with each quartile increase of the thyroid-stimulating hormone [2]. And just as compelling, 358 Nepalese patients with MetS, 29 % were found to have subclinical hypothyroidism detected by laboratory testing [3].

Other hormonal problems involve testosterone. Low total testosterone and sex hormone-binding globulin (SHBG) levels often seen in men with MetS are best explained by the hyperinsulinism and increased inflammatory cytokines that accompany obesity and increased waist circumference. Low SHBG levels may predict future development of the MetS in patients with some but not all criteria for diagnosis.

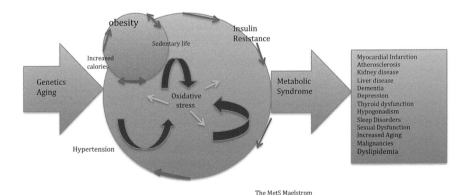

Fig. 8.1   The MetS maelstrom

Childhood obesity is of growing concern, with so many more children being diagnosed with dyslipidemias and carrying a greater risk for MetS as adults. A study of overweight children in Argentina revealed that 74 % of them had a variety of abnormalities, including dyslipidemias, consistent with MetS risk factors [4].

A 23-year study conducted in China demonstrated a strong correlation between childhood obesity and subsequent risk of adult obesity and diabetes. Through the Beijing Blood Pressure Cohort Study, 1209 subjects were followed from childhood through adulthood. The incidence of obesity in adulthood was 13.4 % in those without childhood obesity and 65 % in those adults with history of childhood obesity (documented by both BMI and subscapular skinfold measurement) [5]. Childhood obesity was also associated with an odds ratio of 2.8 for the development of diabetes in adulthood.

Prevention of childhood obesity would certainly be the most cost-effective way to avoid the vicious cycle of MetS.

8.3   The Chicken or the Egg

Several studies from around the world demonstrate strong relationships between lifestyle factors and the incidence of MetS. However, it is often difficult to discern whether certain factors are markers for the disease vs. secondary responses to the condition.

In a 2015 study conducted in India, periodontal disease was found to be associated with MetS, abdominal obesity being most strongly correlated. Gingival index, probing depth, and clinical attachment levels were the three parameters used in comparing the group who had MetS with the group who did not. The authors attribute the higher rate of periodontal disease in the MetS group to oxidative stress [6] (One of the defects in metabolic syndrome and its associated diseases is excess of reactive oxygen species. Reactive oxygen species generated by mitochondria, or from other sites within or outside the cell, cause damage to mitochondrial components and initiate degradative processes.) [1].

In a study using cross-sectional data from the National Health and Nutrition Examination Survey 2005–2008, eligible adults ($n=5511$) were classified into four groups by their number of natural teeth (excluding third molars): full dentition, 21–27 teeth, 1–20 teeth, or edentulous. After adjusting for age, gender, race/ethnicity, ratio of family income to poverty, physical activity, smoking, and energy intake, tooth loss was still significantly associated with metabolic syndrome ($p=0.002$). The number of natural teeth was inversely associated with body mass index, waist circumference, blood pressure, fasting plasma glucose, and insulin concentrations ($p<0.01$ for all); it was positively associated with serum HDL cholesterol concentration ($p=0.003$) [7].

Japanese investigators showed that regular tooth brushing may be protective against MetS. In a review of 12,548 records, self-reported dental hygiene was analyzed along with other lifestyle habits. (Not surprising, as cited in the Oral Health Chapter of this book, men took less care of their teeth and were more likely to have lower frequency of tooth brushing.) Regardless of gender, overall decreased frequency of tooth brushing was correlated to MetS [8]. These conclusions, however, are drawn from self-reported data, which may not reliably prove the correlation or, perhaps, even underestimate the impact of this simple practice.

In another example of potential self-report bias, a study to measure physical activity showed that subject's self-reported data was inconsistent with objective parameters obtained with 7-day accelerometry. Indeed the objective measure correlated more strongly with the inverse relationship between presence of MetS and physical activity [9]. Among the 5580 participants, individuals who did not meet the physical activity guideline had greater odds ratio of MetS.

Speed of eating was shown to increase the rate of developing MetS. In a prospective study, conducted in Japan, nearly 9000 subjects were followed for 3 years. During this period, 647 persons were diagnosed with MetS. This represented 3.1 % of fast eaters vs. 2.3 % of slow eaters. Multivariate-adjusted hazard ratio for the incidence of MetS in fast vs. slow eaters was 1.30 (95 % CI, 1.05–1.60) and also correlated to abnormal waist circumference [10].

The sense of taste may also play a role in MetS. To test this hypothesis, investigators used brain-scanning techniques to measure hypothalamic activation during sweet and bitter taste testing. They compared a group of 15 healthy middle-aged controls with 16 middle-aged persons with MetS, scanning each subject twice—during hunger and after satiety—as they rated pleasantness of sweet and bitter solutions. Participants with higher BMI had greater hypothalamic response during pleasantness evaluation of sucrose in the sated condition. The investigators also observed that middle-aged individuals with MetS responded with significantly less brain activation than controls without MetS during pleasantness evaluation of sweet and bitter tastes in regions involved in sensory and higher-level taste processing [11], which stimulates additional questions about overall brain functioning in the setting of MetS. But once again, did this difference in taste response predispose patients to MetS, or is this finding the consequence of the MetS?

8.4 Gender-Specific Consequences of MetS in Men

8.4.1 Prostate Cancer

Obesity and MetS are associated with increased risk of certain malignancies in men and women. Growing evidence demonstrates a strong correlation between MetS risk factors such as obesity and prostate cancer and more specifically a potentially higher risk of more clinically relevant, higher-grade tumors.

In a group of 668 men, 246 were found to have prostate cancer on biopsy, of which 110 were high grade (Gleason 7 or greater). Logistic regression multivariate analysis showed that BMI (OR 1.05 per unit, 95 % CI 1.00–1.10, $P=0.033$) and waist circumference (WC) (OR 1.02 per cm, 95 % CI 1.00–1.04, $P=0.026$) were significant predictors of prostate cancer diagnosis. BMI (OR 1.11, 95 % CI 1.04–1.18, $P=0.001$) and waist circumference (OR 1.04, 95 % CI 1.02–1.06,

$P=0.001$) were also associated with high-grade CaP. The more compelling result, however, is obesity with central adiposity (BMI $\geq$ 30 kg/m^2 and WC $\geq$ 102 cm), significantly associated with prostate cancer diagnosis (OR 1.66, 95 % CI 1.05–2.63, $P=0.03$) and high-grade disease (OR 2.56, 95 % CI 1.38–4.76, $P=0.003$) [12].

In a series of 195 patients undergoing 12-core prostate biopsy for PSA value $\geq$4 ng/ml and/or positive digital rectal examination, subjects also underwent measurements for BMI, waist circumferences, and blood pressure. Blood samples were also tested for PSA, fasting glucose, triglycerides, and cholesterol HDL. MS presence was defined according to Adult Treatment Panel III criteria. Patients had median age of 69 and median PSA of 5.6 ng/mL. While the presence of MetS was not associated with an increased risk of prostate cancer in this study (OR: 0.97, $P=0.94$), MetS was significantly correlated with an increased risk of Gleason $\geq$7 (OR: 3.82; $P=0.013$) [13].

Meanwhile, a retrospective study from Canadian showed a significant relationship between MetS and prostate cancer [14]. Of 2235 patients, 494 (22.1 %) had MetS. While no individual MetS component was independently associated with CaP, the increasing number of MetS components increased the association with higher-grade prostate cancer ($p<0.001$). Overall, OR between MetS and prostate cancer was 1.54 (95 % confidence interval [CI], 1.17–2.04, $p=0.002$). Odds ratio was 1.56 for high-grade and clinically significant cancer.

8.4.2   Lower Urinary Tract Symptoms

LUTS in men are typically attributed to changes secondary to bladder outlet obstruction caused by prostate enlargement. There is growing evidence of an association between the prevalence of MetS and LUTS in men. However, this association cannot be clearly explained by prostatic enlargement alone. MetS is associated with low testosterone or frank hypogonadism, with diminished stimulation of prostate growth. Bladder function alone may explain the higher incidence of LUTS in this population since LUTS and OAB occur with significantly higher frequency in women with MetS as well. A correlation between weight loss and improved LUTS in both men and women is also becoming better recognized. As comprehensively explained in Chap. 14, "Men have bladders, too," this may be an especially important perspective in the setting of MetS.

In a cohort of 4666 men aged 55–100 years consulting a general practitioner, metabolic syndrome and LUTS were reported in 51.5 % and 47 %, respectively. A significant link was identified between metabolic syndrome and treated LUTS ($P<0.001$). The risk of being treated for LUTS increased with an increasing number of MetS components. Each component, except high-density lipoprotein cholesterol, appeared as an independent risk factor of high IPSS and of LUTS treatment in multivariate analysis. Metabolic syndrome was positively correlated with the severity of the LUTS ($P<0.001$) for overall IPSS and both voiding and storage scores ($P<0.001$) [15]. Another interesting correlation was that between MetS and prostate volume. Taken in light of comorbidities, which could influence bladder function, the enlarged prostate may be a simple marker of age, given this older cohort of men 55–100. On the other hand, voiding and storage scores of the IPSS were affected, thereby implicating the prostate. Without urodynamics, however, we will not know for certain if the voiding component is due to impaired bladder contractility rather than BOO.

In 409 consecutive men seen in urology for LUTS, waist circumference was found to be significantly and positively associated with prostate volume, serum prostate-specific antigen, and International Prostate Symptom Score. Not surprising, increased waist circumference was also significantly associated with a greater prevalence of hypertension, coronary artery disease, DM2, and obesity as well as the presence of erectile dysfunction and ejaculatory dysfunction [16]. The authors promote the use of waist measurement as a correlate to urinary function as well as general health screening, specifically for MetS.

In a very recent 2015 review, however, the authors concluded that MetS and components were determinants of prostate enlargement and MetS "induced metabolic derangements in the development of benign prostate enlargement" [17]. The review of 82 articles led to inclusion of only 8, meeting the criteria for the authors' analysis. The eight studies enrolled 5403 patients, 1426 (26.4 %) of which had MetS. Patients with MetS had significantly higher total prostate volume when compared with those without MetS (+1.8 mL, 95 % confidence interval [CI], 0.74–2.87, $P<0.001$). (**It is important, however, to bear in mind the potentially negligible clinical significance 1.8 mL, especially in such a large cohort of subjects, which predisposes to possible statistical volume bias, whereby clinically insignificant differences are given undeserved statistical significance.**) Surprisingly, there were no differences in IPSS between patients with or without MetS. Meta-regression analysis showed that differences in total prostate volume were significantly higher in older (adjusted $r=0.09$, $P=0.02$), obese patients (adjusted $r=0.26$, $P<0.005$) and low serum high-density lipoprotein cholesterol concentrations (adjusted $r=-0.33$, $P<0.001$). Again, while I do aggressively counsel patients about their weight, diet, and exercise levels, these analyses as such may not have as much clinical relevance in terms of benign prostatic enlargement alone.

From 2009 to 2014, 431 patients of median age 67 years, with median PSA of 3 ng/mL, were evaluated for LUTS in association with BMI, testosterone, as well as the presence of MetS. Twenty-four percent of the patients had MetS, and they were found to have higher IPSS storage subscores. On multivariate analysis, the presence of MetS was associated with an increased risk of an IPSS storage subscore ≥ 4 (odds ratio, 1.782; 95 % confidence interval, 1.045–3.042; $P=.030$) [18]. Again, the storage symptoms may have more to do with the bladder dysfunction, also seen in females with MetS, than with prostatic enlargement.

Although there has not yet been a double-blinded randomized control trial to analyze the effects of testosterone replacement therapy on LUTS, currently available observations demonstrate no increase of LUTS or harm caused by hormone replacement. Indeed, for some, there may be improvement of LUTS with testosterone replacement. This argues against a prostatocentric etiology for LUTS, i.e., the symptoms cannot be solely attributed to prostate enlargement.

From an observational registry study, 261 hypogonadal men treated with testosterone replacement were found to have significant improvement in LUTS after a median follow-up of 42.3 months. The mean IPSS decreased from 10.35 to 6.58, ($P \leq 0.05$). The significant improvement was consistent even after controlling for weight loss and PDE5 inhibitors [19].

A cross-sectional study in a cohort of patients with LUTS-BPH showed an increase of more than fivefold of having a Framingham cardiovascular disease (CVD) risk score of ≥ 10 % (intermediate to high risk) in men with moderate–severe LUTS. For this study, 336 consecutive patients with BPH-related LUTS were prospectively enrolled. The Framingham CVD 10-year risk score was calculated for each patient [20]. Low risk had ≤ 10 % CVD risk at 10 years, with intermediate risk 10–20 % and with high risk ≥ 20 %. Logistic regression analyses were used to identify variables for predicting a Framingham CVD risk score of ≥ 10 % and moderate–severe LUTS using IPSS of 8 or greater. After adjusting for confounding factors, moderate–severe LUTS was independently associated with Framingham CVD risk score of ≥ 10 % (OR 5.91, $P < 0.05$).

8.4.3   Testosterone and Sex

The MetS is strongly correlated with erectile dysfunction and hypogonadism [21] (which are also predictors of future development of MetS). Few studies have addressed treatment of these dysfunctions in the special setting of MetS, other than the observational effects on sexual function after correction of individual risk factors. For example, nonsurgical weight loss has been shown to improve sexual function [22].

In studies of elderly men, low testosterone is frequently associated with erectile dysfunction. However, prevalence of low testosterone and ED is significantly greater among men who are obese or have features of MetS. MetS is also associated with greater incidence of ejaculatory dysfunction including PE as well as delayed ejaculation [22]. One group of 803 consecutive men attending an outpatient medical clinic were evaluated for the incidence and relationship between MetS and sexual dysfunction. Among the 236 patients (29.4 %) who were diagnosed as having MetS, 96.5 % reported ED, 39.6 % hypoactive sexual desire, 22.7 % premature ejaculation, and 4.8 % delayed ejaculation. Patients with MetS were characterized by greater subjective and objective ED parameters and by greater somatized anxiety than the rest of the sample [23]. The prevalence of overt hypogonadism (total testosterone <8 nM) was significantly higher in patients with MetS (11.9 % vs. 3.8 %) and was associated with typical hypogonadism-related symptoms, such as hypoactive sexual desire, low frequency of sexual intercourse, and depressive symptoms.

Diabetes is strongly associated with ED and up to one-third of diabetic men have low testosterone levels. Both conditions, DM and ED, are cardiovascular risk factors. These risk factors are often influenced by comorbidities, which are common in this group of patients, i.e., hypertension, obesity, and dyslipidemia. But as demonstrated in a recent review of the literature, low testosterone may be implicated in each one of these conditions [24].

While hormone replacement therapy in men has been linked to decreased visceral and central body fat [25], patients who engage in weight loss programs with vigorous exercise have been able to improve these parameters and increase their testosterone levels naturally [26].

Viewing the relationship between MetS from a sexual function vantage point also reveals strong links between sexual dysfunction and cardiovascular risk. In one study, after adjusting for comorbid conditions, incident ED alone was associated with a hazard ratio (HR) of 1.25 [95 % confidence interval (CI), 1.04–1.53; $p=0.04$] for subsequent cardiovascular events including MI, coronary revascularization, cerebrovascular accident, transient ischemic attack, congestive heart failure, fatal cardiac arrest, or nonfatal cardiac arrhythmia [27]. Prevalent cases of ED were associated with even higher risk. These observations illustrate the significance of sexual dysfunction as a marker for cardiovascular risk, comparable to the effects of family history of MI, cigarette smoking, or hyperlipidemia!

I agree enthusiastically with the thesis put forth by Miner and Seftel [24], regarding the importance of addressing men's sexual health as a strategy to impact overall health. Traditionally, ED and testosterone levels have been considered mainly, if not exclusively, in the context of sexual health. However, their review and analysis of the literature suggest that these measures provide gender-specific determinants to assess general health in men, including overall cardiovascular and mortality risk.

8.5   Reversing the Trend

Weight loss is the most effective way to manage and reverse the harms associated with MetS. However, as cited by many specialists, recidivism in obesity is high.

Central obesity can be targeted through appetite suppression. Medications used for this purpose include lorcaserin, which has been shown to aid in sustainable weight loss. It may cause, however, attention deficit and other cognitive impairment, as well as headache, dizziness, fatigue, nausea, dry mouth, and constipation [28]. A combination of extended release phentermine and topiramate provides significant appetite reduction and weight loss using a low dose of each chemical to minimize adverse effects. However, there remain concerns about blood pressure elevation, increase pulse rate, potential teratogenicity, and possible neuropathy. Although the mechanism of action of sustained release bupropion with naltrexone for weight reduction is not fully understood, the combination may induce alterations in the hypothalamic melanocortin system as well as brain reward systems that favorably influence mood and food cravings [28].

Thiazolidinedione (TZD) and metformin are examples of insulin sensitizers, targeting one of the most fundamental pathways through which MetS reeks its havoc. TZD reduces the intracellular levels of toxic lipid metabolites, resulting in less lipotoxicity. It also protects against the cytostatic effect of free fatty acids and restores glucose-mediated insulin release. TZD also increases insulin sensitivity in the liver and muscle tissue. While TZD has also been demonstrated to decrease the rate of conversion from prediabetes to diabetes by 72 %, worrisome adverse effects, such as fluid retention, weight gain, and potential urothelial neoplasm, impede its widespread use. Metformin, on the other hand, is recommended as first-line therapy for type 2 diabetes by both the American and the European diabetic associations [28]. Metformin, like TZD, reduces the incidence of new onset diabetes in individuals with metabolic syndrome and should be considered in patients with impaired fasting glucose or impaired glucose tolerance (prediabetes).

Glucagon-like-peptide agonists seem to be a good candidate drug class for metabolic syndrome subjects with hyperglycemia and overweight/obesity since it enhances insulin sensitivity and reduces body weight as well as increases insulin secretory function.

Sodium glucose transporter-2 inhibitors may have the potential to reduce cardiovascular risk not only via glucose-lowering effect but via beneficial effects on body weight, blood pressure, and serum uric acid in patients with metabolic syndrome.

Lipid-lowering agents, such as statins, have been shown to greatly reduce cardiovascular morbidity and mortality in the setting of hyperlipidemia associated with MetS. In some patients with MetS, the treatment for dyslipidemia requires the addition of fibrates in order to target the elevated triglyceride component.

A recent analysis with Cardiovascular Health Study showed that RAS blocking agents reduced cardiovascular events in patients with metabolic syndrome [29]. Thus, renin-angiotensin system blockers are indicated for the treatment of elevated blood pressure in people with metabolic syndrome. ACE inhibitors also have a favorable effect on glucose metabolism as demonstrated by clinical trials such as the HOPE. Besides lowering blood pressure, these medications also decrease oxidative stress and endothelial dysfunction [28].

Recent reports demonstrate dramatic changes in weight, waist circumference, insulin sensitivity, and hemoglobin A1c levels and improvements in each of the components of the MetS induced by testosterone therapy [30]. Multiple cross-sectional studies have found low testosterone and low sex hormone-binding globulin (SHBG) levels in men with MetS, irrespective of age. Normally, 40–50 % of testosterone is bound to SHBG, so reducing SHBG levels will decrease testosterone. Hyperinsulinism, strongly associated with obesity and MetS, suppresses SHBG synthesis and secretion by the liver. This relationship is further supported by the fact that pharmacological correction of hyperinsulinemia improves SHBG levels.

Thirty-two men with MetS, newly diagnosed type 2 diabetes, and low testosterone level were randomized to 52 weeks of treatment with diet and exercise with or without transdermal testosterone (50 mg per day). Addition of testosterone to supervised diet and exercise resulted in greater therapeutic improvement of glycemic control and reversed the MetS in 81 % versus 31 % of controls after 52 weeks [31]. I believe the emphasis here is lifestyle and behavioral intervention, enhanced by replacement therapy, and not just testosterone therapy alone. As mentioned earlier in the chapter, men were able to increase testosterone levels endogenously through vigorous exercise.

While there is growing interest and evidence in disproving harm associated with testosterone [replacement] therapy, large randomized trials are not yet complete. Hopefully, we will gain greater confidence in using hormonal supplementation without fear of increasing cardiovascular risk, increasing prostate size, or increasing risk of prostate cancer. Indeed, there is reason to suspect that replacement therapy may be more beneficial overall.

8.6 Conclusion

The incidence of metabolic syndrome is increasing in the USA and abroad. While the MetS is most frequently associated with increased cardiovascular disease, MetS also predisposes patients to various endocrinopathies besides DM, sexual dysfunction, liver and kidney diseases, as well as depression and dementia. Obesity and sedentary lifestyle appear to be the most potent catalysts in the development of a vicious cycle of declining health and aging.

Using "sexual function" as a screener and incentive for men may be an effective means to address metabolic syndrome and prevent diabetes and cardiovascular disease. If we, as physicians, genuinely wish to make an impact on overall health and life expectancy, we must initiate discussions about obesity and lack of physical activity as well as educating our patients about their sexual problems.

References

1. Bonomini F, Rodella LF, Rezzani R. Metabolic syndrome, aging and involvement of oxidative stress. Aging Dis. 2015;6(2):109–20.
2. Shinkov A, Borissova AM, Kovatcheva R, et al. The prevalence of the metabolic syndrome increases through the quartiles of thyroid stimulating hormone in a population-based sample of euthyroid subjects. Arq Bras Endocrinol Metabol. 2014;58(9):926–32.
3. Gyawali P, Takanche JS, Shrestha RK, et al. Pattern of thyroid dysfunction in patients with metabolic syndrome and its relationship with components of metabolic syndrome. Diabetes Metab J. 2015;39(1):66–73.
4. Casavalle PL, Lifshitz F, Romano LS, et al. Prevalence of dyslipidemia and metabolic syndrome risk factor in overweight and obese children. Pediatr Endocrinol Rev. 2014;12(2):213–23.
5. Liang Y, Hou D, Zhao X, et al. Childhood obesity affects adult metabolic syndrome and diabetes. Endocrine. 2015.
6. Patel SP, Kalra N, Pradeep AR, et al. Association of metabolic syndrome and periodontal disease in an Indian population. J Int Acad Periodontol. 2014;16(4):98–102.
7. Zhu Y, Hollis JH. Associations between the number of natural teeth and metabolic syndrome in adults. J Clin Periodontol. 2015;42(2):113–20.
8. Tsutsumi C, Kakuma T. Regular tooth brushing is associated with a decreased risk of metabolic syndrome according to a medical check-up database. Kurume Med J. 2015.
9. Tucker JM, Welk GJ, Beyler NK, Kim Y. Associations between physical activity and metabolic syndrome: comparison between self-report and accelerometry. Am J Health Promot. 2015.
10. Zhu B, Haruyama Y, Muto T, Yamazaki T. Association between eating speed and metabolic syndrome in a three-year population-based cohort study. J Epidemiol. 2015;25(4):332–6.
11. Green E, Jacobson A, Haase L, Murphy C. Neural correlates of taste and pleasantness evaluation in the metabolic syndrome. Brain Res. 2015. pii: S0006-8993(15)00231-0.
12. De Nunzio C, Albisinni S, Freedland SJ, et al. Abdominal obesity as risk factor for prostate cancer diagnosis and high grade disease: a prospective multicenter Italian cohort study. Urol Oncol. 2013;31(7):997–1002.

13. De Nunzio C, Freedland SJ, Miano R, et al. Metabolic syndrome is associated with high grade Gleason score when prostate cancer is diagnosed on biopsy. Prostate. 2011;71(14):1492–8.
14. Bhindi B, Locke J, Alibhai SMH, et al. Dissecting the association between metabolic syndrome and prostate cancer risk: analysis of a large clinical cohort. Eur Urol. 2015;67(1):64–70.
15. Pashootan P, Ploussard G, Cocaul A, de Gouvello A, Desgrandchamps F. Association between metabolic syndrome and severity of lower urinary tract symptoms (LUTS): an observational study in a 4666 European men cohort. BJU Int. 2014;17.
16. Lee RK, Chung D, Chughtai B, Te AE, Kaplan SA. Central obesity as measured by waist circumference is predictive of severity of lower urinary tract symptoms. BJU Int. 2012;110(4):540–5.
17. Gacci M, Corona G, Vignozzi L, Salvi M, et al. Metabolic syndrome and benign prostatic enlargement: a systematic review and meta-analysis. BJU Int. 2015;115(1):24–31.
18. De Nunzio C, Cindolo L, Gacci M, et al. Metabolic syndrome and lower urinary tract symptoms in patients with benign prostatic enlargement: a possible link to storage symptoms. Urology. 2014;84(5):1181–7.
19. Yassin DJ, El Douaihy Y, Yassin AA, et al. Lower urinary tract symptoms improve with testosterone replacement therapy in men with late-onset hypogonadism: 5-year prospective, observational and longitudinal registry study. World J Urol. 2014;32(4):1049–54.
20. Russo GI, Castelli T, Privitera S et al. Increase of Framingham cardiovascular disease risk score is associated with severity of lower urinary tract symptoms. BJU Int. 2015.
21. Chughtai B, Lee RK, Te AE, Kaplan SA. Metabolic syndrome and sexual dysfunction. Curr Opin Urol. 2011;21(6):514–8.
22. Wang C, Jackson G, Jones TH, et al. Low testosterone associated with obesity and the metabolic syndrome contributes to sexual dysfunction and cardiovascular disease risk in men with type 2 diabetes. Diabetes Care. 2011;34:1669–75.
23. Corona G, Mannucci E, Schulman C, et al. Psychobiologic correlates of the metabolic syndrome and associated sexual dysfunction. Eur Urol. 2006;50(3):595–604.
24. Miner MM, Seftel AD. Erectile dysfunction and testosterone screening with prostate specific antigen screening at age 40: are these three gender specific determinants additive for overall men's heath and do they improve traditional non-gender specific determinants to lessen cardiovascular risk and all-cause mortality? Int J Clin Pract. 2010;64(13):1754–62.
25. Saad F, Aversa A, Isidori AM, Gooren LJ. Testosterone as potential effective therapy in treatment of obesity in men with testosterone deficiency: a review. Curr Diabetes Rev. 2012;8(1):131–43.
26. Lovell DI, Cuneo R, Wallace J, McLellan C. The hormonal response of older men to submaximum aerobic exercise: the effect of training and detraining. Steroids. 2012;77(5):413–8.
27. Thompson IM, Tangen CM, Goodman PJ, Probstfield JL, Moinpour CM, Coltman CA. Erectile dysfunction and subsequent cardiovascular disease. JAMA. 2005;294:2996–3002.
28. Lim S, Eckel RH. Pharmacological treatment and therapeutic perspectives of metabolic syndrome. Rev Endocr Metab Disord. 2014;15(4):329–41.
29. Zreikat HH, Harpe SE, Slattum PW, et al. Effect of Renin-Angiotensin system inhibition on cardiovascular events in older hypertensive patients with metabolic syndrome. Metabolism. 2014;63(3):392–9.
30. Cunningham GR. Testosterone and metabolic syndrome. Asian J Androl. 2015;17(2):192–6.
31. Heufelder AE, Saad F, Bunck MC, Gooren L. Fifty-two-week treatment with diet and exercise plus transdermal testosterone reverses the metabolic syndrome and improves glycemic control in men with newly diagnosed type 2 diabetes and subnormal plasma testosterone. J Androl. 2009;30:726–33.

Andrology: Puberty-Fertility-Andropause

David P. Guo and Michael L. Eisenberg

9.1 Puberty

Puberty refers to the biological changes that occur as one matures into a young adult. While cognitive, psychological, and social changes may occur during this period of adolescence, puberty in the clinical sense commonly refers to the development of reproductive capacity and secondary sexual characteristics. Specifically, the child begins to secrete increasing amounts of sex hormones and produce mature gametes.

Changes to the hypothalamic-pituitary-gonadal axis bring about the effects of puberty. At puberty, the hypothalamus begins to secrete gonadotropin-releasing hormone (GnRH) in a pulsatile fashion, which leads to pulsatile secretion of luteinizing hormone (LH) and follicle-stimulating hormone (FSH). LH stimulates the Leydig cells in the testes to produce testosterone and other androgens, while FSH stimulates Sertoli cells to produce substances that promote gametogenesis [1].

Puberty normally follows a predictable sequence of events. The first sexual change is an increase in testicular size. Next, there is an increase in penile length and then the development of pubic hair. By convention, sexually maturity is rated according to the Tanner Staging Chart (Table 9.1), which classifies the stages of puberty from 1 to 5 according to genital changes (penile length, testicular volume) and pubic hair distribution. Boys progress from prepubertal stage 1, characterized by the absence of genital growth and pubic hair, to mature adult stage 5, during which the genitalia has reached adult size and pubic hair is robust and extends to the medial thigh. Traditionally, it was thought that nocturnal seminal emissions (spermarche) occur after the development of pubic hair. However, a longitudinal study of 40 boys using spermaturia to evaluate spermarche found a wide variation

D.P. Guo, M.D. • M.L. Eisenberg, M.D. (✉)
Department of Urology, Stanford University School of Medicine,
300 Pasteur Drive, S-287, Stanford, CA 94305, USA
e-mail: davidguo@stanford.edu; eisenberg@stanford.edu

© Springer Science+Business Media New York 2016
J.M. Potts (ed.), *Men's Health*, DOI 10.1007/978-1-4939-3237-5_9

Table 9.1 Tanner stages of puberty

Stage	Pubic hair	Genitalia
I	No pubic hair	Penis, testes similar size/proportion as in early childhood
II	Minimal, downy hair at base of penis	Testes have grown, scrotal texture changes
III	Darker, more coarse hair spreads over pubic region	Penile length increases; testes continue to grow
IV	Adult-type hair distributed across pubic region (does not reach thighs)	Penile length and girth increase; continued testis growth with darkening of scrotum
V	Adult-type hair that extends to medial surface of thighs	Adult size penis and testes

testicular size (median 11.5 mL, range 4.7–19.6 mL) and Tanner stage (median 2.5, range 1–5) [2].

While the sequence of pubertal events is predictable, there are fluctuations in the age of onset and pace of development. In a study of 228 British boys from 1970, Tanner and colleagues found the average onset of puberty to be 11.6 years (range 9.5–13.5 years) and the average time to completion of puberty over 3 years (range 1.8–4.7 years) [3]. More recent data on 4131 American boys indicated an earlier onset of puberty: 9.14 years for African American, 10.14 years for non-Hispanic white males, and 10.04 years for Hispanic males [4]. With this new data, it is possible that the current clinical norm (average age of puberty 11.5 years, range 9–14 years) will undergo an adjustment in the coming years.

In addition to sexual changes, other physiologic transitions occur during puberty. Skeletal maturation is accelerated due to the production of sex hormones. The secretion of testosterone also stimulates the release of growth hormone (GH), and the release of GH influences insulin-like growth hormone (IGF). As a result, there is increased bone growth, along with changes in weight and body composition. In fact, the classic change in voice occurs due to the differential effect of testosterone on the growth of the wide bones of the larynx [5].

Several medical issues may become apparent with the onset of puberty. Gynecomastia may be a bothersome manifestation in about 50 % of boys but is usually self-limited and usually resolves within a year [6]. The development of myopia often occurs during puberty due to changing axial length of the eyes and appears to be most correlated with the growth spurt [7]. The prevalence and severity of acne increases with the onset of puberty [8]. Psychological, emotional, and behavioral issues may also manifest at puberty.

9.1.1   Clinical Implications

The timing of puberty and whether a child is developing normally are frequent areas of concern that a clinician should be prepared to address. The onset of puberty is thought to coincide with central nervous system maturation, which results in the gradual increase of pulsatile secretion of GnRH. The onset of puberty is determined heavily by genetics, but factors including ethnicity, nutritional status, medical conditions, and environmental exposures also affect the timing of puberty. When the onset of puberty occurs 2.5 standard deviations earlier or later than the average age of onset, clinicians should be suspicious for an underlying pathology.

Precocious puberty should be suspected if a male child develops symptoms of puberty prior to age 9 (although this number has been debated due to recent findings that the age of puberty is declining in the USA). Precocious puberty may be central (gonadotropin dependent) or peripheral (gonadotropin independent). Central causes depend on the hypothalamic-pituitary-gonadal (HPG) axis and may result from idiopathic early maturation of the HPG axis or development of a hormone-secreting central tumor. Peripheral causes include hormone-secreting testicular or adrenal tumors and exogenous steroid administration.

Delayed puberty should be suspected if the patient does not show signs of testicular volume growth or pubic hair growth until after age 14. Constitutional delay of puberty, in which there is no pathology and the patient undergoes puberty at the later end of the spectrum, accounted for 63 % of cases of delayed puberty in a large academic series of 158 boys [9]. The other main causes are functional hypogonadotropic hypogonadism, in which puberty is delayed but occurs spontaneously despite an underlying condition; idiopathic delayed puberty, in which a cause is not found; or permanent hypogonadism (hypergonadotropic or hypogonadotropic).

Patients who are suspected to have precocious puberty or delayed puberty should be referred for evaluation by a pediatric endocrinologist, who may provide treatment according to underlying etiology.

9.2 Fertility

Men become fertile after the maturation of their gametes during puberty. In contrast to women, who experience an accelerated rate of fertility decline by age 35, there is no limit to fertility as long as a man still produces sperm. However, recent data does suggest a slight decline in fertility with male age [10].

The World Health Organization (WHO) defines infertility as the failure to achieve a clinical pregnancy after 12 months or more of regular unprotected sexual intercourse [11]. Studies have shown that up to 15 % of couples experience problems with fertility [12]. In 20 % of these situations, there is a male factor that is primarily responsible for infertility. In 30 % of situations, there are both male and female factors involved. Therefore, 50 % of infertility cases involve the male [13, 14].

A useful framework for classifying the causes of male infertility is to consider pre-testicular, testicular, and post-testicular causes. Pre-testicular causes refer mainly to endocrine dysfunction or any medical conditions or exposures that secondarily affect testicular function. Testicular causes refer to the failure of normal sperm production despite a favorable hormonal environment. Factors such as varicocele, cryptorchidism, genetic defects, trauma, infection, or malignancy may cause primary testicular failure. Post-testicular causes refer to anatomic or functional problems with releasing sperm, such as obstruction of the vas deferens or ejaculatory ducts.

9.2.1 Clinical Implications

A thorough medical history is vital to the evaluation of male infertility. It is important to note the age of the female partner, since the age of 35 is considered advanced maternal age, and the woman should also receive a separate evaluation. Aspects of the couple's relationship should be investigated, including the length of time in active attempt to conceive, the timing of coitus in relation to the woman's mid-ovulatory cycle, and whether either partner been involved in a previous pregnancy. The medical history should investigate childhood diseases or urologic problems such as a varicocele, cryptorchidism, hypospadias, and any instances of genitourinary trauma or infection. Surgeries in the inguinal, pelvic or genital region may disrupt the reproductive tract. Medications, most notably exogenous steroids, as well as certain antibiotics can disrupt spermatogenesis. Sexually transmitted diseases may result in scarring and obstruction of the reproductive tract. Exposures, both recreational and environmental, should be recorded. Tobacco [15], marijuana, and alcohol use have been associated with semen abnormalities, as well as certain pesticides [16], sauna exposure [17], and laptop usage [18].

The general physical exam, including stature, distribution of hair, and presence of gynecomastia, may provide clues about the patient's androgen status. The genitourinary exam should focus on the phallus and scrotal contents. Anatomical abnormalities of the phallus, including hypospadias and penile torsion, may hinder fertility. For the scrotal examination, an orchidometer is a useful tool to estimate volume and may diagnose testicular atrophy: the size of the adult testes is on average: 4.6 cm long by 2.6 cm wide and 18–20 mL. In addition, the spermatic cord should be palpated to confirm presence of the vas deferens bilaterally and also to evaluate for a varicocele, which is a testicular engorgement of the veins that supply the testes. While 15 % of the male population has a varicocele, 40 % of men with infertility have a varicocele.

Semen analysis should be performed in a male fertility evaluation. The WHO revised its of standards in 2010 for minimum standards of semen quality consistent with fertility using data from over 4500 men from 14 countries [11]. These 5th edition criteria are ejaculate volume (>1.5 mL), sperm concentration (>15×10^6 sperm/mL), vitality (>58 %), progressive motility (>32 %), total motility (>40 %), and morphology (4 % based on Kruger strict criteria) (Table 9.2). Because semen quality can vary widely for the individual male, two samples taken at least 7 days apart are recommended. While semen analyses are useful for some diagnoses, about half of men from infertile couples do not have abnormalities on standard semen analysis [19]. Moreover, men with abnormal semen parameters often achieve pregnancy.

In addition to a semen analysis, serum testosterone and FSH are routinely sent. Low FSH and low testosterone indicate hypogonadotropic hypogonadism, which

Table 9.2 WHO 5th edition semen parameter guidelines, 2010

Measurement	Lower limit	95 % Confidence intervals
Volume (mL)	1.5	1.4–1.7
Sperm count (million per ejaculate)	39	33–46
Concentration (million/mL)	15	12–16
Vitality (live %)	58	55–63
Progressive motility (PR, %)	32	31–34
Total motility (PR + NP, %)	40	38–42
Normal morphology (%)	4	3.0–4.0

may be congenital or iatrogenic (e.g., steroids). High FSH and low testosterone indicate primary hypogonadism due to testicular failure. Further endocrine studies may be necessary if there are abnormalities in these parameters or if there are additional symptoms suggestive of endocrine dysfunction. These include prolactin, LH, and estradiol levels. For example, hyperprolactinemia may be caused by medications, systemic disease, or a pituitary tumor.

An estimated 15 % of infertile men with azoospermia or severe oligospermia have a genetic abnormality. A family history or congenital absence of the vas deferens (CAVD) may indicate cystic fibrosis, since 2 % of infertile males have cystic fibrosis and 90 % of patients with CAVD have cystic fibrosis. In addition, polymerase chain reaction can detect several deletions on the Y chromosome that have been associated with infertility. Karyotype analysis can identify chromosomal causes of infertility, such as Klinefelter's syndrome, in which there is an extra X chromosome.

9.2.2 Treatment

Modern treatment for fertility has drastically increased the fertility rate for patients.

Medical Therapies

For hypogonadotropic hypogonadism, treatment with human chorionic gonadotropin (hCG) and FSH can induce testosterone and stimulate spermatogenesis [20]. For idiopathic infertility, treatment with clomiphene citrate, an estrogen antagonist, has been attempted, but without successful improvement of pregnancy rate [21]. A large meta-analysis of 48 RCTs that study the effect on infertile men of antioxidants, including zinc, vitamin E, vitamin C, L-carnitine, and N-acetylcysteine, on fertility have suggested an improvement in live birth rate, though the quality of evidence was deemed to be low [22].

Surgical Therapies

A variety of surgical interventions are available, depending on the etiology of infertility. For infertile males with varicocele, a varicocelectomy can be performed via a laparoscopic or open approach (inguinal, subinguinal, or retroperitoneal) as well as through interventional radiologic procedures at some centers. For men who have a prior vasectomy or another cause of vasal obstruction, vasal aspiration may be performed to retrieve sperm for one-time use. Microscopic reconstruction may also be performed, with success rates between 70 and 90 % [23]. The vas deferens may be reconnected (vasovasostomy) or the vas deferens can be connected to the epididymis (epididymovasostomy). For men with nonobstructive azoospermia, the use of microscopic techniques was shown to improve the yield of surgical extracted sperm from 45 to 63 % [24]. Furthermore, a review of 1127 men with azoospermia who underwent microdissection testicular sperm extraction demonstrated comparable successful retrieval rate (55 %) even in severe testicular atrophy (<2 mL) [25].

Assisted Reproductive Therapies

The three main assisted reproductive strategies are intrauterine insemination (IUI), in vitro fertilization (IVF), and intracytoplasmic sperm injection (ICSI). The selection of technique depends on the number of viable sperm available and anatomic considerations for the female partner (Table 9.3).

IUI refers to the manual injection of a sperm pellet within the uterus, bypassing the cervical mucosa; this normally requires 5–40 million motile sperm. The success rate per cycle has been reported to be 5–16 % per cycle. IVF requires an intensive and coordinated process involving both partners. The woman undergoes hormonal stimulation, and subsequently her eggs are harvested transvaginally via ultrasound guidance. Sperm are provided by the male partner (ejaculated or surgically retrieved) or from a sperm donor. The eggs and sperm are mixed in vitro, the embryos are incubated for several days, and the best quality embryos are transferred to the uterus. When sperm counts are low (as in surgical retrieval), ICSI is employed. In this procedure, a single viable sperm may be microinjected into an oocyte, and then the fertilized egg is implanted into the uterus. This advanced technique has revolutionized treatment for infertile men previously considered sterile.

Table 9.3 Three primary assisted reproductive technologies

Technique	Description	Sperm required
Intrauterine insemination (IUI)	Manual injection of sperm pellet into uterus	5–40 million
In vitro fertilization (IVF)	Mixing egg and sperm outside of body, using eggs harvested via ultrasound aspiration and ejaculated or surgically retrieved sperm	0.5–5 million
Intracytoplasmic sperm injection (ICSI)	Single viable sperm (often surgically retrieved) is microinjected into the oocyte, and fertilized egg is implanted	1 or more

9.3   Andropause

The term "andropause" has become popularized in the media as the male equivalent of "menopause." Menopause refers to the cessation of ovulation, which arrives with a significant decrease in estrogen and multiple medical implications for aging women. Men do not undergo a parallel process, although they do undergo changes in hormone levels as they age. The mechanism and etiology of declining testosterone levels in men are not completely clear, but epidemiologic data suggests that total testosterone level appears to decline at a relatively constant rate of 3.2 ng/dL (about 0.5–1 %) per year after age 30 [26].

As a clinical entity, andropause may be referred to as "late onset hypogonadism" (LOH), although this has also been termed testosterone deficiency syndrome (TDS). According to the American Endocrine Society guidelines, this is defined as the signs and symptoms of testosterone deficiency confirmed by two early morning measurements of total serum testosterone level that fall below the normal range of 300–950 ng/dL (10.4 to 32.9 nmol/L) [27]. The prevalence of testosterone deficiency syndrome is highly influenced by age: an epidemiological study of 1475 black, Hispanic, and white men found symptomatic androgen deficiency in 3.1–7.0 % of men from ages 30–69, in comparison to 18.4 % of men from ages 70–79 [28].

9.3.1   Clinical Implications

The symptoms of low testosterone are varied and nonspecific, including decreased sexual function, fatigue, diminished neurologic function, decreased mobility, and other physical changes. Changes in sexual function are the most specific and include low libido, erectile dysfunction, and decreased pleasure. The patient may exhibit neurologic symptoms: increased irritability, decreased concentration, or inability to sleep. Decreased muscle mass, energy level, and bone mineralization may result from decreased testosterone levels, and these conditions may translate to decreased mobility or activity level.

In order to diagnose testosterone deficiency syndrome, a total serum testosterone and a serum free testosterone should be measured. Testosterone is normally bound by sex hormone-binding globulin (SHBG), which is produced by the liver. Testosterone is active only in its free form. Depending on the assay used, a level of 300–950 ng/dL (10.4 to 32.9 nmol/L) is considered normal. Testosterone should be performed early in the morning; after the recording of a low level, this should be repeated on a separate occasion due to the inherent variability. Although the symptoms of testosterone deficiency are nonspecific, the association of these symptoms with a low serum testosterone measurement is adequate to diagnose clinical testosterone deficiency. Following diagnosis, the patient should be screened for chronic illnesses including hypertension, hyperlipidemia, obesity, and diabetes. He should also be screened for obstructive sleep apnea and thyroid disease. His mobility and activity level should be assessed.

Next, the etiology should be considered. The first principle of treatment is to rule out reversible causes of low testosterone. These include obstructive sleep apnea, hyperthyroidism, the use of certain medications (e.g., opiates, cimetidine, ketoconazole), depression, and excessive alcohol intake. In particular, the disorder may also have to do with an alteration in the amount of SHBG, which may be affected by the liver or the thyroid. Obesity may lower SHBG levels and therefore lower total testosterone levels. When other causes of low testosterone have been ruled out, the clinician may begin discussion regarding testosterone replacement.

9.3.2 Treatment

There are many forms of testosterone supplementation. We highlight the most commonly used. Testosterone supplementation therapy (TST) may be administered in the form of intramuscular injections in either short- or long-term formulations. It may also be administered transdermally in gel or patch form. This must be applied in a nonexposed area to prevent transfer to other people (especially intimate partners or young children). An alternative formulation is the testosterone pellet (Testopel™), which is injected beneath the skin in an office procedure on a monthly basis. Other formulations include intranasal gel, buccal patches, and oral therapies.

Controversies of Testosterone Treatment

Testosterone treatment has been shown to increase libido [29], muscle strength [30], and bone mineral density [31] while decreasing waist circumference [32]. However, known risks also exist including erythrocytosis, infertility, acne, gynecomastia, balding, and worsening obstructive sleep apnea [27]. Overall, the use of testosterone replacement was formerly seen as beneficial in older men, but it has lately has been controversial due to reports of a negative cardiovascular impact. While some observational studies have demonstrated an overall benefit with testosterone supplementation, other studies have suggested harm.

An observational study of veterans age 40 and above with low testosterone demonstrated a lower all-cause mortality rate (10.3 % vs. 20.7 %, $p < 0.0001$) for men who had received testosterone supplementation therapy versus those who had not [33]. However, in a randomized control trial of men over age 65 with limited mobility and low testosterone, a higher number of cardiovascular events were seen in men who received testosterone gel, resulting in the early termination of the trial [34]. While this study had accrued limited numbers and applied to select group of chronically ill elderly men, the findings raised strong concerns about the usage of testosterone supplementation with regard to cardiovascular risk. Subsequent large database studies were conducted that also raised concern of increased risk of mortality in men who had undergone coronary angiography [35] and increased risk of nonfatal myocardial infarction in men who were receiving testosterone supplementation [36].

Our understanding of the impact of testosterone on prostate cancer has also evolved with time. The current guidelines of the American Endocrine Society recommend against the usage of testosterone replacement in men with prostate cancer [27]. Because androgen deprivation therapy is used to treat high-risk prostate cancer, it is inferred that increased testosterone levels may increase the risk of prostate cancer development or progression. Furthermore, trials of 5-alpha reductase inhibitors, which lower intracellular dihydrotestosterone (DHT) levels, reduce the risk of prostate cancer diagnosis (PCPT and REDUCE trials) and reduce the progression of prostate cancer in men on active surveillance (REDEEM trial) [37–39]. TST, which increases intracellular DHT, might increase the risk of prostate cancer.

However, no large, prospective trials have demonstrated an increased prostate cancer-specific mortality with TST in men on active surveillance, post-prostatectomy, or postradiation setting [40]. One theory that has been advanced has been the "saturation hypothesis" [41]. In this model, prostate cancer is thought only to be responsive to a threshold level of testosterone, and an increased amount would not necessarily result in the development of prostate cancer. In practice, the use of testosterone replacement, even in men with a history of prostate cancer both treated and untreated, has been acceptable to urologists and patients with no signs of adverse consequences [42–45].

The long-term effects of testosterone are incompletely characterized. The results from prior studies are at times in conflict, and the numbers in clinical trials have been small. Therefore, testosterone, as with all medical therapies, should be prescribed with consideration of the patient's individual risk factors after a thorough discussion of the risks and benefits.

References

1. Bordini B, Rosenfield RL. Normal pubertal development. Part I: The endocrine basis of puberty. Pediatr Rev. 2011;32(6):223–9.
2. Nielsen CT, Skakkebaek NE, Richardson DW, Darling JA, Hunter WM, Jørgensen M, et al. Onset of the release of spermatozoa (spermarche) in boys in relation to age, testicular growth, pubic hair, and height. J Clin Endocrinol Metab [Internet]. 1986 Mar [cited 2015 Feb 7];62(3):532–5. Available from: http://www.ncbi.nlm.nih.gov/pubmed/3944237
3. Marshall WA, Tanner JM. Variations in the pattern of pubertal changes in boys. Arch Dis Child. 1970;45:13–23.
4. Herman-Giddens ME, Steffes J, Harris D, Slora E, Hussey M, Dowshen SA, et al. Secondary sexual characteristics in boys: data from the pediatric research in office settings network. Pediatrics. 2012;130:e1058–68.
5. Kahane JC. Growth of the Human Prepubertal and Pubertal Larynx. J Speech Hear Res. 1982;25(3):446–55.
6. Biro FM, Lucky AW, Huster GA, Morrison JA. Hormonal studies and physical maturation in adolescent gynecomastia. J Pediatr [Internet]. 1990 Mar [cited 2015 Feb 7];116(3):450–5. Available from: http://www.ncbi.nlm.nih.gov/pubmed/2137877
7. Yip VC-H, Pan C-W, Lin X-Y, Lee Y-S, Gazzard G, Wong T-Y, et al. The relationship between growth spurts and myopia in Singapore children. Invest Ophthalmol Vis Sci [Internet]. 2012 Dec [cited 2015 Jan 28];53(13):7961–6. Available from: http://www.ncbi.nlm.nih.gov/pubmed/23150611
8. Lucky AW, Biro FM, Huster GA, Morrison JA, Elder N. Acne vulgaris in early adolescent boys: correlations with pubertal maturation and age. Arch Dermatol [Internet]. 1991 Feb [cited 2015 Feb 7];127(2):210–6. Available from: http://www.ncbi.nlm.nih.gov/pubmed/1825016

9. Sedlmeyer IL, Palmert MR. Delayed puberty: analysis of a large case series from an academic center. J Clin Endocrinol Metab [Internet]. 2002 Apr [cited 2015 Feb 7];87(4):1613–20. Available from: http://www.ncbi.nlm.nih.gov/pubmed/11932291

10. Dunson DB, Baird DD, Colombo B. Increased infertility with age in men and women. Obstet Gynecol [Internet]. 2004 Jan [cited 2015 Feb 19];103(1):51–6. Available from: http://www.ncbi.nlm.nih.gov/pubmed/14704244

11. Cooper TG, Noonan E, von Eckardstein S, Auger J, Baker HWG, Behre HM, et al. World Health Organization reference values for human semen characteristics. Hum Reprod [Internet]. 2009 Jan [cited 2014 Sep 3];16(3):231–45. Available from: http://www.ncbi.nlm.nih.gov/pubmed/19934213

12. Gunnell DJ, Ewings P. Infertility prevalence, needs assessment and purchasing. J Public Health Med [Internet]. 1994 Mar [cited 2015 Feb 7];16(1):29–35. Available from: http://www.ncbi.nlm.nih.gov/pubmed/8037949

13. Mosher WD, Pratt WF. Fecundity and infertility in the United States: incidence and trends. Fertil Steril [Internet]. 1991 Aug [cited 2015 Jan 17];56(2):192–3. Available from: http://www.ncbi.nlm.nih.gov/pubmed/2070846

14. Thonneau P, Marchand S, Tallec A, Ferial ML, Ducot B, Lansac J, et al. Incidence and main causes of infertility in a resident population (1,850,000) of three French regions (1988-1989). Hum Reprod [Internet]. 1991 Jul [cited 2015 Jan 7];6(6):811–6. Available from: http://www.ncbi.nlm.nih.gov/pubmed/1757519

15. Künzle R, Mueller MD, Hänggi W, Birkhäuser MH, Drescher H, Bersinger NA. Semen quality of male smokers and nonsmokers in infertile couples. Fertil Steril [Internet]. 2003 Feb [cited 2015 Feb 7];79(2):287–91. Available from: http://www.ncbi.nlm.nih.gov/pubmed/12568836

16. Whorton D, Krauss RM, Marshall S, Milby TH. Infertility in male pesticide workers. Lancet [Internet]. 1977 Dec 17 [cited 2015 Feb 7];2(8051):1259–61. Available from: http://www.ncbi.nlm.nih.gov/pubmed/73955

17. Jurewicz J, Radwan M, Sobala W, Ligocka D, Radwan P, Bochenek M, et al. Lifestyle and semen quality: role of modifiable risk factors. Syst Biol Reprod Med [Internet]. 2014;60(1):43–51. Available from: http://www.ncbi.nlm.nih.gov/pubmed/24074254

18. Sheynkin Y, Jung M, Yoo P, Schulsinger D, Komaroff E. Increase in scrotal temperature in laptop computer users. Hum Reprod [Internet]. 2005 Feb [cited 2015 Feb 7];20(2):452–5. Available from: http://www.ncbi.nlm.nih.gov/pubmed/15591087

19. McLachlan RI, Baker HWG, Clarke GN, Harrison KL, Matson PL, Holden CA, et al. Semen analysis: its place in modern reproductive medical practice. Pathology [Internet]. 2003 Feb [cited 2015 Feb 7];35(1):25–33. Available from: http://www.ncbi.nlm.nih.gov/pubmed/12701680

20. Kim ED, Crosnoe L, Bar-Chama N, Khera M, Lipshultz LI. The treatment of hypogonadism in men of reproductive age. Fertil Steril [Internet]. 2013 Mar 1 [cited 2015 Feb 19];99(3):718–24. Available from: http://www.ncbi.nlm.nih.gov/pubmed/23219010

21. Breznik R, Borko E. Effectiveness of antiestrogens in infertile men. Arch Androl [Internet]. 1993 Jan [cited 2015 Feb 7];31(1):43–8. Available from: http://www.ncbi.nlm.nih.gov/pubmed/8373285

22. Showell MG, Mackenzie-Proctor R, Brown J, Yazdani A, Stankiewicz MT, Hart RJ. Antioxidants for male subfertility. Cochrane database Syst Rev [Internet]. 2014 Dec 15 [cited 2015 Jan 19];12:CD007411. Available from: http://www.ncbi.nlm.nih.gov/pubmed/25504418

23. Matthews GJ, Schlegel PN, Goldstein M. Patency following microsurgical vasoepididymostomy and vasovasostomy: temporal considerations. J Urol [Internet]. 1995 Dec [cited 2015 Feb 7];154(6):2070–3. Available from: http://www.ncbi.nlm.nih.gov/pubmed/7500460

24. Schlegel PN. Testicular sperm extraction: microdissection improves sperm yield with minimal tissue excision. Hum Reprod [Internet]. 1999 Jan [cited 2015 Feb 7];14(1):131–5. Available from: http://www.ncbi.nlm.nih.gov/pubmed/10374109

25. Bryson CF, Ramasamy R, Sheehan M, Palermo GD, Rosenwaks Z, Schlegel PN. Severe testicular atrophy does not affect the success of microdissection testicular sperm extraction. J Urol [Internet]. Elsevier Ltd; 2014;191(1):175–8. Available from: http://dx.doi.org/10.1016/j.juro.2013.07.065

26. Harman SM, Metter EJ, Tobin JD, Pearson J, Blackman MR. Longitudinal Effects of Aging on Serum Total and Free Testosterone Levels in Healthy Men [Internet]. Endocrine Society; 2013 [cited 2015 Feb 20]. Available from: http://press.endocrine.org/doi/full/10.1210/jcem.86.2.7219

27. Bhasin S, Cunningham GR, Hayes FJ, Matsumoto AM, Snyder PJ, Swerdloff RS, et al. Testosterone therapy in men with androgen deficiency syndromes: an Endocrine Society clinical practice guideline. J Clin Endocrinol Metab. 2010;95:2536–59.

28. Araujo AB, Esche GR, Kupelian V, O'Donnell AB, Travison TG, Williams RE, et al. Prevalence of symptomatic androgen deficiency in men. J Clin Endocrinol Metab [Internet]. Endocrine Society; 2007 Nov 2 [cited 2015 Feb 12];92(11):4241–7. Available from: http://press.endocrine.org/doi/abs/10.1210/jc.2007-1245

29. Isidori AM, Giannetta E, Gianfrilli D, Greco EA, Bonifacio V, Aversa A, et al. Effects of testosterone on sexual function in men: results of a meta-analysis. Clin Endocrinol (Oxf) [Internet]. 2005 Oct [cited 2015 Feb 19];63(4):381–94. Available from: http://www.ncbi.nlm.nih.gov/pubmed/16181230

30. Ottenbacher KJ, Ottenbacher ME, Ottenbacher AJ, Acha AA, Ostir G V. Androgen treatment and muscle strength in elderly men: A meta-analysis. J Am Geriatr Soc [Internet]. 2006 Nov [cited 2015 Feb 19];54(11):1666–73. Available from: http://www.pubmedcentral.nih.gov/articlerender.fcgi?artid=1752197&tool=pmcentrez&rendertype=abstract

31. Behre HM, Kliesch S, Leifke E, Link TM, Nieschlag E. Long-term effect of testosterone therapy on bone mineral density in hypogonadal men. J Clin Endocrinol Metab [Internet]. 1997 Aug [cited 2015 Feb 19];82(8):2386–90. Available from: http://www.ncbi.nlm.nih.gov/pubmed/9253305

32. Corona G, Monami M, Rastrelli G, Aversa A, Tishova Y, Saad F, et al. Testosterone and metabolic syndrome: a meta-analysis study. J Sex Med [Internet]. 2011 Jan [cited 2015 Feb 19];8(1):272–83. Available from: http://www.ncbi.nlm.nih.gov/pubmed/20807333

33. Shores MM, Smith NL, Forsberg CW, Anawalt BD, Matsumoto AM. Testosterone treatment and mortality in men with low testosterone levels. J Clin Endocrinol Metab [Internet]. 2012;97:2050–8. Available from: http://www.ncbi.nlm.nih.gov/pubmed/22496507

34. Pasquié J, Scavée C, Bordachar P, Clémenty J, Haïssaguerre M. New Engl J. 2010;2373–83. http://www.nejm.org/doi/full/10.1056/NEJMoa1000485

35. Vigen R, O'Donnell CI, Barón AE, Grunwald GK, Maddox TM, Bradley SM, et al. Association of testosterone therapy with mortality, myocardial infarction, and stroke in men with low testosterone levels. JAMA [Internet]. 2013;310(17):1829–36. Available from: http://jama.jamanetwork.com/article.aspx?articleid=1764051

36. Finkle WD, Greenland S, Ridgeway GK, Adams JL, Frasco MA, Cook MB, et al. Increased risk of non-fatal myocardial infarction following testosterone therapy prescription in men. PLoS One. 2014;9(1):1–7.

37. Andriole GL, Bostwick DG, Brawley OW, Gomella LG, Marberger M, Montorsi F, et al. Effect of dutasteride on the risk of prostate cancer. N Engl J Med [Internet]. 2010 Apr 1 [cited 2015 Feb 6];362(13):1192–202. Available from: http://www.ncbi.nlm.nih.gov/pubmed/20357281

38. Thompson IM, Goodman PJ, Tangen CM, Parnes HL, Minasian LM, Godley PA, et al. Long-term survival of participants in the prostate cancer prevention trial. N Engl J Med [Internet]. 2013 Aug 15 [cited 2015 Feb 6];369(7):603–10. Available from: http://www.pubmedcentral.nih.gov/articlerender.fcgi?artid=4141537&tool=pmcentrez&rendertype=abstract

39. Fleshner NE, Lucia MS, Egerdie B, Aaron L, Eure G, Nandy I, et al. Dutasteride in localised prostate cancer management: the REDEEM randomised, double-blind, placebo-controlled trial. Lancet [Internet]. 2012 Mar 24 [cited 2015 Feb 6];379(9821):1103–11. Available from: http://www.ncbi.nlm.nih.gov/pubmed/22277570

40. Kovac JR, Pan MM, Lipshultz LI, Lamb DJ. Current state of practice regarding testosterone supplementation therapy in men with prostate cancer. Steroids [Internet]. Elsevier Inc.; 2014;89:27–32. Available from: http://dx.doi.org/10.1016/j.steroids.2014.07.004

41. Morgentaler A, Traish AM. Shifting the paradigm of testosterone and prostate cancer: the saturation model and the limits of androgen-dependent growth. Eur Urol [Internet]. 2009 Feb [cited 2015 Jan 2];55(2):310–20. Available from: http://www.ncbi.nlm.nih.gov/pubmed/18838208

42. Khera M, Crawford D, Morales A, Salonia A, Morgentaler A. A new era of testosterone and prostate cancer: from physiology to clinical implications. Eur Urol [Internet]. European Association of Urology; 2014;65(1):115–23. Available from: http://dx.doi.org/10.1016/j.eururo.2013.08.015

43. Pastuszak AW, Pearlman AM, Lai WS, Godoy G, Sathyamoorthy K, Liu JS, et al. Testosterone replacement therapy in patients with prostate cancer after radical prostatectomy. J Urol [Internet]. 2013 Aug [cited 2015 Feb 23];190(2):639–44. Available from: http://www.ncbi.nlm.nih.gov/pubmed/23395803

44. Pastuszak AW, Pearlman AM, Godoy G, Miles BJ, Lipshultz LI, Khera M. Testosterone replacement therapy in the setting of prostate cancer treated with radiation. Int J Impot Res [Internet]. 2013 Jan [cited 2015 Feb 23];25(1):24–8. Available from: http://www.ncbi.nlm.nih.gov/pubmed/22971614

45. Morgentaler A, Lipshultz LI, Bennett R, Sweeney M, Avila D, Khera M. Testosterone therapy in men with untreated prostate cancer. J Urol [Internet]. 2011 Apr [cited 2015 Feb 23];185(4):1256–60. Available from: http://www.ncbi.nlm.nih.gov/pubmed/21334649

Genital Dermatology

10

Alok Vij, Sarah C. Vij, and Kenneth J. Tomecki

10.1 Inflammatory

10.1.1 Fixed Drug Eruption

Fixed drug eruption is a common hypersensitivity reaction to medications, most commonly analgesics, including ibuprofen, aspirin, and paracetamol. The reaction occurs more commonly in men [1] and can occur as a "sexually transmitted" eruption if the patient's partner has ingested the suspected allergen [2]. Repeated ingestion of the allergen induces recurrence of the eruption in the same distribution.

The eruption is usually a well-defined, oval or circular, violaceous, or red-brown plaque (Fig. 10.1). Upon ingestion of the offending agent, the eruption recurs in the same location, commonly the genitalia, lips, trunk, and hands [3]. Occasionally, a vesicle or bulla may arise within the plaque, but ulceration and necrosis are uncommon [4].

The eruption may be painful or itchy and may be accompanied by systemic symptoms, including fever, chills, malaise, nausea, and vomiting. Treatment relies on identifying and discontinuing the causative agent. Antihistamines and topical corticosteroids help to reduce pruritus and hasten the resolution of the eruption, which typically fade within 2–3 weeks followed post-inflammatory hyperpigmentation [3].

A. Vij, M.D. (✉) • K.J. Tomecki, M.D.
Department of Dermatology, Cleveland Clinic Foundation, Dermatology and Plastic Surgery Institute, 9500 Euclid Avenue, Desk A61, Cleveland, OH 44195, USA
e-mail: vija@ccf.org

S.C. Vij, M.D.
Department of Urology, Cleveland Clinic, Cleveland, OH USA

© Springer Science+Business Media New York 2016
J.M. Potts (ed.), *Men's Health*, DOI 10.1007/978-1-4939-3237-5_10

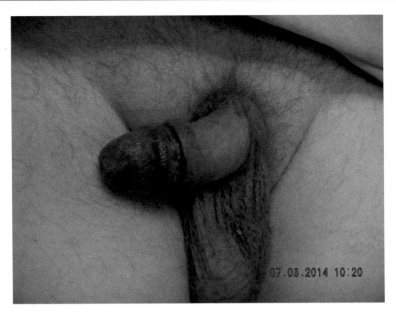

Fig. 10.1 Ulcerative fixed drug eruption. Upon ingestion of ibuprofen, this patient developed a painful red plaque of the glans that ulcerated with further doses of ibuprofen. A second course of ibuprofen months later caused a recurrence of the ulcer

10.1.2 Allergic/Irritant Contact Dermatitis

Contact dermatitis can be allergic or irritant in nature. Causes of allergic contact dermatitis of the male genitalia include sensitivity to condoms, diaphragms, spermicides, lubricants, and topical medications. Sensitivity to other allergens, including industrial or plant allergens, may induce genital dermatitis by "hand transfer." Affected patients usually have sharply demarcated erythematous and edematous plaques on the glans, penile shaft, scrotum, and occasionally the thighs or mons pubis (Fig. 10.2). The eruption of allergic contact dermatitis is pruritic more commonly than painful; irritant dermatitis is more commonly painful than itchy.

The most common contact allergens in condoms are tetramethylthiuram, mercaptobenzothiazole, and dithiocarbamates [5]. Patients allergic to tetramethylthiuram and mercaptobenzothiazole should use Trojan brand condoms or nonrubber condoms made from sheep or lamb intestines. Patients using the latter should be counseled on the reduced efficacy of preventing the spread of sexually transmitted infections compared to latex condoms [6]. Other condom-related contact sensitizers include lubricants or anesthetics such as benzocaine [7].

The five most common causes of non-condom-related allergic contact dermatitis of the genitalia are balsam of Peru, fragrance, tolu balsam, phenylmercuric acetate, and neomycin [8]. The preservatives methylisothiazolinone and methylchloroisothiazolinone are increasing in frequency and severity as cause of genital contact

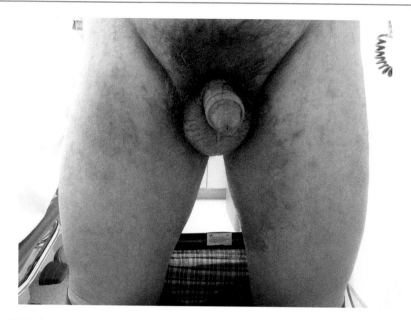

Fig. 10.2 Impetiginized allergic contact dermatitis. After using triple antibiotic ointment to prevent an infection, this patient developed a symmetric, pruritic eruption. Note the honey-colored crusting, suspicious for secondary impetiginization, superimposed upon the erythematous plaques

dermatitis [9]. Less common causes include topical medications such as corticosteroids, antibiotics other than neomycin, or diphenhydramine [10].

Propylene glycol is the relevant allergen in K-Y Jelly, while parabens are the allergens in other lubricants [11, 12]. Alternative products include the aqueous lubricant Surgilube, which does not contain propylene glycol, or SKYN brand condoms, containing non-sensitizing silicone-based lubricant [13].

One allergen frequently transferred from the hands to the genitalia is urushiol, the allergen responsible for Rhus dermatitis, commonly known as "poison ivy" [13]. Urushiol, present in poison ivy, oak, and sumac, can be transferred over 2–3 weeks after initial exposure by oil remaining under the fingernails, clothing, or from pets that had contact with the plants.

Affected patients should wash thoroughly with soap and water within 60 min of plant contact, and clothing should be promptly laundered. Topical steroids can alleviate limited outbreaks, but systemic steroids are needed for generalized or severe outbreaks. Prednisone 1 mg/kg body weight tapered slowly over 2–3 weeks usually suffices; secondary infection is common and may be detected by foul odor, pain, or increasing discharge.

Irritant contact dermatitis is a common cause of chronic or recurrent balanitis that may occur after physical or chemical damage to the skin. Detergents and soaps more commonly than antiseptics or disinfectants cause skin irritation after their use to prevent sexually transmitted infections. Atopic history or frequent washing of the genitalia can induce or aggravate balanitis [14, 15].

10.1.3 Plasma Cell Balanitis (Zoon's Balanitis)

Plasma cell balanitis (Zoon's balanitis) is an inflammatory disease of the penis named after its histologic findings. The balanitis is a persistent, shiny, red plaque on the glans, corona, or mucosal surface of the prepuce in older uncircumsized men. Hemosiderin deposition may yield specks of "cayenne pepper" within the larger plaque (Fig. 10.3) [16]. Usually asymptomatic, the plaques may occasionally be itchy, tender, or painful. Predisposing factors include infection with human papillomavirus (HPV) or *Mycobacterium smegmatis*, heat, occlusion, friction, and poor hygiene [17, 18].

Biopsy is important to differentiate the benign inflammation of Zoon's balanitis from the premalignant or malignant conditions of erythroplasia of Queyrat and squamous cell carcinoma [19]. Histopathology of Zoon's balanitis displays an abundant infiltrate of plasma cells without squamous atypia [20]. In rare cases of long-standing balanitis with coinfection with HPV, squamous cell carcinoma may arise [21].

Definitive treatment is circumcision. Alternative treatments include topical corticosteroids, topical calcineurin inhibitors, cryotherapy, and ablative laser therapy [17, 18, 22].

10.1.4 Vitiligo

Vitiligo is an inflammatory skin disease marked by autoimmune destruction of melanocytes. The resultant depigmented patches can be accentuated by Wood's light examination or by sun exposure, increasing the contrast between normal and

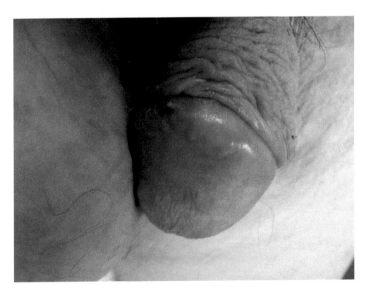

Fig. 10.3 Zoon's balanitis with focal squamous cell carcinoma in situ. The erythematous, shiny plaque persisted despite topical steroids and topical calcineurin inhibitors. A keratotic papule developed at the margin of the plaque; biopsy revealed squamous cell carcinoma in situ

Fig. 10.4 Vitiligo. This patient had generalized depigmented patches of the face, trunk, extremities, and genitals. He responded to UV-B phototherapy

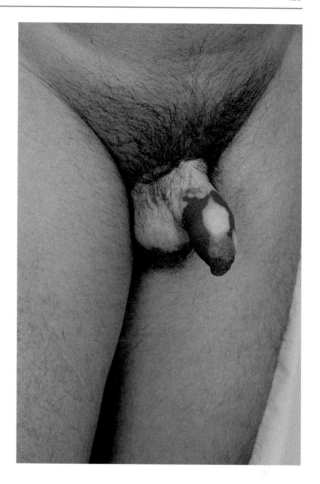

affected skin. Vitiligo has several classic patterns: genital (Fig. 10.4), perioral, segmental, linear, and a "confetti-like" distribution of the extremities [23]. Vitiligo must be differentiated from chemical leukoderma, which may be induced by occupational exposures [24] or immunomodulatory therapy [25].

Treatment of vitiligo is based on the distribution. Several effective brands of camouflage cosmetics can be used in the absence of other therapies. Focal disease can be treated with a combination of topical calcineurin inhibitors and vitamin D analogues. Topical steroids can be used when cost is a limiting factor, but corticosteroid use has been associated with iatrogenic hypopigmentation [26].

Sun protection is advised due to the increased risk of ultraviolet (UV) damage to the skin due to loss of the pigment network [27]. However, UV-B phototherapy or 308 nm xenon chloride (excimer) laser therapy can be used for large areas or as adjunctive therapy for resistant disease [28]. Repigmentation typically begins around the hair follicles, creating a salt-and-pepper-like distribution at the periphery of the affected areas.

10.2 Papulosquamous Diseases

10.2.1 Lichen Simplex Chronicus

Lichen simplex chronicus (LSC) is an overarching term that encompasses pruritus scroti and chronic dermatitis. It is a benign but uncomfortable condition which may arise from pruritus of neuropathic origin [29]. Known as "the itch that rashes," LSC often results from chronic itching or rubbing that leads to lichenification of the skin and an ever-worsening itch-scratch cycle [30]. Primary LSC starts on normal skin, while secondary LSC begins on skin affected by another primary process, such as atopic dermatitis.

Examination reveals lichenified plaques of the scrotum with broken hairs and dyspigmentation; history should focus on hygienic practices and the current use of topical medications, which may be inciting or aggravating factors. Acute pruritus scroti is more commonly caused by infections than neurodermatitis. Allergic/irritant contact dermatitis should be considered in the differential diagnosis [31], and gentle care with hypoallergenic products should be recommended.

Treatment is difficult, including topical steroids or topical calcinuerin inhibitors [32], systemic antihistamines, and inhibition of manipulation with occlusion. Refractory or recalcitrant disease may require antidepressant medications [31] or injection of botulinum toxin [33].

10.2.2 Psoriasis

Psoriasis is a chronic, multisystem inflammatory disorder most commonly affecting the skin and joints, with a known risk of associated obesity and cardiovascular disease [34]. Psoriasis of the genitalia, or inverse psoriasis, affects approximately 50 % of men with psoriasis in the course of their disease [35].

Psoriasis is the most common inflammatory disease of the penis [36], typically exhibiting pink, shiny patches or plaques (Fig. 10.5). Patients are usually asymptomatic, except for occasional sensitivity during intercourse. Genital psoriasis has a negative impact on quality of life due to this sexual dysfunction [37, 93].

Treatment consists of mild topical corticosteroids often with adjuvant vitamin D analogues, topical calcinuerin inhibitors, or coal tar preparations for recalcitrant disease [35]. Widespread or severe disease may benefit from systemic therapy, including methotrexate, retinoids, or biologic agents.

10.2.3 Lichen Planus/Lichen Nitidus

Lichen planus (LP) is an inflammatory disease of squamous epithelia characterized by pruritic, purplish, polygonal papules with an overlying fine, white, reticulated striations. LP affects less than 1 % of the population, but 25 % of affected patients have isolated genital disease, and 20–25 % have both oral and genital disease [38].

Fig. 10.5 Penile psoriasis.
Inverse psoriasis typically
lacks induration and scale
classic for psoriatic plaques
elsewhere on the body

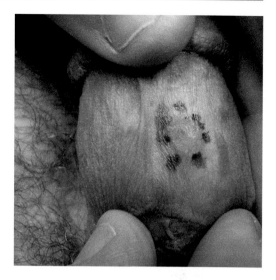

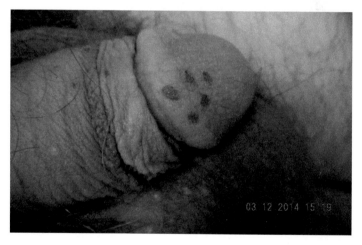

Fig. 10.6 Lichen planus. Wickham's striae are lacy, reticulated thin white plaques that overlie purplish papules and plaques of lichen planus and can be helpful to clinically distinguish lichenoid eruptions from other papulosquamous diseases

Genital LP has a varied morphology, from polygonal papules to annular plaques (Fig. 10.6). Erosive disease is common, with a rare risk of transformation into SCC [39]. Symptoms include pruritus, burning, and sensitivity during intercourse. Exacerbation of pain in concert with enlarging papules or ulceration may indicate the development of malignancy.

Aggressive treatment is indicated given the negative effect on quality of life, including skin disease-related stress and depression [40]. Treatment starts with topical steroids [41]. Topical pimecrolimus is an appropriate steroid-sparing agent; tacrolimus should be avoided as it can induce a burning sensation [42].

Lichen nitidus is an uncommon inflammatory skin disease that exhibits small, monomorphous skin-colored to white papules, which are usually asymptomatic but may be pruritic and may be a significant cosmetic concern to patients or their partners.

Treatment consists of topical steroids for the pruritus and appearance [43]. Cryotherapy, retinoids, or UV-B phototherapy have also been beneficial [44].

10.2.4 Balanitis Xerotica Obliterans

Balanitis xerotica obliterans (BXO) is the rarer, male variant of lichen sclerosus et atrophicus. Characterized by white, atrophic plaques on the glans penis, prepuce, and coronal sulcus, progressive BXO may lead to phimosis and urethral stenosis. Affected patients have a 5 % risk of developing SCC within long-standing plaques [45].

BXO starts insidiously with a burning or stinging pain, often with urethral discharge. Later, phimosis, dysuria, or voiding difficulties may occur [46]. Treatment involves potent topical steroids. Ablative laser therapy may help resistant disease of the glans [47]. Phimosis requires circumcision. Urinary symptoms merit urologic evaluation, especially for urethral stenosis. Interventions may include meatotomy, meatoplasty, or urethroplasty [46, 48].

10.2.5 Miscellaneous Inflammatory Diseases

Patients with a widespread or generalized skin disease may have genital involvement. For example, tense bullae or erosions may be present in bullous pemphigoid (Fig. 10.7), pemphigus vulgaris (Fig. 10.8), or cicatricial pemphigoid.

Additionally, systemic diseases may affect the genitalia. Crohn's disease may present with episodic swelling and induration of the penis or scrotum, particularly in pediatric patients (Fig. 10.9). Sarcoidosis or IgG4-related disease may present with similar periodic infiltration of the genitalia. Histopathology would help to differentiate these conditions.

10.3   Infectious

10.3.1 Human Papillomavirus

Human papillomavirus (HPV) is the cause of genital warts, a condition that affects 1 % of the US population. The prevalence of genital warts is highest among adults ages 18–28 years, with HPV serotypes 6 and 11 accounting for 90 % of warts [49]. Warts are typically asymptomatic, but can be pruritic, painful, and occasionally may cause bleeding and discharge if the urethra is affected.

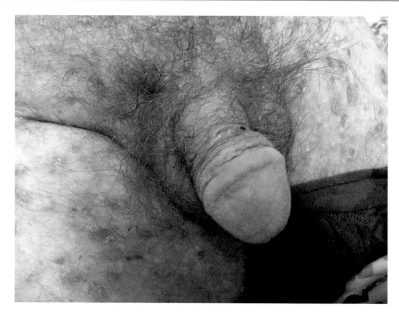

Fig. 10.7 Bullous pemphigoid. Tense bullae and urticarial plaques erupted diffusely over this patient's body. Due to friction, many of the bullae were eroded. Image courtesy of Dr. Sean Condon

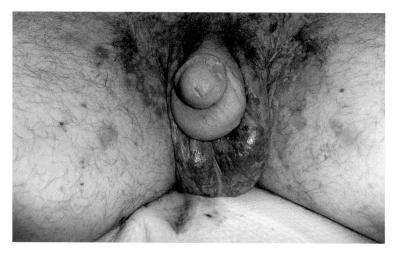

Fig. 10.8 Pemphigus vulgaris. Erosions with crusting affect the skin and mucosae of this patient. Scrotal involvement is common in pemphigus vulgaris

HPV warts are skin-colored to dark brown verrucous papules that may be sessile or pedunculated, distributed on the glans penis, scrotum, perineum, and perianal skin (Fig. 10.10). Clinical morphology usually establishes the diagnosis; biopsy may be diagnostic and therapeutic in certain circumstances.

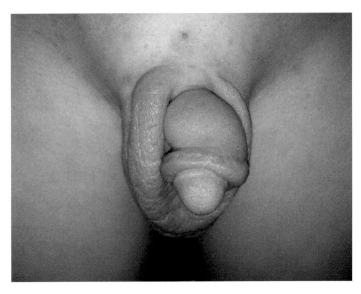

Fig. 10.9 Metastatic Crohn's disease. This patient had several episodes of painful swelling of his penis and scrotum. Biopsy revealed granulomatous infiltration suggestive of Crohn's disease. Esophagogastroduodenoscopy and colonoscopy revealed stricture formation and granulomatous inflammation in several locations throughout the GI tract

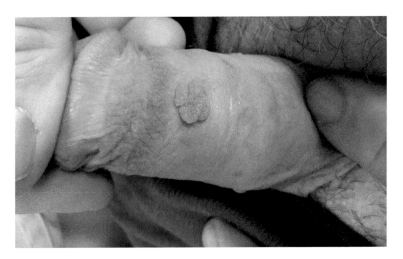

Fig. 10.10 Genital warts. This pedunculated verrucous papule was removed by shave biopsy, a potentially diagnostic and therapeutic procedure

Treatment options are chemical or physical destruction, immunologic therapy, and surgical therapy. Chemical options include the application of podophyllotoxin and 80 % trichloroacetic acid; physical treatments include cryotherapy and curettage. Topical 5-fluorouracil and imiquimod can be used for field therapy. Surgical options include shave excision and CO_2 laser ablation, with caution related to the aerosolization of viral particles.

Two vaccines, one bivalent (Cervarix, GlaxoSmithKline) and the other quadrivalent (Gardasil, Merck & Co., Inc), offer protection against HPV types 6 and 11. The quadrivalent vaccine also protects against serotypes 16 and 18, which account for approximately 70 % of cervical cancers.

10.3.2 Herpes Simplex Virus

Herpes simplex virus (HSV) can produce oral and genital ulcerative disease. Historically, HSV1 caused oral disease, while HSV2 caused genital disease. Today, both types produce disease in both locations, and the incidence of genital HSV1 disease is increasing [50]. HSV infection presents as shallow, well-circumscribed, painful ulcers often with adenopathy (Fig. 10.11), but 85–90 % of infected individuals are asymptomatic [51].

Morphology suggests the diagnosis, but viral culture or direct fluorescent antibody screen can be used to confirm the diagnosis. Treatment for the initial episode is with either acyclovir 200 mg five times per day, valacyclovir 1 g twice daily, or famciclovir 250 mg three times daily, each for 10 days. For recurrent episodes, acyclovir 400 mg three times per day for 5 days, valacyclovir 500 mg twice daily for 3–5 days, or a single dose of famciclovir 1000 mg is recommended. Chronic suppression for patients with more than six outbreaks per year consists of acyclovir 400 mg twice daily, valacyclovir 500 mg once to twice daily, or famciclovir 250 mg daily. These three antivirals have shown to be equivalent in their efficacy in presenting recurrences [52]; medication cost and expected compliance with the prescribed regimen may dictate the choice of therapy.

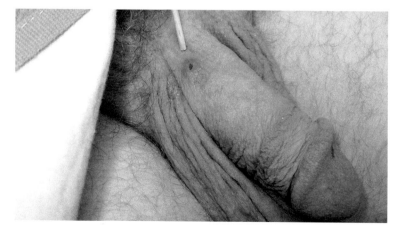

Fig. 10.11 Herpes simplex virus. This patient developed a painful ulcer on the shaft of the penis. Viral culture confirmed HSV-1 infection

Fig. 10.12 Syphilitic chancre. The chancre is a painless, indurated ulcer that often presents with regional lymphadenopathy

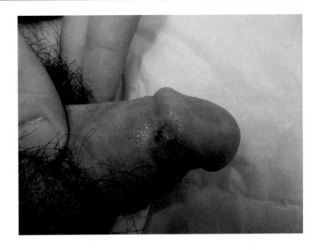

10.3.3 Syphilis

Syphilis is a venereal disease caused by the spirochete *Treponema pallidum*. The rate of reported primary and secondary syphilis in the United States is 5.3 cases per 100,000, double the rate in 2001 [53]. When untreated, syphilis proceeds through three stages: primary, secondary, and tertiary.

The primary infection occurs 10–90 days after exposure, initially presenting with a well-circumscribed, painless, indurated ulcer with regional lymphadenopathy (Fig. 10.12). Most commonly, the ulcer occurs on the prepuce or glans penis, but extragenital presentation may occur depending on the site of inoculation. The secondary stage occurs 3–10 weeks later and manifests classically as copper-colored macules and papules on the trunk, palms, and soles, along with oral ulcers, "moth-eaten" alopecia, condyloma lata, and flu-like symptoms.

The genital ulcer should suggest primary syphilis, which can be confirmed by dark-field examination and rapid plasma regain (RPR) or Venereal Disease Research Laboratory (VDRL) assay. A second confirmatory test for treponema-specific antibodies such as the fluorescent treponemal antibody absorption (FTA-ABS) assay or biopsy can help to confirm the diagnosis. Anti-treponemal immunohistochemical stains are available to aid in the histopathologic diagnosis.

A single dose of 2.4 million units benzathine penicillin is the treatment of choice for primary syphilis. In the setting of penicillin allergy, a single dose of azithromycin 2 g by mouth or doxycycline 200 mg daily for 14 days should be administered.

10.3.4 Candida

Candida albicans is a common cause of balanitis. Approximately 15–20 % of males are asymptomatic carriers, although sexual transmission of *Candida* is not implicated in the pathogenesis of *Candida* vulvovaginitis [54, 55]. True *Candida* balanitis accounts for approximately one-third of all cases of balanitis [56, 57].

Fig. 10.13 Candidal balanitis. Punch biopsy of this red plaque with a satellite papule revealed Candidal forms in the stratum corneum, confirming the diagnosis of Candidal balanitis. Oral fluconazole was an effective treatment

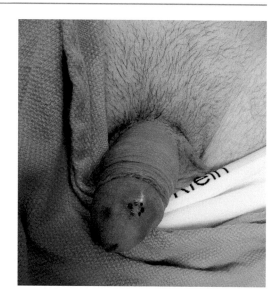

Risk factors include uncircumcised state, phimosis, incontinence, poor hygiene, advanced age, malnutrition, antecedent use of antibiotics, diabetes, obesity, and intercourse with women with *Candida* vulvovaginitis [58]. Patients complain of pain, pruritus, or burning.

Physical examination reveals glazed, red plaques of the penis, scrotum, or thighs with "satellite papules or pustules" at the periphery (Fig. 10.13). Erosions, crusting, and maceration may occur secondarily. In severe, untreated disease or in immunocompromised individuals, phimosis or ulceration can occur. Diagnosis can be confirmed by potassium hydroxide (KOH) examination, which will reveal pseudohyphae [57].

Treatment includes optimization of hygiene, using compresses followed by an anti-yeast cream (e.g., clotrimazole) two to three times a day for 2–3 weeks. Oral fluconazole, 150–200 mg, in a single dose is beneficial [59]. Recalcitrant or recurrent disease may warrant culture with sensitivities, as resistant species of *Candida glabrata* are emerging [60].

10.4   Neoplasia

A variety of growths or tumors can affect the genitalia, and certain entities have a predilection for the penis or scrotum. Pearly penile papules and angiokeratomas are two of the most common benign neoplasms with localization to the penis and scrotum, respectively.

Squamous cell carcinoma and melanoma occur infrequently on the genitalia [61]. Extramammary Paget's disease and Buschke-Lowenstein tumor occur almost exclusively on the genitalia [62]. Cutaneous metastases from genitourinary or gastrointestinal cancers commonly affect the genitalia.

10.4.1 Pearly Penile Papules

Pearly penile papules affect young men, with incidence decreasing with age. They are asymptomatic, 1–2 mm, dome-shaped, pink to skin-colored, smooth papules. They usually arise in a single row on the coronal sulcus of the penis, although they can arise in doubles, on the glans or penile shaft. They may vary in shape, size, and color from person to person, but are invariably uniform in an individual [63].

Pearly penile papules are benign and do not represent a venereal infection, although patients often believe they are genital warts. Biopsy can differentiate those entities, but treatment is based on reassurance of the noninfectious, benign nature of the neoplasms [14].

10.4.2 Angiokeratomas

Angiokeratomas are proliferations of capillaries within the papillary dermis and epidermis that appear as dark red to black papules, usually on the scrotum, penile shaft, or medial thigh (Fig. 10.14). Angiokeratomas may occur in adults in association with varicocele, inguinal hernia, or thrombophlebitis. Bleeding may occur spontaneously or after trauma [64].

Treatment is not necessary unless bleeding, discomfort, or cosmetic concern dictate otherwise. Papules can be treated with excision, cryotherapy, electrocautery, or laser techniques [65].

Fig. 10.14 Angiokeratomas. This patient's partner requested dermatologic examination because she was concerned that these papules were warts

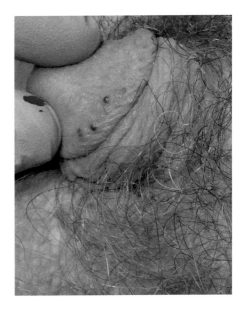

10.4.3 Erythroplasia of Queyrat and Squamous Cell Carcinoma

Erythroplasia of Queyrat (EQ), akin to SCC in situ, is a precancerous condition that may evolve into invasive SCC. EQ affects uncircumcised men in the fifth decade or later as solitary or multiple, well-circumscribed, moist, erythematous plaques covering the glans or prepuce [66]. Pain, itching, or bleeding can occur, and retraction of the foreskin may be painful or difficult. High-risk HPV types and chronic irritation from poor hygiene, friction, trauma, and retained smegma may be causative or aggravating factors [66–68].

Penile cancer is rare in circumcised men and in the United States, but represents 10–20 % of all cancers in men in South America, Asia, and Africa [69, 70]. Risk factors for penile cancer include smoking, psoralen treatment, genital warts, phimosis, multiple sexual partners, delayed or absent circumcision, lichen planus, or balanitis xerotica obliterans [71–73]. Increasing pain or ulceration may herald malignant invasion (Fig. 10.15).

Scrotal SCC, usually a slow-growing papule that ulcerates, is rare domestically; however, specific exposures account for the high incidence in certain African tribesmen, chimney sweepers, and industrial oil workers around the globe [74].

Treatment is based on size and location of the cancer. Treatment options include circumcision, cryosurgery, excision, and Mohsmicrographicsurgery [66, 75].

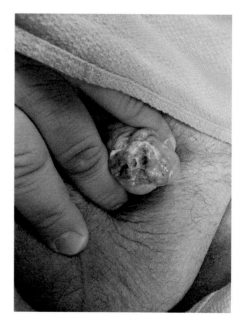

Fig. 10.15 Squamous cell carcinoma of the penis. This patient required penectomy for this long-standing indurated ulcer of the penis

10.4.4 Melanoma

Genital melanoma is rare, most commonly occurring in the sixth or seventh decade. Genital melanoma begins as an enlarging pigmented patch or plaque with variegated color (blue-black, black, brown, or reddish brown) that often ulcerates [76]. It represents less than 10 % of all genitourinary cancers and less than 10 % of all melanomas [77]. Two-thirds of all cases occur on the glans and less frequently on the prepuce, urethral meatus, penile shaft, or coronal sulcus [78–81].

At the time of diagnosis, 60 % of patients have distant metastases [82]. Treatment is wide excision or Mohs micrographic surgery, followed by adjunctive radiotherapy or chemotherapy. Lymph node resection remains controversial [78]. Genitourinary melanoma has the lowest survival rate of all melanomas.

10.4.5 Extramammary Paget's Disease

Extramammary Paget's disease (EMPD) primarily affects women, except in eastern Asians [83]. EMPD begins innocuously as a solitary, well-demarcated, moist eczematous plaque that is often likened to "strawberries and cream" (Fig. 10.16) [84]. The differential diagnosis includes lichen simplex chronicus, psoriasis, SCC, and cutaneous T-cell lymphoma [85].

Primary EMPD is an adnexal adenocarcinoma of the skin without underlying malignancy; secondary EMPD is related to an adjacent internal cancer. About 75 %

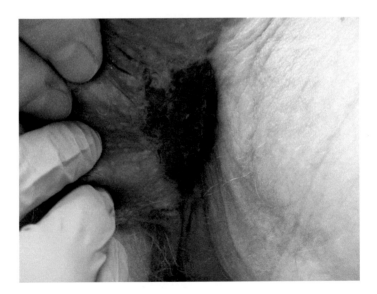

Fig. 10.16 Extramammary Paget's disease. After work-up, this tumor was confined to the skin only. Immunomodulatory therapy with imiquimod initially cleared the plaque, but disease recurrence was noted 1 year later. Mohs micrographic surgery was performed, and the patient has remained disease free after 3 years. Images courtesy of Dr. Jon Meine

of EMPD is primary, and 25 % is secondary [86]. Affected patients deserve screening for distant cutaneous disease as well as underlying visceral malignancy.

Primary EMPD can be treated with topical chemotherapy, e.g., 5-fluorouracil, or topical immunomodulatory therapy, e.g., imiquimod, or Mohs micrographic surgery, although the disease tends to recur [87, 88]. Treatment of secondary EMPD is directed at the underlying malignancy.

10.4.6 Verrucous Carcinoma (Buschke-Lowenstein Tumor)

Buschke-Lowenstein tumor is a rare neoplasm of the anogenital region with a benign histological appearance but locally aggressive behavior. HPV type 6 and 11, traditionally thought to be low risk for malignant potential, are the causative agents [89]. The exact pathogenesis of the locally aggressive tumor is unknown. Radical surgical excision with close follow-up is considered standard of care [62].

10.5 Traumatic

Any cause of trauma to the genitalia can have devastating sequelae. Self-induced lacerations follow accidental or factitious trauma. Penile tourniquet syndrome usually occurs in boys when a hair encircles the penis, causing pain, swelling, and erythema of the glans. If untreated, urethral fistula and amputation of the glans can result [90].

Factitial dermatitis (dermatitis artefacta) is a self-inflicted, often mutilating disease characterized by cuts, excoriations, and sharply demarcated ulcers created by self-induced trauma. Associated guilt, embarrassment, or psychological disturbance are common and may make diagnosis and treatment difficult.

10.5.1 Idiopathic Calcinosis of the Scrotum

Persistent, asymptomatic, pale to yellow-white papules of the scrotum represent idiopathic calcification. Most patients are boys or young men with normal serum calcium, phosphate, and uric acid levels. The papules are usually asymptomatic, but may discharge a chalky white material or may increase in number to cause scrotal deformity. If warranted, excision is usually curative [91, 92].

10.6 Summary

Skin disease of the male genitalia has a wide variety of presentation and etiologies, from self-inflicted trauma to malignancy. Inflammatory skin disease may be a primary process, extension of a generalized disorder, or a manifestation of systemic disease. Diagnosis and treatment may be hindered by patient embarrassment or guilt, but a thorough history and physical examination coupled with interdisciplinary management are sufficient to manage any condition.

References

1. Gendernalik S, Galeckas K. Fixed drug eruptions: a case report and review of the literature. Cutis. 2009;84(4):215–9.
2. Maatouk I, Moutran R, Fahed M, Helou J. A "sexually transmitted" fixed drug reaction. Sex Transm Dis. 2014;41:10.
3. Flowers H, Brodell R, Brents M, Wyatt J. Fixed drug eruptions: presentation, diagnosis, and management. South Med J. 2014;107(11):724–7.
4. Patell R, Dosi R, Shah P, Joshi H. Widespread bullous fixed drug eruption. BMJ Case Rep. 2014. pii: bcr2013200584.
5. Blyumin M, Rouhani P, Avashia N, Jacob S. Acquiring allergen information from condom manufacturers: a questionnaire survey. Dermatitis. 2009;20(3):161–70.
6. Lytle C, Carney P, Vohra S, Cyr W, Bockstahler L. Virus leakage through natural membrane condoms. Sex Transm Dis. 1990;17(2):58–62.
7. Muratore L, Calogiuri G, Foti C, Nettis E, Leo ED, Vacca A. Contact allergy to benzocaine in a condom. Contact Dermatitis. 2008;59(3):173–4.
8. Bhate K, Landeck L, Gonzalez E, Neumann K, Schalock P. Genital contact dermatitis: a retrospective analysis. Dermatitis. 2010;21(6):317–20.
9. Uter W, Geier J, Bauer A, Schnuch A. Risk factors associated with methylisothiazolinone contact sensitization. Contact Dermatitis. 2013;69(4):231–8.
10. Bauer A, Oeheme S, Geier J. Contact sensitization in the anal and genital area. Curr Probl Dermatol. 2011;40:133–41.
11. Fisher A, Brancaccio R. Allergic contact sensitivity to propylene glycol in a lubricant jelly. Arch Dermatol. 1979;115(12):1451.
12. Jones S. Anaphylaxis from rectal lubricant jelly. Am J Med. 1988;85(6):890.
13. Smith G, Sharma V, Knapp J, Shields B. The summer penile syndrome: seasonal acute hypersensitivity reaction caused by chigger bites on the penis. Pediatr Emerg Care. 1988;14(2):116–8.
14. Keller E, Tomecki K. Genitourinary dermatology. In: Potts JM, editor. Essential urology: a guide to clinical practice. Current Clinical Urology. New York, NY: Humana Press; 2012.
15. Birley H, Walker M, Luzzi G, Bell R, Taylor-Robinson D, Byrne M, et al. Clinical features and management of recurrent balanitis; association with atopy and genital washing. Genitourin Med. 1993;69(5):400–3.
16. Kavanagh G, Burton P, Kennedy C. Vulvitis chronica plasmacellularic (Zoon's vulvitis). Br J Dermatol. 1993;129:92–3.
17. Pastar Z, Rados J, Lipozencic J, Skerlev M, Loncaric D. Zoon plasma cell balanitis: an overview and role of histopathology. Acta Dermatovenereol Croat. 2004;12(4):268–73.
18. Retamar R, Kien M, Chouela E. Zoon's balanitis: presentation of 15 patients, five treated with a carbon dioxide laser. Int J Dermatol. 2003;42(4):305–7.
19. Fernandez-Acenero M, Cordova S. Zoon's vulvitis (vulvitis circumscripta plasmacellularis). Arch Gynecol Obstet. 2010;282:351–2.
20. Albers SE, Taylor G, Huyer D, Oliver G, Krafchik B. Vulvitis circumscripta plasmacellularis mimicking child abuse. J Am Acad Dermatol. 2000;42(6):1078–80.
21. Balato N, Scalvenzi M, Bella SL, Costanzo LD. Zoon's balanitis: benign or premalignant lesion? Case Rep Dermatol. 2009;1(1):7–10.
22. Virgili A, Mantovani L, Lauriola M, Marzola A, Corazza M. Tacrolimus 0.1% ointment: is it really effective in plasma cell vulvitis? Report of four cases. Dermatology. 2008;216:243–6.
23. Speeckaert R. Geel Nv. Distribution patterns in generalized vitiligo. J Eur Acad Dermatol Venereol. 2014;28(6):755–62.
24. Broding H, Monse C, Bruning T, Fartasch M. Induction of occupational leucoderma and vitiligo. Can butylated hydroxytoluene induce vitiligo similarly to p-tert-butylphenol? Hautarzt. 2011;62(3):209–14.
25. Zhang R, Zhu W. Genital vitiligo following use of imiquimod 5% cream. Indian J Dermatol. 2011;56(3):335–6.

26. Silverberg N. Update on childhood vitiligo. Curr Opin Pediatr. 2010;22(4):445–52.
27. Tamesis M, Morelli J. Vitiligo treatment in childhood: a state of the art review. Pediatr Dermatol. 2010;27(5):437–45.
28. Mehraban S, Feily A. 308nm excimer laser in dermatology. J Lasers Med Sci. 2014;5(1): 8–12.
29. Cohen A, Andres I, Medvedovsky E, Peleg R, Vardy D. Similarities between neuropathic pruritus sites and lichen simplex chronicus sites. Isr Med Assoc J. 2014;16(2):88–90.
30. Rajalakshmi R, Thappa D, Jaisankar T, Nath A. Lichen simplex chronicus of anogenital region: a clinico-etiological study. Indian J Dermatol Venereol Leprol. 2011;77(1):28–36.
31. Weichert G. An approach to the treatment of anogenital pruritus. Dermatol Ther. 2004;17(1): 129–33.
32. Aschoff R, Wozel G. Topical tacrolimus for the treatment of lichen simplex chronicus. J Dermatolog Treat. 2007;18(2):115–7.
33. Heckmann M, Heyer G, Brunner B, Plewig G. Botulinum toxin type A injection in the treatment of lichen simplex: an open pilot study. J Am Acad Dermatol. 2002;46(4):617–9.
34. Romero-Talamas H, Aminian A, Corcelles R, Fernandez A, Berthauer PSS. Psoriasis improvement after bariatric surgery. Surg Obes Relat Dis. 2014;10(6):1155–9.
35. Meeuwis K, de Hullu J, Massuger L, van de Kerkhof P, van Rossum M. Genital psoriasis: a systematic literature review on this hidden skin disease. Acta Derm Venereol. 2011;91(1): 5–11.
36. Kohn F, Pflieger-Bruss S, Schill W. Penile skin diseases. Andrologia. 1993;31 Suppl 1:3–11.
37. Meeuwis K, de Hullu K, van de Nieuwenhof H, Evers A, Massuger L, van de Kerkhof P, et al. Quality of life and sexual health in patients with genital psoriasis. Br J Dermatol. 2011;164(6): 1247–55.
38. Schmidt H. Frequency, duration, and localization of lichen planus. A study based on 181 patients. Acta Derm Venereol. 1961;41:164–7.
39. Matoso A, Ross H, Chen S, Allbritton J, Epstein J. Squamous neoplasia of the scrotum: a series of 29 cases. Am J Surg Pathol. 2014;38(7):973–81.
40. Lundqvist E, Wahlin Y, Bergdahl M, Bergdahl J. Psychological health in patients with genital and oral erosive lichen planus. J Eur Acad Dermatol Venereol. 2006;20(6):661–6.
41. Mirowski G, Goddard A. Treatment of vulvovaginal lichen planus. Dermatol Clin. 2010;28:717–25.
42. Lonsdale-Eccles A, Velangi S. Topical pimecrolimus in the treatment of genital lichen planus: a prospective case series. Br J Dermatol. 2005;153:390–4.
43. Fox B, Odom R. Papulosquamous diseases: a review. J Am Acad Dermatol. 1985;12(4): 597–624.
44. Kim Y, Shim S. Two cases of generalized lichen nitidus treated successfully with narrow-band UV-B phototherapy. Int J Dermatol. 2006;45:615–7.
45. Neill S, Lewis F, Tatnall F, Cox N. British association of dermatologists' guidelines for the management of lichen sclerosus. Br J Dermatol. 2010;163:672–82.
46. Das S, Tunuguntla H. Balanitis xerotica obliterans – a review. World J Urol. 2000;18(6): 382–7.
47. Aynaud O, Plantier F. Genital lichen sclerosus treated by carbon dioxide laser. Eur J Dermatol. 2010;20(3):387–8.
48. Neuhaus I, Skidmore R. Balanitis xerotica obliterans and its differential diagnosis. J Am Board Fam Pract. 1999;12(6):473–6.
49. Koutsky L. Epidemiology of genital human papillomavirus infection. Am J Med. 1997; 102(5Z):3–8.
50. Roberts C, Pfister J, Spear S. Increasing proportion of herpes simplex virus type 1 as cause of genital herpes infection in college students. Sex Transm Dis. 2003;30(10):797–800.
51. Leone P. Reducing the risk of transmitting genital herpes: advances in understanding and therapy. Curr Med Res Opin. 2005;21(10):1577–82.
52. Lebrun-Vignes B, Bouzamondo A, Dupuy A, Guillaume J, Lechat P, Chosidow O. A meta-analysis to assess the efficacy of oral antiviral treatment to prevent genital herpes outbreaks. J Am Acad Dermatol. 2007;57(2):238–46.

53. Patton M, Su J, Nelson R, Weinstock H. Primary and secondary syphilis--United States, 2005-2013. MMWR Morb Moral Wkly Rep. 2014;63(18):402–6.
54. Rodin P, Kolator B. Carriage of yeasts on the penis. Br Med J. 1976;1(6018):1123–4.
55. Lisboa C, Costa A, Ricardo E, Santos A, Azevedo F, Pina-Vaz C, et al. Genital candidosis in heterosexual couples. J Eur Acad Dermatol Venereol. 2011;2011(25):145–51.
56. Abdullah A, Drake S, Wade A, Walzman M. Balanitis (balanoposthitis) in patients attending a department of genitourinary medicine. Int J STD AIDS. 1992;3(2):128–9.
57. Dockerty W, Sonnex C. Candidal balano-posthitis: a study of diagnostic methods. Genitourin Med. 1995;71(6):407–9.
58. Mayser P. Mycotic infections of the penis. Andrologia. 1993;31 Suppl 2:13–6.
59. Stary A, Soeltz-Szoets J, Ziegler C, Kinghorn G, Roy R. Comparison of the efficacy and safety of oral fluconazole and topical clotrimazole in patients with candida balanitis. Genitourin Med. 1996;72(2):98–102.
60. Farmakiotis D, Tarrand J, Kontoyiannis D. Drug-resistant Candida glabrata infection in cancer patients. Emerg Infect Dis. 2014;20(11):1833–40.
61. Suyama T, Teramoto Y, Yamamoto A, Kuroda I, Yoshikawa S, Kiyohara Y. Case of giant basal cell carcinoma around the base of the penis in an elderly patient. J Dermatol. 2014;41(5):439–42.
62. Sandhu R, Min Z, Bhanot N. A gigantic anogenital lesion: Buschke-Lowenstein tumor. Case Rep Dermatol Med. 2014;2014:650714.
63. Agarwal S, Bhattacharya S, Singh N. Pearly penile papules: a review. Int J Dermatol. 2004;43(3):199–201.
64. Taniguchi S, Inoue A, Hamada T. Angiokeratoma of Fordyce: a cause of scrotal bleeding. Br J Urol. 1994;73(5):589–90.
65. Odezmir M, Baysal I, Engin B, Odezmir S. Treatment of angiokeratoma of Fordyce with long-pulse neodymium-doped yttrium aluminum garnet laser. Dermatol Surg. 2009;35:92–7.
66. Graham J, Helwig E. Erythroplasia of Queyrat. A clinicopathologic and histochemical study. Cancer. 1973;32(6):1396–414.
67. Cupp M, Malek R, Goellner J, Smith T, Espy M. The detection of human papillomavirus deoxyribonucleic acid in intraepithelial, in situ, verrucous and invasive carcinoma of the penis. J Urol. 1995;154(3):1024–9.
68. Sarkar F, Miles B, Plieth D, Crissman J. Detection of human papillomavirus in squamous neoplasm of the penis. J Urol. 1992;147(2):389–92.
69. Burgers J, Badalament R, Drago J. Penile cancer: clinical presentation, diagnosis, and staging. Urol Clin North Am. 1992;19(2):247–56.
70. Narayana A, Olney L, Loening S, Weimar G. Carcinoma of the penis: analysis of 219 cases. Cancer. 1982;49(10):2185–91.
71. English H, Laws R, Keogh G, Wilde J, Foley J, Elston D. Dermatoses of the glans penis and prepuce. J Am Acad Dermatol. 1997;37(1):1–24.
72. Campus G, Alia F, Bosincu L. Squamous cell carcinoma and lichen sclerosus et atrophicus of the prepuce. Plast Reconstr Surg. 1992;89(5):962–4.
73. Johnson D, Fuerst D, Ayala A. Carcinoma of the penis. Experience with 153 cases. Urology. 1973;1(5):404–8.
74. Lowe F. Squamous cell carcinoma of the scrotum. J Urol. 1983;130(3):423–7.
75. Lai K, Mercurio M. Medical and surgical approaches to vulvar intraepithelial neoplasia. Dermatol Ther. 2010;23:477–84.
76. An J, Li B, Wu L, Lu H, Li N. Primary malignant amelanotic melanoma of the female genital tract: report of two cases and review of literature. Melanoma Res. 2009;19(4):267–70.
77. Piura B. Management of primary melanoma of the female urogenital tract. Lancet Oncol. 2008;9:973–81.
78. Schellhammer P, Jordan G, Robey E, Spaulding J. Premalignant lesions and nonsquamous malignancy of the penis and carcinoma of the scrotum. Urol Clin North Am. 1992;19(1):131–42.

79. Rashid A, Williams R, Horton L. Malignant melanoma of penis and male urethra: is it a difficult tumor to diagnose? Urology. 1993;41(5):470–1.
80. Zurrida S, Bartoli C, Clemente C, Palo GD. Malignant melanoma of the penis. A report of four cases. Tumori. 1990;76(6):599–602.
81. Manviel J, Fraley E. Malignant melanoma of the penis and male urethra: 4 case reports and literature review. J Urol. 1988;139(4):813–6.
82. Johnson D, Ayala A. Primary melanoma of penis. Urology. 1973;2(2):174–7.
83. Lee S, Choel Y, Jung H, et al. A multicenter study on extramammary Paget's disease in Korea. Int J Dermatol. 2011;50:508–15.
84. Smith D, Handy F, Evans J, Falzon M, Chapple C. Paget's disease of the glans penis: an unusual urological malignancy. Eur Urol. 1994;25(4):316–9.
85. Lam C, Funaro D. Extramammary Paget's disease: summary of current knowledge. Dermatol Clin. 2010;28:807–26.
86. Lowe E, Schmitt A, Bordeaux J. Management of unusual cutaneous malignancies: atypical malignant fibroxanthoma, fibrous histiocytoma, sebaceous carcinoma, extramammary Paget disease. Dematol Clin. 2011;29:201–16.
87. Hegarty P, Suh J, Fisher M. Penoscrotal extramammary Paget's disease: The University of Texas M. D. Anderson Cancer Center Contemporary Experience. J Urol. 2011;186:97–102.
88. Kitagawa K, Bogner P, Zeitouni N. Photodynamic therapy with methyl-aminolevulinate for the treatment of double extramammary Paget's disease. Dermatol Surg. 2011;37:1043–6.
89. Martin J, Molina I, Monteagudo C, Marti N, Lopez V, Jorda E. Buschke-Lowenstein tumor. J Dermatol Case Rep. 2008;2(4):60–2.
90. Sallami S, Rhouma SB, Cherif K, Noura Y. Hair-thread tourniquet syndrome in an adult penis: case report and review of the literature. Urol J. 2013;10(2):915–8.
91. Pak K, Takayama H, Tomoyoshi T. Idiopathic calcinosis of scrotum. Urology. 1983;21(5):521–3.
92. Yahya H, Rafindadi A. Idiopathic scrotal calcinosis: a report of four cases and review of the literature. Int J Dermatol. 2005;44(3):206–9.
93. Molina-Leyva A, Almodovar-Real A, Ruiz-Carrascosa J, Naranjo-Sintes R, Serrano-Ortega S, Jimenez-Moleon J. Distribution pattern of psoriasis affects sexual function in moderate to severe psoriasis: a prospective case series study. J Sex Med. 2014;11(12):2882–9.

Male Sexual Concerns

11

Jeannette M. Potts

11.1 The Importance of the Sexual History

The combination of cultural openness and the availability of treatments for sexual dysfunction has led to a permissive environment for these types of discussions.

The growing attitude of normalcy toward sexual concerns provides health-care professionals with a new and perhaps even better means to assess patient well-being, while prescribing more compelling interventions to improve patient health.

Sexual health in men is comprised of an intricate web of biochemical factors influenced by weight gain and insulin resistance; vascular and inflammatory changes; hormonal factors that can become altered by lifestyle, medications, or age; and psychosocial issues which include quality of partner relationship, job satisfaction, and stressful life events. I believe that an open query about a man's sex life provides more answers and valuable insights about his overall health and psychosocial well-being. By incorporating a simple screening phrase like "Now tell me about your sex life?" into the standard Review of Systems, the health-care provider can demonstrate the importance of this topic while creating a comfortable environment for further discussion.

Because medical education in sexual health in the United States and Canada is believed to be lacking, a summit was held to address the depth of the problem and formulate solutions. "Medical students and practicing physicians report being underprepared to adequately address their patients' sexual health needs" [1]. As many of us can attest, there was little instruction about this topic during medical school or residency training. Indeed, findings presented at the summit demonstrated high rates of inadequate sexual health training. Ageism may prevent us from acknowledging sexual function concerns in older patients. People are living longer,

J.M. Potts, M.D. (✉)
Vista Urology and Pelvic Pain Partners, 2998 South Bascom Avenue,
Suite 100, San Jose, CA 95124, USA
e-mail: DrPotts@VistaUrology.com

© Springer Science+Business Media New York 2016
J.M. Potts (ed.), *Men's Health*, DOI 10.1007/978-1-4939-3237-5_11

well beyond their reproductive years. And although comorbidities that can impact sex increase with age, our growing elderly population is generally healthy and active. Research has shown that 40 % of men between 75 and 85 are sexually active [2]. Surveys of older married men demonstrated significant rise in the percentage of men enjoying an active sex life in this era as compared to their peers from 20 years ago: 68 % vs. 52 %. Among unmarried men, the increase was likewise impressive: 54 % vs. 30 % [3].

I would also add that some health-care providers erroneously assume that they would make patients uncomfortable, especially if they don't share the same age, gender, or sexual orientation of the patient. This in fact may reflect the discomfort of the health-care provider. Hopefully, through education and introspection, we can assuage this discomfort in our colleagues and improve care for our patients.

11.2   Just Ask!

Consider this, if you are already conducting a thorough Review of Systems by asking about eating and exercise habits, sleep, micturition, and bowel habits, wouldn't it gracefully follow to ask about sexual well-being or concerns?

By revealing that he has noticed a decrease in sexual frequency and desire, one might find out that a healthy-appearing middle-aged man is having financial problems and consuming more alcohol. By sharing his recent discomfort after intercourse, a patient may reveal symptoms of pelvic floor neuromuscular dysfunction. Recent onset of sexual dysfunction in men may be considered a sentinel event for cardiovascular disease, diabetes, metabolic syndrome, hyperlipidemia, hyperthyroidism, depression, alcoholism, spousal abuse, domestic violence, etc. By opening a dialogue about sex with patients, health-care providers may be better able to implement earlier interventions for some conditions while providing more compelling education about diet, exercise, weight loss, stress management, individual psychotherapy, and couple's counseling.

Among men, sexual dysfunction has been shown to be associated with significantly lower health-related quality of life. In a study from Iran, two groups of subjects (mean age 49 years) were compared: 95 patients (69 % men) with sexual dysfunction versus 111 controls (69.30 % men). Men most frequently complained of premature ejaculation, while the most common complaint in women was decreased libido. The presence of sexual dysfunctions was associated with greater social dysfunction, sleep issues, mood, and overall quality of life [4].

Sexual desire within a relationship is a key determinant of the quality of the nonsexual aspects of the relationship. Both men and women reporting a discrepancy between their own and their partner's sexual desire have lower relationship satisfaction, and individuals in sexually inactive marriages report less marital happiness [5].

Obviously, as a quality of life parameter alone, sex is an extremely important health issue; but as a marker for serious chronic disease, sexual functioning should be in the forefront of our patient assessments.

11.3   Questionnaires and Surveys

Validated questionnaires and surveys are essential for research of sexual dysfunction, but they are unnecessary in purely clinical practice. In other words, just because you don't use the latest "approved" sex questionnaire in your office doesn't mean you can't conduct a review of systems that should include a question pertaining to sexual function. None of us have specially printed pamphlets to ask patients if they become short of breath with exertion or have regular bowel movements without bleeding.

On the other hand, a written questionnaire prior to office visits may provide some patients and their doctors with an "icebreaker" with which to introduce the topic during the face-to-face consultation. The SHIM is one of the most widely used and tested.

But again, be aware that although many questionnaires are adequate for their own purposes (research of a specific parameter), some investigators have found "a serious lack of standardized, internationally (culturally) acceptable questionnaires that are truly epidemiologically validated in general populations" [6]. Therefore, some questionnaires are not applicable to persons who are single, currently not sexually active, or involved in same-sex relationships.

11.4   Recognizing His Concerns within the Context of His Relationship

Though I wish to emphasize the importance of evaluating and treating patients in the context of their relationship to their sexual partner, sexual health and well-being should be addressed in single patients and those not currently involved in a sexual relationship. Men's sense of desire, arousal, and attractiveness can continue to play an important part of their health and sense of well-being even when they choose not to be involved in a sexual relationship.

I frequently ask single patients if they have any worries or concerns that could arise if they were to contemplate a sexual relationship. Some patients identify themselves as asexual. Other patients may explain that their dysfunction or worries actually prevent them from seeking a relationship or socializing in general. If not for the direct query by the physician, these concerns and health issues would be often overlooked among single patients. This is also important among recently widowed or divorced men. I always include sexual functioning questions along with queries regarding grief and bereavement in these individuals.

For couples, things may not always be what they seem either. Some men may develop erectile dysfunction as a result of fear of "hurting" their postmenopausal wife who has recently complained of discomfort during intercourse. ("Doc, someone prescribed Viagra – it didn't help. I would've hurt her even more.") Some men lose their desire because they cannot achieve an erection. ("I just started avoiding sex, and I am just used to not feeling this way anymore.") Conversely, some women may misinterpret their partner's erectile dysfunction as their fault, believing it is a result of their own lack of sexual attractiveness. ("He doesn't think I am sexy any-more!") This may lead to further performance anxiety and fuel a vicious cycle of miscommunication and sexual dysfunction.

Fostering healthy communication for men is one important way to address sexual concerns; this should include the sexual partner whenever possible.

Decline in sexual desire is observed in older patients and in those in longer relationships. But women also report lower desire when their partner experienced a sexual dysfunction [7]. Female partners of men with ED have also been shown to suffer a range of emotions from frustration to hopelessness, while others have (creatively) focused on nonsexual intimacy strategies [8].

Sexual dysfunction in one partner is also associated with sexual dysfunction in the other partner. Conversely, successful treatment of sexual dysfunction may improve sexual functioning parameters in the partner. Sexual life satisfaction, for example, improved in female partners of men receiving PDE-5 inhibitortreatment for erectile dysfunction [9]. In one study, the favorable effects of erectile dysfunction therapy in men were enhanced by the "couple global caring" parameter, again, emphasizing the importance of the relationship and a shared intention.

Investigators in Australia and New Zealand observe that while drugs like Viagra impact on both individuals and interpersonal relationships, the social and psychological aspects of treatment are absent from the majority of research on the drug. "The advent of Viagra has seen diminishing sexual capacities once linked with normal aging now viewed as dysfunctional, with possible alternative psychological factors largely ignored" [10].

In a similar study involving in-depth interviews, three issues and concerns for women regarding the use of Viagra by their male partners were identified: the neglect of women by those producing and prescribing Viagra, the embodied relationship (which encompasses physical and psychosocial effects of Viagra use), and broader sociocultural implications (e.g., the impact of "the culture of Viagra" on understandings about sexuality in older age and on ideas about male and female sexuality) [11].

Both studies remind us of the importance of, including the partner, both the discussion about the problem and the strategies to address mutual concerns.

Other sexual dysfunctions are also associated with distress for the partner. Issues of climax and orgasm affect both partners even when only one partner manifests the disorder. Premature ejaculation is associated with low sexual satisfaction in men and their partners [12]. This in turn, obviously, adversely affects the overall quality of the relationship.

It is important to remind couples that sex is an important part of communication. Although relationship dynamics change over time and partners may not have stereotypical roles, many of my patients have found the following written prescription helpful:

Women need to feel emotionally connected in order to be sexual… Men need sex in order to feel emotionally connected.

Table 11.1 Interest in sexual activity

	Men	Women
Never	6.7 %	46.7 %
1/month	26.7	33.3
1/week	40.0	10.0
Daily	23.3	0

As described by Kalra [13]

A common complaint among heterosexual married men is the incompatibility of desired frequency of sex with their partner.

A study from India illustrates these differences [13]. Men and women were queried about their ideal frequency of sex, which varied greatly (see Table 11.1). Perhaps a little education can be provided to men about female health issues and vice versa. This can go a long way in sensitizing men about their spouse's needs, resulting in overall improvement of their relationship, which often translates into better sex for both.

Experts agree that a woman's motivation and ability to find and respond to sexual stimuli is largely influenced by her emotional intimacy with her partner [14]. Partners need to understand that a woman's emotional and relationship well-being contributes more to her sexual enjoyment than does her physiological response. Likewise, partners of men need to understand the need for physical sexual connectivity and how strongly this is linked to men's emotional well-being.

11.5   Opportunity and Libido

Sexual desire in men (and women) arises from their intrinsic hormonal, emotional, and biochemical milieu as well as extrinsic factors of sexual attraction and social opportunity.

Patients should be asked about opportunity, which may be limited due to shift work or adult children moving back home.

According to Dr. Berman of Berman Center for Sexual Health and other experts, couples should never allow more than two-week gaps in their sexual activity, for risk of creating an unhealthy pattern and decreasing emotional connectivity.

Risk factors for low libido have been linked to age; however, this may reflect increased prevalence of comorbid conditions and diminished opportunity.

In men, risks factors for diminished libido include alcohol and drug abuse, chronic illness such as COPD or renal failure, sleep apnea, cardiovascular disease, depression, diabetes, hyperlipidemia, hypertension, hypogonadism, hyperprolactinemia, neurological disease (multiple sclerosis), obesity, sedentary lifestyle, smoking, thyroid disease, surgery (GU or vascular), trauma, and medications [15].

Over the past decade, significant strides have been made in recognizing the adverse effects of obesity, diabetes, and sleep deprivation on testosterone levels. The metabolic syndrome is a risk factor for sexual dysfunction, but sexual dysfunction has been found to be predictive of subsequent metabolic syndrome as well [16]. A separate discussion regarding metabolic syndrome is included as a separate chapter in this book.

Bereavements, economic problems, retirement, children leaving or returning home, divorce and personal illness, or illness of their partner or close relative may impact sexual functioning. For some older persons, their most significant obstacles to sexuality are their adult children. Cultural biases and ageism can prevent many mature adults from seeking or nurturing sexual relationships after death of a spouse or divorce, and children may be the most prejudiced or restrictive of their parents.

A change in a partner's sexual function, which may be diminished or enhanced by medication, may alter the dynamics and sexual functioning in a relationship.

Male self-esteemissues that can affect libido arise from stability in career or financial matters, as well as the respect and fulfillment derived from their vocations. Therefore, it is essential to address these issues as part of a sexual history.

Impaired sexual function is a common feature of depression as well as antidepressant therapy. Ironically, adverse effects of most commonly prescribed antidepressants such as serotonin reuptake inhibitors manifest as diminished libido, impaired arousal, and/or delayed or absent orgasm [17].

As discussed earlier, hormonal factors in men can occur with aging but are strongly linked to other conditions such as obesity and diabetes. In contrast to the decline in estrogen in women following menopause, testosterone levels in men do not change abruptly, but diminish gradually with age.

Thyroid dysfunction is associated with erectile dysfunction and low libido. Sexual dysfunction has been demonstrated as significantly more prevalent among men with either hypo- or hyperthyroidism when compared to age-matched controls [18]. Hypothyroidism is also associated with sleep apnea, which alone is also a risk factor for sexual dysfunction.

11.6   Erectile Dysfunction

While there is certainly strong evidence correlating age and erectile dysfunction, the increasing prevalence of comorbidities over time, along with pharmacological therapies. may play a more significant role.

Aging alone is associated with compromised blood flow to the erectile tissue, endothelial dysfunction with decreased release and availability of nitric oxide (which relaxes the vascular tone), decreased smooth muscle cells, and increased collagen deposition, all of which are enhanced by androgen deficiency—also linked to aging [19]. However, among younger men, these phenomena can be frequently observed in association with obesity, hypertension, and diabetes.

Although erectile dysfunction is not the most common form of male sexual dysfunction, it is the most common sexual complaint prompting medical consultation. It is defined as the persistent inability to attain and maintain penile erection sufficient for sexual intercourse. Among elderly men, it is cited as the "main reason" for sexual inactivity.

As mentioned earlier, obesity, diabetes, and metabolic syndrome are strongly linked to sexual dysfunction in men.

I believe the increasing prevalence of obesity and metabolic syndrome will have a greater impact on global sexual health than the apparent concern over the advancing age in the general population.

11.7   Disorders of Climax

Although erectile dysfunction receives so much greater public and medical attention, disorders of ejaculation are far more prevalent than ED across all ages. According to one survey, nearly half of men reported an ejaculatory "disturbance" during the prior 4 weeks [20].

The ejaculatory process is mainly mediated by the autonomic nervous system and consists of two main phases: emission and expulsion. The organs involved in the emission phase comprise the epididymis, vas deferens, seminal vesicles, prostate gland, prostatic urethra, and bladder neck. The organs participating in the expulsion phase include the bladder neck and urethra, as well as the pelvic striated muscles [20]. Anatomical changes, neurological disorders, or functional impairment of these structures may cause ejaculatory dysfunction.

Ejaculatory dysfunctions include premature ejaculation (PE), delayed ejaculation, retrograde ejaculation, anorgasmia, and dysorgasmia (see Table 11.2 for definitions). Depending upon his or his partner's perceptions, men may feel extremely dissatisfied with their ejaculatory function. However, what one man perceives as frustrating (e.g., delayed or retarded ejaculation), another may perceive with pride.

Some investigators have observed a relationship between hormonal levels and the spectrum of orgasmic disorders. For example, in an Italian cohort, men with most severe symptoms of PE had highest levels of testosterone and lowest levels of TSH and prolactin, while those with increasing delay in ejaculation up to anorgasmia had correspondingly lower testosterone levels and higher average prolactin and TSH levels [21]. Others believe there exists a potential genetic link for PE as seen in a Finnish study of twin pairs. Genetics was observed to be a consistent factor in 30 % of men with lifelong PE [22]. And still others would argue that some

Table 11.2 Defining ejaculatory dysfunction

Premature: brief ejaculatory latency (usually <2 min), associated with feeling of lack of control and/or distress for the patient or his partner
Delayed: orgasm/ejaculation which does not occur in >20–30 min and causes distress to the man and/or his partner
Anorgasmia: inability to achieve an orgasm despite long and adequate sexual stimulation
Retrograde: ejaculation which "falls" back into the bladder rather than being expelled through the urethra due to anatomical or functional decrease in bladder neck tone
Dry ejaculation: climax without semen may be due to retrograde ejaculation or decreased semen production resulting from radiation therapy of medication, for example
Dysorgasmia: climax or ejaculation which are uncomfortable or painful

ejaculatory variations are not disorders at all. For example, some believe PE should not be considered a dysfunction, since upper mammalian species, including primates, ejaculate almost immediately on penetration of the vagina [23]. One can imagine the evolutionary advantage of being able to inseminate the female quickly. Perhaps increasing delay of ejaculation posed a risk to copulating couples, making them more vulnerable or less successful in achieving conception.

PE affects 4–39 % of men as a primary disorder. This range reflects the variation in definitions, regional and cultural differences in prevalence, as well as degree of patient bother [24]. Female partners of men with PE report significantly greater sexual problems, with reduced satisfaction, increased distress and interpersonal difficulty, and more orgasmic problems than partners of non-PE men [12].

Criteria have been published that define any ejaculation occurring in 1 min, 2 min, 3 min, or even 7 min from penetration, or 8–15 penile thrusts, as premature. Even more confusing is the historical perspective by Masters and Johnson, who suggested that a man has PE if he is unable to delay his ejaculation until his partner is sexually satisfied in at least 50 % of their sexual approaches [25]. (This definition certainly overestimates the number of women who are able to climax with vaginal penetration alone.) And yet another inadequate definition, in my opinion, is found in The European Association of Urology disorders of ejaculation guidelines, published in 2004, which defines PE as the inability to control ejaculation for a "sufficient" length of time before vaginal penetration.

Taking into account these criteria and the various ways men respond to PE, the International Society of Sexual Medicine, in 2009 [26], proposed this more meaningful and clinically useful definition:

…a male sexual dysfunction characterized by ejaculation which always or nearly always occurs prior to or within about 1 minute of vaginal penetration, and the inability to delay ejaculation on all or nearly all vaginal penetrations, and negative personal consequences, such as distress, bother, frustration and/or the avoidance of sexual intimacy.

The controversy about whether PE is behavioral or biomedical is reflected in the two differing approaches to therapy (i.e., behavioral or psychotherapy versus pharmacological therapy). Psychological causes include anxiety, novelty of partner or situation, and low frequency in sexual activity. Biological causes include endocrinopathy such as hyperthyroidism, substance abuse, opiate withdrawal, and perhaps UTI or prostatitis. Lifelong or primary PE may be due to certain physiological factors such as penile hypersensitivity, hyperexcitable ejaculatory reflex, hyperarousability, genetic predisposition, or dysfunction of the 5-hydroxytryptamine (5-HT) receptor [25].

Lifelong PE is best managed with pharmacotherapy [selective serotonin reuptake inhibitor (SSRI) and/or topical anesthetics]. According to investigators at the Brazilian Cochrane center, there is overall weak and inconsistent evidence regarding the effectiveness of psychological interventions for the treatment of PE, especially primary PE [20].

The management of acquired PE is etiology specific and may include erectile dysfunction pharmacotherapy, for example, in men with comorbid ED. Behavioral therapy is indicated when psychogenic or relationship factors are present. Counseling combined with pharmacotherapy in an integrated treatment program may be helpful as an integrated PE management strategy.

Nonmedical therapies include start and stop methods as well as squeeze technique; however, long-term management of PE using these methods has not been observed in the majority of patients studied. For younger men, precoital masturbation has been helpful in diminishing penile sensitivity [26], but again, if this is confirmed to be lifelong PE, pharmacotherapy should be recommended.

In contrast to PE, primary lifelong delayed ejaculation is less common (estimated 4 % prevalence) and has not been well studied. As mentioned earlier, men with premature vs. delayed ejaculation may have hormonal profiles reflecting this spectrum. However, in one of very rare studies looking at delayed ejaculation, testosterone and prolactin levels were similar between 19 men with delayed ejaculation and 19 age-matched controls [27]. But a few significant differences were noted. Lifelong delayed ejaculation was associated with higher and idiosyncratic masturbatory activity. Men with lifelong delayed ejaculation were also more likely to have lower incidence of night emissions, infertility, longer ejaculation latency times, lower orgasmic and intercourse satisfaction domains of International Index of Erectile Function, as well as higher anxiety and depression scores [27].

Retrograde ejaculation is defined as semen entering the bladder during orgasm, instead of emerging through the meatus and out of the penis. Men with this condition report little or no semen even though they have reached sexual climax. This poses no medical problems except in younger men who wish to impregnate their partner. The condition, however, can cause some distress in any man and his partner.

Retrograde ejaculation may occur as an adverse effect of alpha-blocking drugs used in the treatment of BPH/LUTS and occurs more commonly with tamsulosin [28]. The phenomenon is reversible upon discontinuation of the drug; however, I have found that most patients can accept this side effect if they are provided with a detailed description of the anatomy along with thorough explanation of the mechanism which causes the semen to flow into the bladder rather than forward through the urethra. Understanding that the bladder neck relaxation achieved to relieve voiding symptoms is allowing for a path of less resistance at the time of ejaculation, assuages patients' fears, and extinguishes the misconception that semen is actually being blocked or "backed up." Transurethral resection of the prostate gland for BPH is associated with a >70 % incidence of retrograde ejaculation. And again, even though this poses no health risk to the patient, appropriate counseling and preparation are required prior to the procedure, as the absence of ejaculation during orgasm can be very distressing to the patient and his partner. Neurological conditions or neuropathies (e.g., diabetic neuropathy) can also lead to decreased tone of the bladder neck, facilitating retrograde ejaculation.

Some men notice decreased volumes of semen during ejaculation, but this may not be the result of retrograde ejaculation, but rather diminished semen production associated with age or use of 5-alpha-reductase inhibitors, which shrink the glandular component of the prostate. Many men also experience a decrease in semen volume after radiation or brachytherapy of the prostate gland. It may diminish to completely dry orgasm, which often correlates to lowest PSA nadirs reached many months after treatment.

Delayed ejaculation, anejaculation, and/or anorgasmia may have a biogenic and/ or psychogenic etiology. Men with age-related penile hypoanesthesia should be educated, reassured, and instructed in revised sexual techniques, which maximize arousal [29].

Because sexual function studies involve mostly heterosexual persons or activities, there may be some concern regarding interpretation within the context of homosexual relationships. Potential effects of sexual orientation on ejaculatory function, for example, have been overlooked in the literature. In preparation of the fifth edition of DSM, efforts were made to use universally suitable definitions of ejaculatory dysfunction. To that end, a recent study from Finland aimed to investigate effects of sexual orientation on premature and delayed ejaculation. When differences in frequencies and patterns of sexual activities were controlled for, there remained no significant effects of sexual orientation on ejaculatory dysfunction [30]. This suggests similar prevalence and concerns among same-sex couples and the importance of addressing sexual issues in all patients, regardless of gender or sexual orientation.

Dysorgasmia is a poorly understood condition, which is often misdiagnosed as prostatitis. Investigation of sexually active men with BPH, revealed discomfort associated with ejaculation [31]. While it is important to rule out an infection, one must be aware that men who experience pain during ejaculation are more likely to have a noninfectious cause for this symptom, such as pelvic floor myalgia or pelvic floor myofascial pain syndrome or pudendal neuralgia. In rare cases, this symptom is the manifestation of ejaculatory duct obstruction, requiring transrectal ultrasound confirmation and endoscopic intervention. Alpha-blocking agents have been shown to ameliorate symptoms of dysorgasmia.

11.8 Evaluation

A thorough history obtained during a comfortable interview cannot be overemphasized. All facets of the patient's life should be considered for query: childhood, sexual awakening/awareness, sexual education and experience, stress and psychosocial issues, family dynamics, religion, relation(s), fidelity, and career and employment (see Table 11.3).

A complete physical examination is warranted and must include a more comprehensive examination of the genitalia. This includes a sensory exam of the lower abdomen and saddle area and by testing for anal wink and bulbocavernosa reflex. The pelvic floor either via the rectum should be palpated for masses, muscle spasm, myofascial trigger points, and laxity.

The penis should be examined for evidence of plaques due to Peyronie's disease, which causes curvature of the penis and is sometimes associated with painful erection. The meatus and shaft should be examined for signs of inflammation or trauma.

Table 11.3 Managing sexual dysfunction in men

Biopsychosocial assessment
Partner status
Employment
Sexual experiences, history of abuse
Sexual stimulation, mental and physical arousal
Medical history, medications, drug/alcohol use
Exercise, smoking, and sleep
Comprehensive physical evaluation
Special attention to genital and pelvic exam
Vascular: BP, pulses, fundi, etc.
Neurosensory
Understand psychosocial or contextual issues
Body image and self-esteem
Financial issues and job stress
Inhibitions and anxieties, cultural/religious beliefs
Screen for depression

Testicles are examined for signs of atrophy or neoplasm. Large hydroceles or spermatoceles may pose a physical or aesthetic obstacle to intercourse.

Neurosensory and vascular assessment should be carried out, testing sensation, temperature, and pulses.

The prostate should be examined. Although it is rare, aggressive prostate cancers in younger men can manifest as erectile dysfunction without any other symptoms or cause. In one of my clinics, several years ago, a healthy 53-year-old man was referred to me because of a mildly elevated PSA level. As part of my routine history, I ask about sexual function and was surprised that this man had become impotent 4 years earlier and had never pursued further workup as he and his wife were not distressed by this. When I examined his prostate, I encountered a very bumpy piece of cement—prostate cancer, Gleason 10, which had already metastasized.

Laboratory tests to consider include hormonal levels: testosterone, LH, prolactin, and thyroid-stimulating hormone (TSH). As dictated by history and physical findings, patients may require additional testing, such as lipid profile, cardiac stress test, sleep lab studies, or imaging.

For a comprehensive summary of questionnaires and algorithms for evaluation and treatment, I would refer the reader to "Summary of the Recommendations on Sexual Dysfunctions in Men," a consensus by Lue and colleagues, cited in the references.

11.9   First-Line Therapy: Lifestyle Modifications

Obesity, sedentary lifestyle, and cigarette smoking are the most common lifestyle factors that cause or contribute to ED and/or decreased libido. These issues should be addressed as primary management strategies.

The heart-healthiest recommendations have consistently served as the safest and most potentially effective options in urology for benign prostatic hyperplasia, chronic nonbacterial prostatitis, interstitial cystitis, multiple urologic cancers, male infertility, *sexual dysfunction*, kidney stones, and Peyronie's disease [32, 33]. In other words, anything that is good for the heart (and the colon) is most probably good for sexual health (and everything else).

Dietary and pharmacological management of dyslipidemia should be among the first steps in managing sexual functioning in men. Statins, for example, have been shown to improve sexual function [34]. A single center prospective randomized placebo-controlled parallel-group trial was conducted. One hundred sixty male patients with ED and dyslipidemia were randomized in a one-to-one ratio to receive up to 1500 mg oral niacin daily or placebo for 12 weeks. Among patients with moderate to severe erectile dysfunction, niacin afforded improvements as measured by the erectile function of the International Index of Erectile Function and Sexual Health Inventory for Men [35]. Niacin alone may be helpful in improving both erectile functioning and lipid profiles in some men.

Along with diet and lipid profiles, exercise is positively correlated to sexual health. Regular aerobic exercise is associated with a significant risk reduction of future erectile dysfunction in men. While hormone replacement therapy in men has been linked to decreased visceral and central body fat [36], patients who engage in weight loss programs with vigorous exercise have been able to improve these parameters and increase their testosterone levels naturally [37].

Although I have had numerous long distance cyclist in my practice, only a few have had sexual complaints or chronic pelvic pain syndrome related to cycling. Through careful observation of their riding techniques and physical therapy, we have recommended appropriate bicycle seats and corrected riding style and seat positioning.

It is important to keep these parameters in mind as preventive measures for those patients about to embark in a new exercise or weight loss program. Similarly, when prescribing exercise to patients, counseling should include the importance of proper technique, proper footwear, and stretching.

I prescribe specialized PT for the management of men with CP/CPPS with or without dysorgasmia. Frequently, patients volunteer an improvement in the quality of their erections and increase in pleasure during climax after a period of PT and exercise. Anderson and colleagues have also observed significant improvement in sexual functioning after specialized PT and progressive relaxation sessions prescribed for the treatment of CP/CPPS [38].

Eliminating risk factors, such as smoking, is another valuable health intervention. A group of male smokers, irrespective of erectile dysfunction status, who were motivated to stop smoking ("quitters") were enrolled in an 8-week smoking cessation program involving a nicotine patch therapy and adjunctive counseling. Participants were assessed at baseline (while smoking regularly), at mid-treatment (while using a high-dose nicotine patch), and at a 4-week post-cessation follow-up. At each visit, penile plethysmography, sexual arousal indices, and self-reported sexual functioning were assessed. Despite this relatively short time interval, quitters compared to relapsed smokers showed enhanced erectile tumescence responses and faster onset to reach maximum subjective sexual arousal [39]. These results may serve as a novel means to motivate men to quit smoking.

To me, sleep is an obvious correlate to sexual functioning and should be addressed anyway, as part of general health maintenance. In a compelling review, investigators addressed the interrelationships between testosterone, sexual function, and sleep, including sleep-disordered breathing in both sexes. Hormonal changes in testosterone were associated with sleep apnea and chronic sleep deprivation, with negative ramifications on sexual life [40].

11.10 Prescribed Therapies for Sexual Dysfunction

Hypogonadism in men is associated with low sexual desire, erectile dysfunction, arousal disorders, and orgasmic/ejaculation disorders. Hormonal measures should be done to exclude deficiencies of testosterone in men. Replacement therapies should be carefully weighed against the individual's risk factors. Sex hormone replacement therapies remain controversial for both sexes; however, there is growing evidence showing overall health benefits of testosterone given to hypogonadal men, with minimal to no increased risk of prostate cancer [41]. However, high doses of testosterone can increase cardiovascular events, possibly due to polycythemic effects.

Individual and/or couples counseling should be encouraged for most patients as sexual dysfunction is rarely a purely physical phenomenon, and the consequences, regardless of cause, can be emotionally devastating for individuals and their partners. Even in cases that appear to be purely organic, such as ED after prostatectomy, psychological counseling is recommended while recovering sexual functioning.

Replacement or ablative therapies should be prescribed accordingly, for hypo- or hyperthyroidism, a not uncommon cause of sexual dysfunction.

Sildenafil citrate (Viagra) is a potent PDE 5 inhibitor. By inhibiting this enzyme, sildenafil citrate results in larger concentrations of cGMP and improved smooth muscle relaxation and erections provided that sexual stimulation occurs. Vardenafil's (Levitra) mechanism of action is similar. Some men appreciate fewer AEs with vardenafil; however, Viagra has continued to be the favorite among my patients until the arrival of tadalafil (Cialis). With its longer half-life, Cialis has afforded many patients with greater romantic and sexual spontaneity. Given the high prevalence of cardiac conditions in the aging man, one needs to be cautious when prescribing these medications. They are contraindicated in anyone taking nitrates or nitrate donor medications and are relatively contraindicated in patients with unstable angina pectoris, recent myocardial infarction, certain arrhythmias, and poorly controlled hypertension. In patients taking alpha-blockers, the addition of PDE5 inhibitor may cause postural hypotension.

Other ED treatments can be administered as injections. The most commonly utilized substances include prostaglandin E1 (PGE1), phentolamine, and papaverine. PGE1 and papaverine cause cavernous smooth muscle relaxation by elevation of the intracellular concentration of the second messengers, cGMP and cyclic adenosine monophosphate. Phentolamine is an alpha-adrenergic antagonist. PGE1 is also available as an intraurethral administrated pellet (medicated urethral system/suppository for erection, MUSE). Urethral and intracavernosal administration of vasoactive substances results in erection within several minutes, which may last 30 min to 2 h [15].

Adverse events from these therapies include priapism, variable degrees of pain with injection in about half of patients, and penile fibrosis after long-term use. MUSE has been associated with hypotension, syncope, urethral burning or pain, and vaginal irritation in the partner. Relative contraindications to injection therapy include men who have a history of priapism and those with bleeding disorders.

For men who are unable to take PDE5 inhibitors or have inadequate response to nonsurgical therapies, the vacuum constriction devices provide a relatively safe alternative and may help some patients to avoid or postpone surgical implantation of penile prosthetics. It may seem awkward or cumbersome for some patients and their partners, and couples need to be prepared for the less natural appearance of the penis, which may become cool and cyanotic. Maintenance of erection is facilitated by application of a rubber cuff applied around the penile base, which may cause some instability as the firmness of the penis will be distal to this ring [15].

For more details regarding treatment options, I strongly recommend the article, "Evaluation and Treatment of Erectile Dysfunction in the Aging Male: A mini-review," cited in the references.

Medications for PE include alpha-blockers and antidepressants. Adverse effects are important considerations for the use of these medications especially because efficacy in treatment of PE is best with consistent daily regimens. While on-demand therapy seems most appealing and minimizes adverse effects, most men would prefer daily treatment because of its affording sexual spontaneity. On the other hand, with regard to off-label use of antidepressants for PE, men may be uncomfortable with the stigma of an antidepressant prescription.

Based upon the observations of delayed orgasm or anorgasmia among patients treated with SSRIs, this group of antidepressants has been most frequently used for PE. Sertraline is the most commonly prescribed SSRI prescribed in the United States, both as daily or on-demand regimens. Side effects, however, include fatigue, yawning, mild nausea, loose stools, and perspiration [17]. Decreased libido and mild erectile dysfunction may occur with SSRIs as well. The most serious concern is increased suicide risk observed in depressed patients treated with SSRIs especially paroxetine.

Dapoxetine is a drug specifically developed for the on-demand treatment of PE, not currently licensed in the United States. It has been extensively evaluated in five randomized, placebo-controlled phase III clinical trials involving more than 6000 men with PE. This is the largest and most comprehensive clinical trial program to date for a drug therapy to treat PE. It is a short-acting SSRI designed to be taken as needed, 1–3 h before sexual intercourse, which is currently available in Europe [24]. As of 2015, it has not yet been approved by the FDA.

Treatment of PE with PDE5 inhibitors remains controversial although some have theorized that the decreased sexual latency period observed with this drug could facilitate immediate repeat intercourse of possibly increased duration, but this has never been studied. Because one-third of men with ED also have PE, the use of PDE5 inhibitors may be the treatment of choice, especially if the PE occurred secondarily to ED.

Desensitizing creams have also been shown to be effective in treating PE. Prilocaine-lidocaine may be administered as a cream or aerosol spray. There are local and rarer systemic adverse effects associated with this topical therapy. Desensitizing creams and sprays can cause side effects including hypoanesthesia of the penile shaft and numbing of the vaginal vault of the partner, unless a condom is used [24].

In cases of delayed ejaculation, the use of bupropion-SR in a daily dosage of 150 mg provided statistically significant benefits to the patients: improvement in ejaculation control, improved orgasmic and intercourse satisfaction, and improved depression scores [27].

Management and therapies are summarized in Table 11.4.

11.11 Depression and Therapy

Because depression and antidepressant use are so prevalent in the general population, it is important to bear in mind that untreated depression and antidepressant medications can both cause sexual dysfunction. The incidence of sexual dysfunction caused by antidepressants may be as high as 93 %; side effects from SSRIs occur in 67 % of patients, manifest as decreased desire, arousal difficulties (lack of erection), or inability to climax or ejaculate [17].

Because up to 40 % of patients complaining of sexual adverse effects were found to have had sexual dysfunction prior to initiating therapy, I strongly recommend assessing sexual functioning prior to prescribing antidepressants, particularly those which have greater risk such as SSRIs 17. One must also bear in mind that antidepressant medication therapy is associated with a relatively high noncompliance rate (30 %), which may be due in part to the sexual side effects.

Management strategies for antidepressant-induced sexual dysfunction include investigating pre-tx function (which, again, is much better achieved by assessing at the time just prior to prescribing medication), investigating noncompliance, reassessment for comorbidities or other medications that may cause sexual dysfunction, and counseling about adaptation, which may help a small number of patients who can resume normal activity after a brief period of adjustment 17. The majority of patients, however, will not be able to "adapt"; therefore, one might consider decreasing the dose or switching, for example, from sertraline to nefazodone. In one study, 67 % of men taking sertraline reported ejaculatory difficulties compared with 19 % of the nefazodone-treated group. In women, nefazodone was superior to sertraline with regard to the ability to achieve orgasm. Bupropion may also be an appropriate alternative. In another study, sexual dysfunction developed in 15 % of men taking

Table 11.4 Management and treatment

Clinical testing and labs
Metabolic syndrome, diabetes, hypertension, etc.
Consider hormonal abnormalities
Testosterone, thyroid replacement
Rule out medication side effects esp. antihypertensives and antidepressants
Prescribe or modify drug regimens
Penile ultrasound and Doppler
Lifestyle
Diet and exercise
Weight loss
Smoking cessation
Sleep hygiene
Coordination of schedules and bedtime
Integrative approaches
Counseling or life coaching
Yoga
Specialized physical therapy
Marriage retreats (spiritual/religious)
Prescribed therapies
Low libido
Testosterone, bupropion
ED
Sildenafil, vardenafil, MUSE
Alprostadil injection, vacuum device
Premature ejaculation
Sertraline, PDE-5 inhibitor, topical anesthetics
Retrograde ejaculation
Adrenergic agonists
Delayed ejaculation/anorgasmia
Testosterone, bupropion
Dysorgasmia
Alpha-adrenergic blockers
Antibiotics, low-dose benzodiazepine
Specialized pelvic floor physiotherapy

bupropion as compared to 63 % taking sertraline. Bupropion is an important alternative for the treatment of depressed patients who are concerned about maintaining their sexual functioning.

Alternatively, patients may be prescribed bupropion in addition to the primary antidepressant to "reverse" the adverse effect. Some experts also debate the implementation of drug holidays, perhaps for weekends [17]. While this may be helpful in some patients with less severe depression or in those using drugs with shorter half-life, caution is needed for possible drug withdrawal symptoms and perhaps lack of spontaneity with unreasonable time constraints imposed by the "holiday" schedule.

11.12 Summary

While sexual dysfunction is classified into components of desire, arousal, and climax, treatments targeting one of these can improve other aspects and overall sexual function. Emotional and marital factors should not be discounted in male sexual health. The subject of sexual functioning should be a "natural" part of general health maintenance, and caregivers should strive to provide a comfortable environment in which to approach this topic.

References

1. Coleman E, Elders J, Satcher D, et al. Summit on medical school education in sexual health: report of an expert consultation. J Sex Med. 2013;10(4):924–38.
2. Lindau ST, Gavrilova N. Sex, health, and years of sexually active life gained due to good health: evidence from two US population based cross sectional surveys of ageing. BMJ. 2010;340:c810.
3. Kleinplatz PJ. Sexuality and older people. BMJ. 2008;337:a239.
4. Naeinian MR, Shaeiri MR, Hosseini FS. General health and quality of life in patients with sexual dysfunctions. Urol J. 2011;8:127–31.
5. Brezsnyak M, Whisman MA. Sexual desire and relationship functioning: the effects of marital satisfaction and power. J Sex Marital Ther. 2004;30:199–217.
6. Giraldi A, Rellini A, Pfaus JG, Bitzer J, Laan E, Jannini EA, Fugl-Meyer AR. Questionnaires for assessment of female sexual dysfunction: a review and proposal for a standardized screener. J Sex Med. 2011;8:2681–706.
7. McCabe MP, Goldhammer DL. Demographic and psychological factors related to sexual desire among heterosexual women in a relationship. J Sex Res. 2012;49(1):78–87. Epub 2011 May 24.
8. O'Connor E, McCabe M, Conaglen H, Conaglen J. Attitudes and experiences: qualitative perspectives on erectile dysfunction from the female partner. J Health Psychol. 2012;17(1):3–13.
9. Chevret-Méasson M, Lavallée E, Troy S, Arnould B, Oudin S, Cuzin B. Improvement in quality of sexual life in female partners of men with erectile dysfunction treated with sildenafil citrate: findings of the index of sexual life (ISL) in a couple study. J Sex Med. 2009;6(3):761–9. Epub 2009 Jan 7.
10. Barnett ZL, Robleda-Gomez S, Pachana NA. Viagra: the little blue pill with big repercussions. Aging Ment Health. 2012;16(1):84–8.
11. Potts A, Gavey N, Grace VM, Vares T. The downside of Viagra: women's experiences and concerns. Sociol Health Illn. 2003;25(7):697–719.
12. Graziottin A, Althof S. What does premature ejaculation mean to the man, the woman, and the couple? J Sex Med. 2011;8 Suppl 4:304–9.
13. Kalra G, Subramanyam A, Pinto C. Sexuality: desire, activity and intimacy in the elderly. Indian J Psychiatry. 2011;53(4):300–6.
14. Walsh KE, Berman JR. Sexual dysfunction in the older woman: an overview of the current understanding and management. Drugs Aging. 2004;21(10):655–75.
15. Lue T, Giuliano F, Montorsi F, et al. Summary of the recommendations on sexual dysfunctions in men. J Sex Med. 2004;1(1):6–23.

16. Esposito K, Giugliano D. Obesity, the metabolic syndrome, and sexual dysfunction in men. Clin Pharmacol Ther. 2011;90(1):169–73.
17. Higgins A, Nash M, Lynch A. Antidepressant-associated sexual dysfunction: impact, effects, and treatment. Drug Healthc Patient Saf. 2010;2:141–50.
18. Krassas GE, Tziomalos K, Papadopoulou F, Pontikides N, Perros P. Erectile dysfunction in patients with hyper- and hypothyroidism: how common and should we treat? J Clin Endocrinol Metab. 2008;93(5):1815–9.
19. Albersen M, Orabi H, Lue TF. Evaluation and treatment of erectile dysfunction in the aging male: a mini-review. Gerontology. doi:10.1159/000329598.
20. Melnik T, Althof S, Atallah AN, Puga ME, Glina S, Riera R. Psychosocial interventions for premature ejaculation. Cochrane Database Syst Rev. 2011;10(8):CD008195.
21. Corona G, Jannini EA, Lotti F, Boddi V, De Vita G, Forti G, Lenzi A, Mannucci E, Maggi M. Premature and delayed ejaculation: two ends of a single continuum influenced by hormonal milieu. Int J Androl. 2011;34(1):41–8.
22. Jern P, Santtila P, Johansson A, Sandnabba NK. Genetic and environmental effects on the continuity of ejaculatory dysfunction. BJU Int. 2010;105(12):1698–704. Epub 2009 Oct 26.
23. Wainberg J. Essai d'interpretation ontogene-tique de l'ejaculation prematuree, In: Buvat J, Jouaunnet P, editors. L'ejaculation et ses perturbances. Simep: Lyon-Villeurbanne; 1984. p. 112–6. As cited in Bettochi et al. and Mohee et al.
24. Mohee A, Eardley I. Medical therapy for premature ejaculation. Ther Adv Urol. 2011;3(5):211–22.
25. Bettocchi C, Verze P, Palumbo F, Arcaniolo D, Mirone V. Ejaculatory disorders: pathophysiology and management. Nat Clin Pract Urol. 2008;5(2):93–103.
26. Althof S, Abdo C, Dean J, Hackett G, McCabe M, McMahon C, et al. (2009) International Society for Sexual Medicine's guidelines for the diagnosis and treatment of premature ejaculation. http://www.issm.info/v4/. Accessed 23 Sept 2011.
27. Abdel-Hamid IA, Saleh S. Primary lifelong delayed ejaculation: characteristics and response to bupropion. J Sex Med. 2011;8(6):1772–9.
28. Wolters JP, Hellstrom WJG. Current concepts in ejaculatory dysfunction. Rev Urol. 2006;8 Suppl 4:S18–25.
29. Rowland D, McMahon CG, Abdo C, Chen J, Jannini E, Waldinger MD, Ahn TY. Disorders of orgasm and ejaculation in men. J Sex Med. 2010;7(4 Pt 2):1668–86.
30. Jern P, Santtila P, Johansson A, Alanko K, Salo B, Sandnabba NK. Is there an association between same-sex sexual experience and ejaculatory dysfunction? J Sex Marital Ther. 2010;36(4):303–12.
31. Müller A, Mulhall JP. Sexual dysfunction in the patient with prostatitis. Curr Urol Rep. 2006;7:307–12.
32. Moyad MA. Heart health = urologic health and heart unhealthy = urologic unhealthy: rapid review of lifestyle changes and dietary supplements. Urol Clin N Am. 2011;38(3):359–67.
33. Esposito K, Giugliano D. Lifestyle/dietary recommendations for erectile dysfunction and female sexual dysfunction. Urol Clin N Am. 2011;38(3):293–301.
34. Gupta BP, Murad MH, Clifton MM, Prokop L, Nehra A, Kopecky SL. The effect of lifestyle modification and cardiovascular risk factor reduction on erectile dysfunction: a systematic review and meta-analysis. Arch Intern Med. 2011;171(20):1797–803.
35. Ng C-F, Lee C-P, Ho AL, Lee VWY. Effect of niacin on erectile function in men suffering erectile dysfunction and dyslipidemia. J Sex Med. 2011;8:2883–93.
36. Saad F, Aversa A, Isidori AM, Gooren LJ. Testosterone as potential effective therapy in treatment of obesity in men with testosterone deficiency: a review. Curr Diabetes Rev. 2012;8(1):131–43.
37. Lovell DI, Cuneo R, Wallace J, McLellan C. The hormonal response of older men to sub-maximum aerobic exercise: the effect of training and detraining. Steroids. 2012;77:413–8.
38. Anderson RU, Wise D, Sawyer T, Chan CA. Sexual dysfunction in men with chronic prostatitis/chronic pelvic pain syndrome: improvement after trigger point release and paradoxical relaxation training. J Urol. 2006;176(4 Pt 1):1534–8.

39. Harte CB, Meston CM. Association between smoking cessation and sexual health in men. BJU Int. 2011;109:888–96.
40. Andersen ML, Alvarenga TF, Mazaro-Costa R, Hachul HC, Tufik S. The association of testosterone, sleep, and sexual function in men and women. Brain Res. 2011;1416:80–104.
41. Corona G, Rastrelli G, Forti G, Maggi M. Update in testosterone therapy for men. J Sex Med. 2011;8(3):639–54.

Benign Prostatic Hyperplasia and LUTS

12

Harcharan Gill

12.1 Etiology and Pathophysiology

BPH is a histopathologic finding in the aging prostate characterized by an increase in epithelial and stromal cells in the area of the prostate surrounding the urethra [1]. The precise molecular etiology of this hyperplastic process is uncertain, but androgens, estrogens, stromal-epithelial interactions, growth factors, and neurotransmitters may play a role. Their action is through the combination of increased cell proliferation and impairing cell death, apoptosis. Although androgens do not cause BPH, the development of BPH requires the presence of testicular androgens during early prostate development, puberty, and aging [2]. Patients castrated before puberty or who are affected by a variety of genetic diseases that impair androgen action or production do not develop BPH. In the prostate the enzyme 5α-reductase converts the hormone testosterone into DHT, which makes it the principal prostate androgen [3]. There are two subtypes of 5α-reductase inhibitor enzymes. Type 1 5α-reductase is predominant in extraprostatic tissues, such as the skin and liver; Type 2 5α-reductase is predominant in the prostate, although it is also slightly expressed in extraprostatic tissues. Neural factors, specifically sympathetic signaling pathways, are also important in the etiology and pathophysiology of LUTS through modulation of the smooth muscle cell phenotype in the prostate [4]. Inflammation, which is commonly seen in BPH specimens, may play a role in the pathogenesis of the disease through cytokines that promote cell growth or lead to smooth muscle contraction. Genetic and familial factors are also associated with the development of BPH.

H. Gill, M.D. (✉)
Department of Urology, Stanford University Hospital,
875 Blake Wilbur Avenue, Stanford, CA 94305, USA
e-mail: hgill@standford.edu

© Springer Science+Business Media New York 2016
J.M. Potts (ed.), *Men's Health*, DOI 10.1007/978-1-4939-3237-5_12

The pathophysiology of BPH is complex and seldom is the prostate alone in the causation of LUTS. The basic concept of mechanical obstruction causing an increase in urethral resistance, although logical, is rare in isolation. The size of the prostate does not correlate with the symptoms, but the tone in the smooth muscles in the prostate and bladder neck is important. In addition, the bladder compensates to the outlet obstruction and results in further urinary symptoms making LUTS more bothersome. LUTS are also compounded by age-related changes in both bladder and nervous system function which lead to increased urinary frequency, urgency, and nocturia.

12.2   Epidemiology and Natural History

There are no standardized definitions of prevalence of BPH or LUTS. The prevalence of BPH thus can be calculated based on histologic criteria (autopsy prevalence) or on clinical criteria (LUTS). There are a large number of descriptive epidemiologic studies, both cross-sectional and longitudinal in the literature [5]. The use of International Prostate Symptom Score (IPSS) has been a pivotal in the clinical research of LUTS and BPH and has standardized most of the recent epidemiological studies. In multiple international studies, despite the significantly different proportion of men with moderate-to-severe symptoms, a clear trend toward an increase in symptom scores with advancing age is evident. Approximately 30 % of American men older than 50 years have moderate-to-severe LUTS [6, 7]. The Urologic Diseases in America BPH Project examined the prevalence of moderate-to-severe LUTS reported in US population-based studies. They defined moderate-to-severe LUTS as men with an American Urological Association (AUA) Symptom Index (SI) score of ≥ 7. They reported a progressive increase in the prevalence of moderate-to-severe LUTS, rising to nearly 50 % by the eighth decade of life. The presence of moderate-to-severe LUTS was also associated with the development of acute urinary retention (AUR) as a symptom of BPH progression, increasing from a prevalence of 6.8 episodes per 1000 patient years of follow-up in the overall population to a high of 34.7 episodes in men aged 70 and older with moderate-to-severe LUTS. Based on the demographics of the US population, 6.5 to 8.7 million men are eligible to discuss BPH treatment options [7, 8]. Also, in all cross-sectional studies, prostate volume as assessed by TRUS has been found to increase slowly but steadily with advancing age. With the exception of age, correlations between various measures, including BMI and metabolic syndrome, LUTS, and BPH, are modest in community-based population studies and weak in BPH clinic and trial populations. The relationship between serum PSA and prostate volume is moderate and influenced by age, race, and ethnic origin. Age, symptom severity, flow rate, prostate size, and serum PSA are useful predictors of the risk of progression. Complications of LUTS and BPH such as mortality, urinary tract infections, bladder decompensation, bladder stones, hematuria, urinary incontinence, and upper urinary tract deterioration with renal insufficiency are rare in properly followed-up patients. The two most significant progression events are AUR and the need for BPH-related surgery.

12.3 Evaluation

The clinical manifestations of BPH include LUTS, poor bladder emptying, urinary retention, overactive bladder, UTI, hematuria, and renal insufficiency. The American Urological Association (AUA) BPH guidelines updated in 2014 has detailed evaluation recommendations [9].

In the initial evaluation, a detailed medical history should be obtained to identify other causes of voiding dysfunction or comorbidities that may complicate treatment. The symptoms are quantified using the International Prostate Symptom Score (IPSS), a symptom-scoring instrument to assess the baseline assessment of symptom severity in men presenting with LUTS and also to monitor response to treatment. Bother and interference with activities of daily living due to LUTS are equally if not more important than the enumeration of symptom frequency and severity alone [10]. A digital rectal exam, urinalysis, and PSA are also part of the initial evaluation. Cystoscopy is not indicated unless the patient has hematuria. Urinary flow rate and post-void residual (PVR) urine volume are basic office evaluations that should be done on all patients. Flow rate is only diagnostic if the voided volume is at least 150 cm^3. Although neither subjectively assessed symptoms nor quantified symptom score analysis correlates strongly with uroflowmetry measurements, each is an independent assessment. PVR urine volume does not correlate well with other signs or symptoms of clinical BPH, but large PVR urine volumes may predict bladder decompensation. Complex pressure-flow urodynamic studies are only appropriate tests to consider in the evaluation of men with severe symptoms, neurologic disorder history, or failed surgical treatment. Pressure-flow studies differentiate between patients with a low PFR secondary to obstruction and those whose low PFR is caused by impaired detrusor contractility [11].

12.4 Treatment

Major changes have been made in the last two decades and there are a number of new procedures and drugs that may be available in the future. A large number of options are available to the physician and patient. The treatment decision is often made based on the severity of symptoms, options available, and patient preference. The following options are currently available:

Watchful waiting (active surveillance)
Medical therapy
Minimally invasive therapy
Surgical treatment

12.4.1   Watchful Waiting

Rationale   This option is based on multiple natural history studies that show 15–30 % of patients have spontaneous improvement in their symptoms in the non-treatment arms of these studies. A significant number of men with LUTS will choose this option because the symptoms are not bothersome or the complications or side effects of treatment are perceived to be greater than the inconvenience of the symptoms. Patients often make minor lifestyle changes such as decreasing total fluid intake, especially before bedtime, and moderating the intake of alcohol- and caffeine-containing products. Patients with mild symptoms, IPSS < 8, are ideal for watchful waiting. Patients on surveillance should be followed up at least annually.

12.4.2   Medical Treatment

The primary objective of medical therapy is to improve LUTS and improve the quality of life index.

Rationale   The presence of α_1-adrenergic receptors associated with prostatic smooth muscle [12] and 5α-reductase in the prostate stroma and glands leads to the development of drugs that block the alpha receptors or inhibit the enzyme 5α-reductase. The importance of this dynamic obstruction was supported by morphometric studies demonstrating that smooth muscle is one of the dominant cellular constituents of BPH, accounting for 40 % of the area density of the hyperplastic prostate [13]. The rationale for androgen suppression is based on the observation that the embryonic development of the prostate is dependent on androgen dihydrotestosterone (DHT).

Classification of Medical Treatments

1. Alpha-blockers
2. 5α-reductase inhibitors

Classification of Alpha-Blockers

Nonselective	Phenoxybenzamine
Short-acting alpha 1	Prazosin
Long-acting alpha 1	Terazosin, doxazosin
Prostate-specific a1a	Alfuzosin, silodosin, tamsulosin

Multiple randomized, double-blind, multicenter, placebo-controlled studies have demonstrated the efficacy and safety of alpha-blockers for BPH [14]. Side effects that are bothersome, especially in the elderly, are dizziness and orthostatic hypotension. In population studies of elderly men, the presence of moderate and severe LUTS independently increased the 1-year risk of falls, and there was a modest increase in risk associated with exposure to α-adrenergic blockers [15].

Thus, caution should be taken in elderly men before starting alpha-blockers. Erectile dysfunction (ED) can occur in some patients without clear differences between the different alpha-blockers. Ejaculatory dysfunction during treatment occurs more frequently with tamsulosin and silodosin than with other drugs of this class. Often young men find it most bothersome.

Classification of 5 Alpha Reductase Inhibitors

Type 2	Finasteride
Type 1 and Type 2	Dutasteride

Multicenter, randomized, double-blind, placebo-controlled studies support the role of this group of drugs in the treatment of BPH. Both these drugs reduce the prostate volume by approximately 20 %. The overall treatment-related improvements in symptom score and peak flow rate (PFR) relative to placebo are modest, and long-term safety and durability of efficacy have been demonstrated. This group of drugs is best used in patients with prostates greater than 30 cm³ in volume [16]. The adverse clinical events associated with finasteride and dutasteride are minimal and are related primarily to sexual function.

Combination Therapy
The results of the MTOPS trial suggest that the combination of doxazosin and finasteride exerts a clinically relevant, positive effect on rates of disease progression. Men who received combination therapy were significantly less likely to experience BPH progression than those receiving either monotherapy or placebo, with risk reduction rates of 39 % for doxazosin, 34 % for finasteride, and 67 % for combination therapy compared with placebo [17]. The combination of an alpha-blocker and a 5-ARI is an appropriate and effective treatment for patients with LUTS associated with demonstrable prostatic enlargement based on volume measurement (>30 cm³), PSA level as a proxy for volume (>1.5).

Anticholinergics
There is an overlap between symptoms traditionally regarded as being due to BPH and those ascribed to the syndrome of over active bladder (OAB). OAB symptoms may coexist with BPH and LUTS complex. Short-term trial data suggest antimuscarinic agents can be safely given to carefully selected men with OAB and BPH. The combination of antimuscarinic agents and α-adrenergic blocker therapy may improve both storage and voiding symptoms. Men with large PVR urine volumes (≥200 mL) should not be treated with antimuscarinic agents.

12.4.3 Minimally Invasive Treatment

Minimally invasive techniques have been introduced in the last 2 decades with the hope that they will have less complications than transurethral resection of the prostate (TURP), less requirement for anesthesia, and a shorter and therefore potentially less expensive hospital stay. These have been popularized by urologists, patients, and the industry, but there have been many disappointments along the way. Many of these FDA-approved therapies were introduced based on a series of poorly constructed short-term trials. In spite of the fact that they were originally welcomed as a significant advance in the treatment of BPH, in the longer term they have not turned out to be so. However, the demise of some of the earlier technologies has led to the strengthening and evolution of newer ones, all of which has been beneficial for patients with BPH.

Minimally Invasive Treatments
Prostate balloon dilatation
Prostate stents
Transurethral needle ablation
Microwave therapy
Water-induced thermotherapy
Implant: UROLIFT

Prostate balloon dilatation was introduced based on knowledge gained from cardiovascular angioplasties; however, it was rapidly abandoned due to lack of efficacy, durability, and complications. Prostate stents were the natural evolution to the balloons. Thus, in an attempt to find less traumatic methods of treating symptomatic BPH, either temporary or permanent, intraprostatic stents were developed, and both permanent and biodegradable material used. There have been many small trials of a number of these devices. Originally, permanent prostatic stents were introduced as a definitive treatment for prostatic obstruction for patients unfit for prostatic surgery who presented with urinary retention. Although patients were able to void satisfactorily in most cases, the complications were relatively high. UroLume stent has been the most frequently investigated and reported but has now been removed from the market [18].

Transurethral needle ablation (TUNA) uses low-level radio frequency to cause thermal necrosis of the prostate adenoma. The TUNA device can be used under local anesthesia. The needle delivers radio-frequency pulses to raise the temperature to 60 °C; however, there is a quick decline in temperature as the distance increases from the treatment needle. Although good outcomes were reported in the US randomized trial comparing TUNA with TURP in 65 patients treated by TUNA and 56 by TURP [19], other studies have shown lack of durability. The most common reported side effect of TUNA was urinary retention ranging from 13 to 45 %.

Transurethral microwave therapy (TUMT) has been greatly investigated in the last two decades. The technology of TUMT has also evolved from low-energy to high-energy application as has our knowledge of patient selection for this technique. The current devices heat the prostate up to 70 °C, and the mechanism of action for improving LUTS is thought to be through damage to the sympathetic nerve endings and induction of apoptosis. TUMT has less morbidity than TURP but is not as effective as TURP in improving symptoms or reducing LUTS. TUMT is associated with a lengthy period of catheterization after treatment, thus causing higher rates of urinary tract infection and urinary retention. The durability of TUMT is poor, with only 23 % of patients remaining satisfied after 4 years with a single such treatment [20].

Water-induced thermotherapy (WIT) was introduced and tested as a cost-effective form of thermotherapy; however, it has not gained popularity due to limited efficacy, lack of durability, and a number of competitive products on the market.

UROLIFT is the latest minimally invasive technology approved for the treatment of LUTS and BPH. The implant is delivered transurethrally to separate encroaching lateral prostate lobes and relieve obstruction without thermal injury or resection of prostatic tissue. This is an outpatient procedure done under local anesthesia. In a recent multicenter randomized controlled and blinded study of 206 men (prostatic urethral lift 140 vs. sham 66), prostatic urethral lift subjects experienced AUASI reduction from 22.1 baseline to 11.1 at 12 months, and peak urinary flow rate increased by 4.0 ml per second at 12 months [21]. Long-term data is pending.

Surgical Treatment
Incision: TUIP
Coagulation: TUILC, VLAP, TUILC

Vaporization:
    Lasers: PVP, HoLAP
    Electric: TUVP

Resection
    Laser: HoLEP, HoLRP
    Electric: TURP

Simple prostatectomy

Transurethral incision of prostate (TUIP) is a well-established and simple technique generally offered to patients with small symptomatic prostates. These patients are oftentimes also younger. The efficacy is comparable in such patients with TURP, and the results are maintained in the long term.

Lasers: The use of lasers in management of BPH has evolved over the last two decades as our knowledge and experience has expanded. The technology has also evolved with improved fibers and delivery systems. Lasers in urology can be categorized into two basic groups, coagulative or vaporizing. Although the wavelength makes the major difference in these two properties, other factors include the power density of the laser beam itself, the total energy delivered, and the time for which it is applied. The modes of action of common lasers that are used are shown below.

Laser	Wavelength	Main mode of action	Procedure
Neodymium-YAG	1064 nm	Coagulation	VLAP, TULIP
Potassium titanyl phosphate (KTP)	532 nm	Vaporization	PVP
Holmium	2100 nm	Vaporization, cutting	HoLEP, HoLAP, HoLRP
Diode		Vaporization	

Coagulative lasers were the first ones introduced for BPH. Although initially popular, the postoperative symptoms and incidence of retention were high. The efficacy of visual laser ablation of the prostate (VLAP) was reported in a number of large studies [22]. Neither the UK study [23] nor the US study [24] had any patient treated with VLAP requiring a blood transfusion. VLAP caused neither "TURP syndrome" nor any particular effect on serum sodium levels. The retrograde ejaculation rate varied from 27 to 33 %, urethral stricture rate from 0 to 1.8 %, and bladder neck contracture occurred in 4.4 %. Postoperative dysuria rates were high, 15–30 % at 3 months, and posttreatment retention rate was 30.4 % in the patients treated by VLAP [24].

Vaporizing lasers, KTP and holmium, have gained popularity due to their efficacy and durable results. Multiple studies, including randomized, have proven the long-term efficacy of these lasers. A number of different techniques are described and often it is the surgeon's experience that determines what the patient receives. The holmium laser has been used for vaporization (HoLAP), resection (HoLRP), and enucleation (HoLEP) of the BPH adenoma. Multiple studies have shown efficacy and durability of all three techniques [25]. HoLEP has come closest to challenging the gold standard TURP. The KTP laser has a photo-selective wavelength that causes vaporization. Although the initial studies were at low power of 60 W, current techniques utilize 120–180 W. The efficacy and durability of this has also been shown in randomized trials [26]. This laser can be used on anticoagulated patients and those with bleeding disorders. A recent systematic literature review assessed the evidence presented between 2006 and 2008 for PVP and HoLEP, suggesting that both of these techniques are promising alternatives to both TURP and open prostatectomy [27].

Transurethral resection of the prostate has been labeled the gold standard for surgical treatment of BPH due to extensive experience and established durability of results; however, it is constantly challenged by new technology that has fewer side effects but unestablished durability. TURP has undergone multiple modifications from the first time it was introduced in the 1920s. The most recent modification is the introduction of bipolar technology. The previous remarkable change was in the 1960s with the development of a continuous flow resectoscope. Both these modifications have helped in reducing the morbidity of the procedure, especially the TURP syndrome. A large number of reports on the outcomes of TURP are available in published literature. There is a trend over the years of decreasing morbidity, most likely from better patient selection, improved antibiotics, new technology, and better perioperative care including anesthesia. Wasson [28] reported on a prospective randomized study in which patients were assigned to either watchful waiting or TURP. Ninety-one percent of the men had no complications during the first 30 days after surgery. The complications noted were a need for replacement of urinary catheter (4 %), perforation of the prostatic capsule (2 %), and hemorrhage requiring transfusion (1 %), and there was no difference between either groups in the incidence of urinary incontinence or impotence Therefore, in well-trained hands, TURP is a safe and effective way of treating BPH, with an acceptable side-effect profile.

Simple prostatectomy in the USA is restricted to very large glands. It is the most invasive approach to BPH but has the best outcomes. Recent attempts at doing this endoscopically, robotic, have been published. The widespread use of this remains unknown as the outcome complications and outcomes are similar [29].

References

1. McNeal J. Pathology of benign prostatic hyperplasia: insight into etiology [review]. Urol Clin North Am. 1990;17:477–86.
2. Peters CA, Walsh PC. The effect of nafarelin acetate, a luteinizing-hormone-releasing hormone agonist, on benign prostatic hyperplasia. N Engl J Med. 1987;317:599–604.
3. Walsh PC, Hutchins GM, Ewing LL. Tissue content of dihydrotestosterone in human prostatic hyperplasia is not supernormal. J Clin Invest. 1983;72:1772–7.
4. Lin VK, Wang D, et al. Myosin heavy chain gene expression in normal and hyperplastic human prostate tissue. Prostate. 2000;44:193–203.
5. Berry SJ, Coffey DS, et al. The development of human benign prostatic hyperplasia with age. J Urol. 1984;132:474–9.
6. Chute CG, Panser LA, et al. The prevalence of prostatism: a population-based survey of urinary symptoms. J Urol. 1993;150:85–9.
7. Jacobsen SJ, Girman CJ, et al. Natural history of prostatism: longitudinal changes in voiding symptoms in community dwelling men. J Urol. 1996;155:595–600.
8. Wei J, Calhoun E, Jacobsen S. Urologic diseases in America project: benign prostatic hyperplasia. J Urol. 2005;173:1256.
9. McVary KT, Roehrborn CG, Avins AL, Barry MJ, Bruskewitz RC, Donnell RF, Foster HE, Gonzalez CM, Kaplan SA, Penson DF, Ulchaker JC, Wei JT. Update on AUA guideline on the management of benign prostatic hyperplasia. J Urol. 2011;185(5):1793–803.
10. Garraway WM, Armstrong C. Follow-up of a cohort of men with untreated benign prostatic hyperplasia. Eur Urol. 1993;24:313–8.
11. Abrams P. Objective evaluation of bladder outlet obstruction [review]. Br J Urol. 1995;76: 11–5.
12. Caine M, Schuger L: The "capsule" in benign prostatic hypertrophy. Publication No. 87–2881. Bethesda (MD): U.S. Department of Health and Human Services; 1987.
13. Shapiro E, Becich MJ. The relative proportion of stromal and epithelial hyperplasia is related to the development of symptomatic benign prostate hyperplasia. J Urol. 1992;147:1293–7.
14. Roehrborn CG, Schwinn DA. Alpha1-adrenergic receptors and their inhibitors in lower urinary tract symptoms and benign prostatic hyperplasia. J Urol. 2004;171:1029–35.
15. Parsons JK, Kashefi C. Physical activity, benign prostatic hyperplasia, and lower urinary tract symptoms. Eur Urol. 2008;53:1228–35.
16. Lepor H, Williford W, Barry M. The efficacy of terazosin, finasteride, or both in benign prostatic hyperplasia. Veterans Affairs Cooperative Studies Benign Prostatic Hyperplasia Study Group. N Engl J Med. 1996;33:533.
17. McConnell JD, Roehrborn C. The long-term effects of doxazosin, finasteride and the combination on the clinical progression of benign prostatic hyperplasia. N Engl J Med. 2003;349: 2385–96.
18. Oesterling JE, Kaplan SA, Epstein HB. The North American experience with the UroLume endoprosthesis as a treatment for benign prostatic hyperplasia: long-term results. The North American UroLume Study Group. Urology. 1994;44:353–62.
19. Bruskewitz R, Issa M, Roehrborn CG. A prospective, randomised, 1-year clinical trial comparing transurethral needle ablation (TUNA) to transurethral resection of the prostate for the treatment of symptomatic benign prostatic hyperplasia. J Urol. 1998;159:1588–94.

20. Wheelahan J, Scott NA, Cartmill R. Minimally invasive non-laser thermal techniques for prostatectomy: a systematic review. BJU Int. 2000;86:977–88.
21. Roehrborn CG, Gange SN, Shore ND, Giddens JL, Bolton DM, Cowan BE, Thomas Brown B, McVary KT. The prostatic urethral lift for the treatment of lower urinary tract symptoms associated with prostate enlargement due to benign prostatic hyperplasia: The L.I.F.T. study. J Urol. 2013;190(6):2161–7.
22. Kabalin J. Holmium:YAG laser prostatectomy: results of a US pilot study. J Endourol. 1996;10:453–7.
23. Anson K, Nawrocki J, Buckley J. A multicenter randomised prospective study of endoscopic laser ablation versus transurethral resection of the prostate. Urology. 1995;43:305–10.
24. Cowles RS, Kabalin JN, Childs S. A prospective randomised comparison of transurethral resection to visual laser ablation of the prostate for the treatment of benign prostatic hyperplasia. Urology. 1995;46:155–8.
25. Gilling P, Cass C, Cresswell M. The use of the holmium laser in the treatment of benign prostatic hyperplasia. J Endourol. 1996;10:459–61.
26. Sandhu JS, Ng C, Vanderbrink BA. High-power potassium-titanyl-phosphate photoselective laser vaporization of prostate for treatment of benign prostatic hyperplasia in men with large prostates. Urology. 2004;64:1155–9.
27. Naspro R, Bachmann A, Gilling P. A review of the recent evidence (2006–2008) for 532-nm photoselective laser vaporisation and holmium laser enucleation of the prostate. Eur Urol. 2009;55:1345–57.
28. Wasson JH, Reda DJ, Bruskewitz RC. A comparison of transurethral surgery with watchful waiting for moderate symptoms of benign prostatic hyperplasia. N Engl J Med. 1995;332:75–9.
29. Adam C, Hofstetter A, Deubner J. Retropubic transvesical prostatectomy for significant prostatic enlargement must remain a standard part of urology training. Scand J Urol Nephrol. 2004;38:472.

Prostate Cancer Screening

13

Jeannette M. Potts

> *"...we primary care clinicians must ensure there is no more routine, indiscriminate PSA screening and no washing our hands of responsibility once the patient is referred to a specialist for prostate-cancer treatment. We owe it to our patients to provide them with the kind of guidance about this screening test that they need and deserve. That's the way to help put the [PSA] controversy to rest . . . one man at a time."* [1]
>
> Mary F. McNaughton-Collins, M.D., M.P.H.,
> and Michael J. Barry, M.D.

13.1 Introduction

It is clear that prostate cancer represents a major public health concern. With almost 200,000 new cases annually and nearly 30,000 deaths each year, the human toll is substantial [2].

When one recognizes that approximately one man in four who undergoes prostate biopsy is found to have prostate cancer, we can estimate that 800,000 prostate biopsies are being performed annually, subjecting many men to significant morbidity as well. This too has been a major healthcare concern.

Although the detection of prostate cancer has increased since the introduction of PSA screening, more cancers tend to be localized as well as low grade. In the pre-PSA era, 11 % of men were diagnosed with prostate cancer; however, most of these were clinically symptomatic at the time of diagnosis and 75 % eventually died as consequence of prostate cancer. In the current PSA era, more men are diagnosed with prostate cancer; however, only 3 % die from the consequences of prostate cancer. In the pre-PSA era only 27 % of prostate cancers were localized, while today, 98 % of men diagnosed via PSA screening have localized prostate cancer [3]. Currently, it is estimated that 80 % of men diagnosed with prostate cancer will never

J.M. Potts, M.D. (✉)
Vista Urology & Pelvic Pain Partners, 2998 South Bascom Avenue,
Suite 100, San Jose, CA 95124, USA
e-mail: DrPotts@VistaUrology.com

© Springer Science+Business Media New York 2016
J.M. Potts (ed.), *Men's Health*, DOI 10.1007/978-1-4939-3237-5_13

develop symptoms of the disease [4]. Indeed, these diagnoses may be considered false positives, carrying with them unnecessary and enormous costs—physically, emotionally, and economically.

The morbidity associated with treatment is significant; this toll on our male population is even more disturbing when we consider that most men would eventually die from other causes without treatment and die with their diagnosis but not from it.

Based on the review of several trials, the US Preventive Services Task Force concluded in the fall of 2011 that PSA-based screening is associated with detection of more prostate cancers; small to no reduction in prostate cancer-specific mortality after about 10 years; and harms related to false-positive test results, subsequent evaluation, and therapy, including overdiagnosis and overtreatment. They recommended against routine screening of prostate cancer with a D statement [5]. This grade D recommendation applies to healthy men of all ages, regardless of race or family history. The task force's grade D recommendation is intended to "discourage the use of this service."

Tragically, a study done shortly before the USPSTF investigation showed that up until 2010, PSA screening occurred in 69.8 % in the low-risk group, 65.3 % in the intermediate risk, and 56 % in the high risk [6]. This means that doctors were not adherent to the criteria of screening, which had always recommended against screening any person who had less than a 10-year life expectancy. The study showed that 56 % of men screened by PSA were at highest risk and therefore ineligible for screening. (Imagine how many of this group with abnormal PSA went on to have biopsy or worse treatment for prostate cancer!)

13.2 How Have We Justified Screening for Prostate Cancer in the Past?

Preventive healthcare strategies are typically divided into three categories: primary, secondary, and tertiary prevention. Primary prevention involves steps toward avoiding occurrence of disease or trauma. Examples include vaccinations, healthy diet and lifestyle, the use of seat belts, and not smoking. Secondary prevention involves the screening or detection of disease prior to the appearance of symptoms. The objective is to diagnose a problem early, when it is most treatable. Examples included cancer screening programs (PSA, mammography, PAP, and colonoscopy) and measurement of cholesterol to prevent cardiovascular diseases. Tertiary prevention is intended to reduce the negative impact of a symptomatic disease. Examples would include antibiotics to treat pneumonia and surgery to stop the spread or progression of a disease.

Localized prostate cancer exists almost always without symptoms. PSA was introduced in 1986 as a means of screening and detecting cancer early. Although it is frequently recommended that men with obstructive voiding symptoms consider an evaluation for possible prostate cancer, this would be an unusual presenting complaint. The reason: prostate cancer generally arises in the peripheral zone of the prostate and rarely will lead to urethral obstruction. It is only when metastases to bone (pain) or to regional lymph nodes (lower extremity lymphedema or deep vein thrombosis) or to the retroperitoneal lymph nodes (ureteral obstruction, flank pain, and uremia) occur that symptoms develop. I have, however, diagnosed prostate cancer in a supposedly "asymptomatic" 52-year-old man, with minimal PSA elevation, who had noted erectile dysfunction over the previous 4 years. His prostate was a concrete mass, and not surprising, the pathology showed Gleason 10. Unfortunately, he had not had screening for sexual dysfunction nor a digital rectal examination to screen for prostate cancer prior to his urological consultation. The neurovascular bundles involved in erectile function had been clearly destroyed by the malignancy.

Since the advent of prostate-specific antigen (PSA) testing, in combination with digital rectal examination (DRE), prostate cancer diagnosis has been changed in a revolutionary manner. Approximately 10 % of men tested with PSA will be found to have a value >4.0 ng/mL and between 3 and 10 % will have an abnormal DRE. Of men undergoing biopsy, cancer detection rates have been increasing and vary from 25 to 50 %. With PSA screening, more than 97 % of prostate cancer cases diagnosed are clinically confined to the prostate [7].

Clearly, the outcome of treatment is related to the extent of disease. Failures are greater if nodal disease, seminal vesicle involvement, or extracapsular disease is present. For tumors that are confined to the prostate, presumed to be detected early, the progression-free probability at 10 year exceeds 90 % [8]. However, lead time bias may be an important factor in this interpretation.

PSA screening in the USA began in earnest in the late 1980s. In association with this was a dramatic increase in the detection of disease. After a period of almost exponential rise in detection, the incidence rate fell to relatively stable rates. Beginning in 1991, and virtually every year since, a fall in the rate of metastatic disease has been seen [9].

Since the early 1990s when the rate of metastatic disease began to fall, there has been a gradual decrease in prostate cancer mortality [10]. This was in the face of gradually increasing mortality rates in the late 1980s. The increased use of hormonal therapies as injectable LHRH agonists and oral antiandrogens may have also played a role in decreased mortality rates in patients with metastatic disease.

13.3 But Routine Prostate Cancer Screening Went Too Far!

A combination of autopsy data and national statistics suggests that although almost 70 % of men will develop histological evidence of prostate cancer and 16 % will be diagnosed, only 3–4 % will die of the disease. These statistics can be translated to real-life scenario in the recent ERSSPC results, which showed that it was necessary to screen 1410 men [several hundred biopsies] and to treat 48 men to save one life [11].

13.4 We Relied on PSA, Which Lacks Predictive Value

Despite the fact that the combination of regular PSA and DRE testing significantly reduces the stage of prostate cancer at diagnosis, they are not perfect. In those men in the Washington University series who were diagnosed with prostate cancer at the time of their initial PSA, 37 % had clinically or pathologically advanced disease. Among those with serial PSA measurements, 29 % still had advanced disease [12]. These observations suggest that, with time, even those men who are screened repetitively with PSA will be at risk for treatment failure and demise from their disease.

PSA thresholds may also provide false sense of security for men with low levels, while causing anxiety with repeated, often unnecessary, biopsies in those with higher levels.

PSA and histology data, reviewed from 36,316 patients, revealed that prostate cancer incidence among men with PSA 2.5–4.0 ng/mL was the same as in men with PSA levels between 4.0 and 10 ng/mL [13]. Other investigators likewise demonstrated the risk of having prostate cancer with PSA as low as 0.5 ng/mL or less, which was 6.6 % [14].

Others have reported the prevalence of prostate cancer among men with PSA levels <2.0. This led to proposal of lower PSA threshold of 2.6 in 1995, which yielded 22 % cancer detection rate via sextant biopsy [15]. Among men with PSA levels <4.0, other investigators diagnosed 15.2 % of men with prostate cancer, observing that 14.9 % had Gleason 7 score or higher [16]. However, another way of interpreting this result is by acknowledging the fact that 85 % of patients had low-grade cancers, most of which may be clinically insignificant.

In a review conducted over a 15-year period at the Cleveland Clinic, data from 5570 biopsy cases were analyzed and comparisons were made with regard to race and PSA. PSA differences between Blacks and Whites diminished over time. Also, as the levels of PSA declined over time, the association with cancer detection weakened for both races. In most years after 2000, the association between PSA and cancer was not significant—with areas under the ROC curve close to 0.5 [17]. In other words, PSA is as good as a coin toss, simply providing an excuse rather than a valid reason to biopsy men. It is well known that PSA functions well as a BPH or prostate volume surrogate [18, 19]. Therefore, [positive] PSA screening may simply reflect the increase incidence of both BPH and cancer with age.

13.5 Diagnosis Through Transrectal Ultrasound-Guided Prostate Biopsy Carries with It Significant Risks and Complications

As stated by Neulander and colleagues in their letter to editor, "…prostate biopsy is the only means for prostate cancer detection. It is an invasive procedure through a septic cavity and any casual approach to this operation should be avoided…" [20].

Prostate biopsy is associated with risk of infection, sepsis, hematuria, hematospermia, pain, and rectal bleeding, which can be fatal in extremely rare cases.

Prostate biopsy has a relatively high false negative, up to 45 % depending on the number of cores obtained [3]. To avoid this problem, 12–14 cores are recommended for initial biopsy, further increasing the risk of complications.

In a group of 2023 men who underwent TRUS prostate biopsy, the number of cores was correlated to risk of infection. The overall sepsis rate was 3.06 % or 62/2023 patients; but when analyzed according to number of cores taken, the incidence of sepsis was 2.74 % vs. 4.21 % among men who had undergone 8–10-core biopsy vs. 12-core biopsy, respectively ($p < 0.001$) [21]. Nam and colleagues also reported a fourfold increase in hospitalizations due to post-prostate biopsy infection or bleeding, which was related to the increase in number of cores taken during one biopsy session, i.e., sextant biopsy compared with 8-, 10-, or 18-core biopsy [22].

In 2006, Jones and colleagues compared two cohorts of men undergoing initial biopsy. One group, consisting of 139 men, underwent 24-core saturation biopsy and the other group of 87 men underwent 10-core prostate biopsy. To the investigators' surprise, saturation biopsy afforded no advantage in the cancer detection rate and did not significantly increase the rate of complication such as infection [23].

There is growing evidence and concern regarding the overall increasing incidence of post biopsy infection and the increasing proportion of infections caused by organisms resistant to fluoroquinolones. At the 30th Annual Congress of the European Urological Association, researchers presented data demonstrating significant rise in the post biopsy infection rate over the past 10 years. In the USA, there is increasing rate of infection requiring hospitalization [24].

Gross hematuria is a relatively common complication of prostate biopsy, occurring in up to 58 % of patients. While gross hematuria is very distressing to patients, the majority of episodes are short-lived and do not require medical intervention nor hospitalization. When considering adverse effects, some investigators only included gross hematuria that persisted for more than 2 weeks or rare instances that required hospitalization, with reported rate of 6.5 % [25].

Reported incidence of hematospermia is quite variable, ranging from 0.2 % to 84%! The study reporting the highest incidence of hematospermia (84 %, with mean duration of 3.5 weeks) was the only study designed prospectively to research this specific problem and therefore much more compelling to me as a men's health specialist. The researchers were also sensitive to anticipate this problem among men who were able to be sexually active [26]. The otherwise, significantly lower incidence of hematospermia reported in the literature may reflect study design, age, and comorbid conditions of patients, as well as cultural differences between regions and study centers.

Hematochezia is observed in 1.5–37 % of men after TRUS biopsy. Some researchers believe the prevalence of rectal bleeding after TRUS-guided prostate biopsy is underestimated in many cases because the bleeding episode is clinically irrelevant or ceases within a couple of days [27]. Fortunately, severe bleeding is rare but can be fatal.

Other adverse effects of prostate biopsy include pain, psychological stress, and the ongoing risk of all complications secondary to the possibility of requiring repeated biopsies for persistently elevated PSA, PCA3, or other abnormal screening parameters (false-negative screening tests).

13.6   Another Risk of Prostate Biopsy Is the High Rate of "False Positives"

I am defining false positives as the burden of a "cancer" diagnosis, in cases of clinically insignificant malignancy. This may represent approximately 75 % of all cancers detected in the PSA era!

False positives, or the detection of low-grade low-volume cancers, frequently lead to secondary physical harm by way of overtreatment as well as the complications associated with therapies. Options for localized prostate cancer include, generally, radiotherapy with external beam, brachytherapy, and surgery (radical prostatectomy). Each of these carries with it a unique spectrum of complications, including erectile dysfunction, urinary incontinence, urinary obstruction, radiation injury to the rectum or bladder, urethral strictures, and need for secondary therapies. These complications are challenging to justify especially with the recent observations published by ERRSSPC cited earlier, indicating that 48 men need to be treated in order to save one man's life.

Diagnosis of prostate cancer is occurring at much lower PSA levels with much greater likelihood of localized and low-grade cancers. As observed in the Prostate Cancer Prevention Trial, where all men were biopsied for study purposes, regardless of PSA level, high-grade tumors (Gleason 7 or greater) were detected in 10–27 % of men diagnosed with prostate cancer who had PSA levels less than 4.0 ng/mL [13]. Again, using the reciprocal, one can conclude that 73–90 % of cancers are low grade and, therefore, eligible for active surveillance.

Sadly, some experts have found that only 36 % of men surveyed who were diagnosed with low-volume, low-grade disease were offered active surveillance by their urologists, when a doctor's counseling about AS may be the most important factor in a man's decision to pursue this management option [28]. Additional concerns have been raised regarding the pressure hospitals have in promoting robotic prostatectomy in order to pay off the $2 million equipment used for this procedure. Robotics are used in 75 % of US prostatectomy cases, and the rate of prostatectomies has been shown to increase significantly and dramatically, soon after hospitals acquire the robotics. This was even true in regions where the overall incidence of prostate cancer had diminished [29].

Complications of prostatectomy include bladder irritability, incontinence, and erectile dysfunction. Despite improved surgical techniques, the reported stress urinary incontinence rates range between 5 % and 48.0 % [10]. A literature review revealed high prevalence of de novo voiding dysfunction confirmed urodynamically in post-prostatectomy patients. Detrusor overactivity was reported in 2–77 % of patients. Impaired bladder compliance was present in 8–39 % of patients and was de novo in about half. Impaired detrusor contractility was found de novo in 47 % but was recovered in about half of these men after 1 year [30].

The incidence of post-prostatectomy erectile dysfunction is common. Potency rates, as cited by Tal and Mulhall, range from 21 to 62 % of patients after unilateral nerve-sparing prostatectomy and 54 to 86 % of patients after bilateral nerve-sparing prostatectomy. The data reviewed includes patients who underwent radical, laparoscopic, and robotic procedures and were defined as patients with full or partial erections sufficient for intercourse. In some studies, patients were taking medication, such as PDE-5 inhibitors, to treat post-prostatectomy erectile dysfunction. According to the SEER registry, however, 80 % of patients were not able to achieve erections sufficient for intercourse after prostatectomy [31].

In a meta-analysis (26 articles = 8302 patients) comparing quality of life among prostatectomy patients and radiation therapy patients, all treatments were associated with short-term or long-term reductions in urinary, bowel, and sexual domains. Bowel quality of life and bladder irritation were worse for radiation patients. A greater decline in sexual function was observed in surgery patients compared to radiation patients; however, surgery patients had higher levels of sexual functioning at baseline [32]. Using the CaPSURE database, investigators compared the health-related quality life of patients who underwent prostate cancer treatment. Among 3294 men, 1139 (34 %) underwent nerve-sparing radical prostatectomy (NSRP), 860 (26 %) underwent non-NSRP, 684 (21 %) underwent brachytherapy, 386 (12 %) underwent external beam radiotherapy, 161 (5 %) underwent primary androgen deprivation therapy, and only 64 (2 %) pursued watchful waiting/active surveillance. Median follow-up was 74 months. Most treatments resulted in early declines in quality of life, with some recovery over the next 1–2 years and a plateau in scores thereafter. Radiation had the strongest effect on bowel function. Not surprising, surgery had the largest impact on sexual function and bother and on urinary function. Androgen deprivation therapy had the strongest effect on physical function [33]. Rectourethral fistulas are rare but devastating consequences of radiation therapy, specifically combined brachytherapy and external beam regimens. Early- or late-onset bladder or rectal bleeding occurs secondary to mucosal and vascular damage. Unfortunately these cannot be predictive; however, lower dose therapies may decrease this risk.

The European Randomized Study of Screening for Prostate Cancer (ERSSPC), initiated in the early 1990s, showed PSA screening reduced the rate of death due to prostate cancer by 20 %. But what does a 20 % reduction really mean? If an average middle-aged man has a 3 % risk of dying of prostate cancer, would screening decrease this risk to 2.4 %? The study also showed that overdiagnosis and overtreatment are probably the most important adverse effects of prostate cancer screening and are more common than in screening for breast, colorectal, or cervical cancer [34]. Additionally, population observations regarding changes in mortality are subject to numerous confounds and do not clearly demonstrate an effect of screening or treatment.

In another prospective study from Sweden, 20,000 men age 50 to 64 were followed for 14 years. One-half of the men were screened using PSA every 2 years, while the others were not screened. All cause mortality was the same for both groups; however, the prostate cancer mortality was reduced by 44 % in the screened group; however, absolute reduction was determined to be only .34 percentage points. From a public health standpoint, this difference may be too costly given the larger number of men who must submit to biopsy, are over diagnosed, and undergo unnecessary therapy (along with all the comorbidities of treatment) [35].

13.7   What Can Be Done to Enhance the Predictive Value of PSA to Decrease Unnecessary Biopsies and Ultimately Unnecessary Therapies?

PSA coupled with MRI may help to decrease the number of unnecessary biopsies (30th Annual Congress of the EAU). At the 30th Annual Congress of the European Association of Urology (March, 2015), data was presented demonstrating the use of lower PSA thresholds in combination with MRI, resulting in fewer men requiring diagnostic needle biopsy. While decreasing the overdetection of low-grade low-volume prostate cancers is a priority, one immediate benefit of this approach is the decreased risk of TRUS biopsy, which is currently associated with higher rates of infection requiring hospitalization as cited earlier. Significant increases over the past 10 years in infection rates associated with TRUS biopsy have also been reported in Europe.

MRI–TRUS fusion involves prostate ultrasound, as performed for the past several decades. While viewing the prostate, the MRI of that prostate, which is performed beforehand and stored in the device, is fused with real-time ultrasound using a digital overlay, allowing the target(s), previously delineated by a radiologist, to be brought into the aiming mechanism of the ultrasound machine. The fusion results in the creation of a three-dimensional reconstruction of the prostate, and on the reconstructed model, the aiming and tracking of biopsy sites occur. The results are very promising in that more specific targeting and therefore better yield of the procedure are done without increasing number of cores taken. However, differentiating low grade from high grade has not been proven [36]. Other investigators observe that MRI targeted biopsies are more sensitive for detection of prostate cancer than TRUS-guided, systematic biopsies and detect more significant prostate cancers and fewer insignificant cancers than conventional biopsies. However, the same group believes that a negative MRI scan should not defer biopsy [37], which leads us back to the significant risk of over biopsy and overdiagnosis, not to mention higher costs of MRI.

PSA blood tests can be coupled with urine Prostate Cancer Assay 3 (PCA3). It is unclear, however, that PCA3 can help in differentiating clinically significant malignancies among prostate biopsy naïve patients or if it has a role as part of initial screening.

A group of 859 men (mean age, 62 years) from 11 centers scheduled for a diagnostic prostate biopsy between December 2009 and June 2011 were enrolled to test performance of PCA3. Using a score of >60, positive predictive value (PPV) of PCA3 was tested in men undergoing a biopsy for the first time. Negative predictive value was tested using a score <20 among men undergoing repeat biopsy [38]. The addition of PCA3 to individual risk estimation models (which included age, race/ethnicity, prior biopsy, PSA, and digital rectal examination) improved the stratification of cancer and of high-grade cancer. In the setting of repeat biopsy, use of the PCA3 could reduce the number of biopsies performed by half! This reduction could be associated with a 3 % risk of missing high-grade disease; however, as noted in editorial comment, the incidence of high-grade prostate cancer in the setting of low PCA3 is higher at 13 % [39].

For the purposes of initial screening, however, PCA3 may perform too well, predicting all cancers, with an overall detection rate of 80 % [37]. It is unable to differentiate, therefore, leaving us with similar challenges as PSA in overdiagnosis of low-grade disease. So while it has a promising role in preventing the over biopsy and overdiagnosis of those undergoing repeat biopsy, PCA3 may not be helpful for initial screening.

The prostate health index (PHI) may potentially decrease the rate of prostate biopsy by 30 %. Loeb and colleagues used PHI, which is comprised of 3 parameters (total PSA, free PSA and p2PSA, an isoform of free PSA identified as most specific to prostate cancer) to compare predictive value of each screening parameter alone. Among 658 men (median age of 63), PHI was correlated to biopsy results. Clinically significant cancer was defined by Epstein criteria (Gleason 7 or greater, 3 or more positive cores, and >50 % involvement of any core). The PHI outperformed free PSA alone in differentiating clinically significant cancer from indolent cancer or negative biopsies; therefore, PHI may afford a 30 % decrease in number of men requiring biopsy, compared to possible avoidance of biopsy of 21 % with free PSA [40].

13.8 Shared Decision-Making

For decades, family doctors were guided by the American College of Physicians and the American Academy of Family Physicians to counsel men older than 50 years about the "known risks and unknown benefits" of PSA screening and to obtain informed consent from those who wish to proceed with screening [41].

We as primary care physicians have not adhered to this policy of shared decision-making for prostate cancer screening. In one study, 47 % of physicians endorsed "shared decision-making" for prostate cancer screening [42]. However, most doctors surveyed cited lack of time, fear of malpractice, and other barriers as the cause for continued PSA testing without informed or shared decision-making [42, 43], hence the inappropriate counseling and testing of so many men, elderly, infirmed, or just uninformed. And once Pandora's box is opened, in the form of a patient having an abnormal PSA result, it is more challenging to assuage the fear of the patient and to avoid further evaluation even when screening had been inappropriate from the start.

PSA testing decreased significantly after the USPSTF recommendations came out. One group of researchers examined overall trends by facility locations (urban, suburban, or rural), by patient age, and by provider type (primary care or urology). Although decreased PSA screening occurred across all specialties over time, the greatest reductions in such testing were seen among urologists, among patients in the intermediate age group (aged 50–59 years), and at an urban teaching hospital [44]. While this is a favorable trend, consistent with the objectives implicit of the task force recommendation, it is this author's hope that this reflects shared decision-making rather than a simple paucity in the discussion of screening during patient visits.

The American Cancer Society (ACS) recently updated its guideline for the early detection of prostate cancer (http://www.cancer.org/cancer/prostatecancer/moreinformation/prostatecancerearlydetection/prostate-cancer-early-detection-acs-recommendations), recommending that asymptomatic men who have at least a 10-year life expectancy be given an opportunity to make an informed decision with their healthcare provider about screening for prostate cancer. Informed decision implies a discussion about the uncertainties, risks, and potential benefits associated with screening. The ACS asserts that prostate cancer screening should not occur without an informed decision-making process. For far too long, PSA was simply added to a battery of tests which were ordered for any patient when they reached a certain age and annually thereafter. The serious implications of this test were overshadowed by the simplicity and accessibility of the blood test.

The push back by the USPSTF and others was not just the misuse of the blood test, but the further abuse of the results leading to, perhaps, due indiscriminate biopsies followed by costly and morbid radiation therapy or surgery to treat low-grade disease.

Improved education and counseling about watchful waiting and active surveillance may help prevent the conversion of overdiagnosis to overtreatment, mitigating the harms of screening that are so accurately portrayed by the task force.

The grade D recommendation made by the task force once again removes the patient from the decision-making process while swinging the pendulum from broad, uninformed, indiscriminate use of screening to unilateral inaccessibility to screening. Either way, "adherence" to either standard seems like a cop out on the part of primary care doctors and urologists.

This author agrees with McNaughton-Collins and Barry in proposing a modification to the task force's recommendation, from Grade D to a C recommendation. The Grade C recommendation would include the suggestion that physicians "offer/provide this service only if other considerations support offering or providing the service in an individual patient." In keeping with the ACS guidelines, the C recommendation would allow the patient to be involved in the decision of screening by means of digital rectal examination and/or other modalities such as PSA, MRI, or PCA3. The pros and cons would be equally presented and discussed. The patient could then provide his perspective on how he views the trade-off, in short, a genuine shared decision-making process.

We must also accept that shared decision-making will have as many different formulas as there are patient personalities. This, perhaps, may seem the most challenging to already time-restricted and overworked doctors. Ultimately, it will be up to the patient to define the balance of decision-making and the physician to provide the reciprocal or compensatory counterbalance through patient education and compassion.

13.9 Conclusion

Dr. Ian Thompson, a leading oncological urologist, was recently quoted about the PSA dilemma: "….better diagnostic techniques, such as biopsies guided by magnetic resonance imaging tests, along with personalized risk assessment and more informed decision making by men and their doctors [is] a better way to use the PSA test than to screen every man of a certain age."

In treating each patient as individuals, we must set a goal to achieve a reduction in the mortality and morbidity of prostate cancer, while minimizing the risks, cost, complications, and emotional burdens of screening, diagnosing, and overtreating this disease.

References

1. McNaughton-Collins MF, Barry MJ. One man at a time – resolving the PSA Controversy. N Engl J Med. 2011;365:1951–3.
2. Greenlee RT, Hill-Harmon MB, Murray T, et al. Cancer statistics 2001. CA Cancer J Clin. 2001;5:15–36.
3. Shteynshlyuger A, Andriole G. Prostate cancer: to screen or not to screen? Urol Clin North Am. 2010;37:1–9.
4. Yao SL, Lu-Yao G. Understanding and appreciating overdiagnosis in the PSA era. J Natl Cancer Inst. 2002;94(13):958–60.
5. Moyer VA. U.S. Preventive Services Task Force. Screening for prostate cancer: U.S. Preventive Services Task Force recommendation statement. Ann Intern Med. 2012;157(2):120–34.
6. Royce T: MS4 Affiliation: University of North Carolina at Chapel Hill, Chapel Hill, NC. Does Patient Life Expectancy Affect Receipt of Routine Cancer Screening in the United States? A Population-Based Study. Reported by: Abigail Berman, MD Affiliation: The Abramson Cancer Center of the University of Pennsylvania Last Modified: October 31, 2012.
7. Smith DS, Catalona WJ. The nature of prostate cancer detected through prostate specific antigen based screening. J Urol. 1994;152:1732–6.
8. Hull GW, Rabbani F, Abbas F, Wheeler TM, Kattan MW, Scardino PT. Cancer control with radical prostatectomy alone in 1,000 consecutive patients. J Urol. 2002;167:528–34.
9. Hankey BF, Feuer EJ, Clegg LX, et al. Cancer surveillance series: interpreting trends in prostate cancer—Part I: evidence of the effects of screening in recent prostate cancer incidence, mortality, and survival rates. J Natl Cancer Inst. 1999;91:1017–24.
10. Potosky AL, Feuer EJ, Levin DL. Impact of screening on incidence and mortality of prostate cancer in the United States. Epidemiol Rev. 2001;23:181–6.
11. Schroder FH, Hugosson J, Roobol MJ, Tammela TL, Ciatto S, Nelen V, et al. Screening and prostate-cancer mortality in a randomized European study. N Engl J Med. 2009;360:11320.
12. Catalona WJ, Smith DS, Ratliff TL, Basler JW. Detection of organ-confined prostate cancer is increased through prostate-specific antigen-based screening. JAMA. 1993;270:948–54.
13. Gilbert SM, Cavallo CB, Kahane H, et al. Evidence suggesting a PSA cutpoint of 2.5 ng/mL for promoting prostate biopsy: a review of 36,316 biopsies. Urology. 2005;65:549–53.
14. Thompson IM, Pauler DK, Goodman PJ, et al. Prevalence of prostate cancer among men with a prostate-specific antigen level<or =4.0 ng per milliliter. N Engl J Med. 2004;350(22): 2239–46.
15. Krumholtz JS, Carvalhal GF, Ramos CG, Smith DS, Thorson P, Yan Y, Humphrey PA, Roehl KA, Catalona WJ. Prostate-specific antigen cutoff of 2.6 ng/mL for prostate cancer screening is associated with favorable pathologic tumor features. Urology. 2002;60(3):469–73.
16. Thompson IM, Ankerst DP, Chi C, et al. Operating characteristics of prostate-specific antigen in men with initial PSA level of 3.0 ng/mL or lower. JAMA. 2005;294:66–70.
17. Potts J, Lutz L, Walker E, Modlin C, Klein E. Trends in PSA, age and prostate cancer detection among black and white men from 1990-2006 at a tertiary care center. Cancer. 2010;116(16): 3910–5.
18. Roehrborn CG. The utility of serum prostatic-specific antigen in the management of men with benign prostatic hyperplasia. Int J Impot Res. 2008;20 Suppl 3:S19–26.

19. Stamey TA, Johnstone IM, McNeal JE, et al. Preoperative serum prostate specific antigen levels between 2 and 22 ng./ml. correlate poorly with post-radical prostatectomy cancer morphology: prostate specific antigen cure rates appear constant between 2 and 9 ng./ml. J Urol. 2002;167(1):103–11.
20. Neulander EZ, Yusim I, Kaneti J. Letter Re: increasing hospital admission rates for urological complications after transrectal ultrasound guided prostate biopsy: R. K. Nam, R. Saskin, Y. Lee, Y. Liu, C. Law, L. H. Klotz, D. A. Loblaw, J. Trachtenberg, A. Stanimirovic, A. E. Simor, A. Seth, D. R. Urbach and S. A. Narod J Urol 2010; 183: 963-969. J Urol. 2010; 184(5):2216–7.
21. Simsir A, Kismali E, Mammadov R, Gunaydin G, Cal C. Is it possible to predict sepsis, the most serious complication in prostate biopsy?. Urol Int. 2010;84(4):395–9.
22. Nam RK, Saskin R, Lee Y, et al. Increasing hospital admission rates for urological complications after transrectal ultrasound guided prostate biopsy. J Urol. 2010;183(3):963–8.
23. Jones JS, Patel A, Schoenfield L, et al. Saturation technique does not improve cancer detection as an initial prostate biopsy strategy. J Urol. 2006;175(2):485–8.
24. Nam RK, Saskin R, Lee Y, et al. Increasing hospital admission rates for urological complications after transrectal ultrasound guided prostate biopsy. J Urol. 2013;189(1 Suppl):S12–7. discussion S17–8.
25. Ecke TH, Gunia S, Bartel P, Hallmann S, et al. Complications and risk factors of transrectal ultrasound guided needle biopsies of the prostate evaluated by questionnaire. Urol Oncol. 2008;26(5):474–8.
26. Manoharan M, Ayyathurai R, Nieder AM. Soloway MS Hemospermia following transrectal ultrasound-guided prostate biopsy: a prospective study. Prostate Cancer Prostatic Dis. 2007;10(3):283–7.
27. Kilciler M, Erdemir F, Demir E, et al. The effect of rectal Foley catheterization on rectal bleeding rates after transrectal ultrasound-guided prostate biopsy. J Vasc Interv Radiol. 2008;19(9): 1344–6.
28. Gorin MA, Soloway CT, Eldefrawy A, Soloway MS. Factors that influence patient enrollment in active surveillance for low-risk prostate cancer. Urology. 2011;77(3):588–91.
29. Neuner JM, See WA, Pezzin LE, et al. The association of robotic surgical technology and hospital prostatectomy volumes: increasing market share through the adoption of technology. Cancer. 2012;118(2):371–7.
30. Porena M, Mearini E, Mearini L, et al. Voiding dysfunction after radical retropubic prostatectomy: more than external urethral sphincter deficiency. Eur Urol. 2007;52(1):38–45.
31. Tal R, Alphs HH, Krebs P, Nelson CJ, Mulhall JP. Erectile function recovery rate after radical prostatectomy: a meta-analysis. J Sex Med. 2009;6(9):2538–46.
32. Lee TK, Breau RH, Mallick R, Eapen L. A systematic review of expanded prostate cancer index composite (EPIC) quality of life after surgery or radiation treatment. Can J Urol. 2015;22(1):7599–606.
33. Punnen S, Cowan JE, Chan JM, Carroll PR, Cooperberg MR: Long-term health-related quality of life after primary treatment for localized prostate cancer: results from the CaPSURE Registry. Eur Urol. 2014 Sep 18. pii: S0302-2838(14)00844-6.
34. Andriole GL, Crawford ED, Grubb III RL, Buys SS, Chia D, et al. Mortality results from a randomized prostate-cancer screening trial. N Engl J Med. 2009;360:1310–9.
35. Hugosson J, Carlsson S, Aus G, Bergdahl S, Khatami A, et al. Mortality results from the Göteborg randomized population-based prostate-cancer screening trial. Lancet Oncol. 2010;11:725–32.
36. Marks L, Young S, Natarajan S. MRI–ultrasound fusion for guidance of targeted prostate biopsy. Curr Opin Urol. 2013;23(1):43–50.
37. Stephenson SK, Chang EK, Marks LS. Screening and detection advances in magnetic resonance image-guided prostate biopsy. Urol Clin North Am. 2014;41(2):315–26.
38. Wei JT, Feng Z, Partin A, et al. Can urinary PCA3 supplement PSA in the early detection of prostate cancer? J Clin Oncol. 2014;32(36):4066–72.

39. Vickers AJ. Markers for the early detection of prostate cancer: some principles for statistical reporting and interpretation. J Clin Oncol. 2014;32(36):4033–4.
40. Loeb S, Sanda MG, Broyles DL, et al. The prostate health index selectively identifies clinically significant prostate cancer. J Urol. 2015;193(4):1163–9.
41. Gates TJ. Screening for cancer: evaluating the evidence. Am Fam Physician. 2001;63(3): 513–22.
42. Davis K, Haisfield L, Dorfman C, et al. Physicians' attitudes about shared decision making for prostate cancer screening. Fam Med. 2011;43(4):260–6.
43. Dunn AS, Shridharani KV, Lou W, et al. Physician-patient discussions of controversial cancer screening tests. Am J Prev Med. 2001;20(2):130–4.
44. Aslani A, Minnillo BJ, Johnson B, Cherullo EE, Ponsky LE, Abouassaly R. The impact of recent screening recommendations on prostate cancer screening in a large health care system. J Urol. 2014;191(6):1737–42.

Men Have Bladders, Too

14

Christopher K. Payne

14.1 Introduction: It Is Not Always the Prostate

For most of the history of urology, particularly since the introduction of the resectoscope and the transurethral resection of the prostate, it has been assumed that prostatic enlargement, obstruction, and infection were the causes of essentially all lower urinary tract problems in men. It is now obvious that this is not the case. Bladder problems of all types are prevalent in men, generally to a similar degree found in women. Yet men continue to be misdiagnosed, underdiagnosed, mistreated, and undertreated. This may be due in part to residual prejudices in the medical community, but it also relates to reluctance of men to discuss these problems. A great deal of research has documented the stigma of urinary incontinence and how this makes patients reluctant to seek treatment. It is likely that this is magnified for men. At a Simon Foundation Innovating for Continence meeting, a female member of a patient panel reported how relieved she was that adult continence products were placed next to the menstrual pads. Needless to say, this does not provide any shelter to the man with incontinence.

Doctors need to ask all patients, men and women, about their bladder function and be prepared to offer evaluation and treatment. Despite decades of effort at patient education (and some success), the majority of those suffering with bladder disorders remain reluctant to seek help.

What Makes a Normal Bladder? Since lower urinary tract function is rarely taught in medical training, a few words about normal function should precede the discussion of abnormal conditions. The functional classification system detailed

C.K. Payne, M.D. (✉)
Emeritus Professor of Urology, Stanford University, Stanford, CA, USA

Vista Urology & Pelvic Pain Partners, 2998 South Bascom Avenue, Suite 100,
San Jose, CA 95124, USA
e-mail: cpayne59@gmail.com

© Springer Science+Business Media New York 2016
J.M. Potts (ed.), *Men's Health*, DOI 10.1007/978-1-4939-3237-5_14

below was developed decades ago by Alan Wein; it remains the best way to think about lower urinary tract function and dysfunction [1].

Relevant Anatomy The lower urinary tract is conveniently considered to be simply composed of the bladder and the bladder outlet. The urinary bladder has a protective inner transitional cell lining (to prevent absorption of the excreted urine) covered by three layers of smooth muscle. It contracts under parasympathetic stimulation through the pelvic nerve. Relaxation during filling is facilitated by β-adrenergic stimulation via the hypogastric nerve.

In the male, the bladder outlet consists of the bladder neck (internal sphincter), the urethra, the prostate, and the external sphincter. The bladder neck is also composed of smooth muscle, but its primary receptors are α-adrenergic which facilitate closure; the external sphincter is composed of striated muscle and is under somatic control through the pudendal nerve. The primary neurotransmitter is norepinephrine. However, in classification, it helps to initially consider the entire bladder outlet as a single unit.

Overview of Function The normal lower urinary tract has two roles: urine storage and bladder emptying. In order to store urine properly, three things must be present:

1. The bladder must hold urine at low pressure and with appropriate sensation.
2. There must be no involuntary bladder contractions.
3. The bladder outlet must be closed at rest and remain closed against abdominal pressure.

Similarly, emptying is dependent on three basic factors:

1. There must be a coordinated bladder contraction of adequate magnitude and duration.
2. The outlet must open in coordination with the bladder contraction.
3. There cannot be any fixed anatomic obstruction.

All lower urinary tract dysfunction can be attributed to failure of one (or more) of these six properties.

Classification of Lower Urinary Tract Dysfunction Lower urinary tract dysfunctions can thus be classified as *failure to store* (broadly, incontinence) and *failure to empty* (broadly, retention). Furthermore, the dysfunction can either be *because of the bladder* or *because of the outlet*. This leads to a simple Wein classification system (Table 14.1); for example, one type of failure to empty because of the outlet is

Table 14. 1 Classification of lower urinary tract dysfunction

	Failure to store (incontinence)	Failure to empty (retention)
Because of the bladder	Overactive bladder, urgency incontinence, interstitial cystitis	Atonic/hypotonic bladder (e.g., diabetes, sacral injury, peripheral neuropathy)
Because of the outlet	Stress incontinence	Benign prostatic obstruction, sphincter dyssynergia, urethral stricture

urinary retention in males due to enlarged, obstructing prostate. The advantage of this system is that it is intuitive and each classification leads to a potential treatment algorithm. The disadvantage is that patients may have more than one dysfunction combining to produce very complex clinical problems (a woman with impaired bladder contractility and sensation due to diabetes who also has involuntary bladder contractions and stress incontinence).

The Basic Evaluation Sophisticated testing is rarely indicated in the initial evaluation of lower urinary tract symptoms. The essential elements of the work-up are the history, physical exam, urinalysis, post-void residual, and frequency-volume chart (bladder diary). Attention should always be paid to the reversible causes of LUTD as defined in the DIAPPERS mnemonic by Dr. Neil Resnick in 1985 (delirium, infection of urine, atrophic vaginitis, pharmaceuticals, psychological disorders/depression, excessive urine output, restricted mobility, stool impaction).

History As always, a complete history is essential in the evaluation of lower urinary tract dysfunction. However, there are a few items of particular importance to consider in the history.

- Define the problem: Understand the primary complaint, categorize as storage or emptying, and think about the possible problems noted above. However, regardless of the primary complaint, always ask about other lower urinary tract symptoms (LUTS); if complaint is leakage of urine, make sure to define emptying function and vice versa. Ask about urinary tract pain and gross hematuria.
- Onset: Most lower urinary tract problems have a slow, chronic onset. When the onset is abrupt, urinary tract infection must always be considered as a possibility. Acute and subacute onset often suggests a specific, reversible etiology.
- Past medical history: Any neurologic disease, and particularly low back disease, should be considered as a specific cause of lower urinary tract symptoms.
- Medications: A great many medications have anticholinergic properties and thus may affect bladder function. The cumulative effect of multiple anticholinergics is often underestimated.
- Review of symptoms: The colorectal, sexual, and neurologic review of symptoms is particularly relevant to complaints of lower urinary tract disease (LUTD) and should always be included.

Physical Exam A good urologic exam need not take a long time but it does require that patients undress. As patients often mention urinary and sexual problems right at the end of a visit, it is often inconvenient to perform a proper physical examination. In such cases, it is useful to suggest that the patient keep a home bladder diary (see below) to better quantify the LUT function and return for an exam and discussion of the problem. The exam should include a percussion/palpation of the bladder after voiding (reasonably accurate in slender patients to exclude significant urinary retention), resting anal sphincter tone, force and coordination of voluntary sphincter contraction, size and consistency of the prostate, and a basic assessment of sacral sensation (perianal and pedal).

The Bladder Diary The most underutilized tool in the evaluation of LUTD is the bladder diary or frequency-volume chart. The patient simply records the time and volume of each urination for 24–48 h. It is critical to record individual nighttime voids. Other information such as fluid intake, time and cause of incontinent episodes, degree of urgency, and degree of pain all may be helpful, but the key is to understand the typical function of the specific patient. While there is published normative data that is inadequate, consider these guidelines in counseling patients:

- Healthy 24-h urine output: 1500–2500 cm^3 (more urine output puts more stress on the bladder, but we want our patients to be adequately hydrated for overall health)
- Average single urination: 8 oz/1 cup/240 mL
- Maximum single urination: 12–20 oz/2 cups/360–600 mL (almost always the first morning void or a void that wakens the patient from sleep)

Combined with validated symptoms scores, the bladder diary is an important tool to assess a patient's progress over time and response to specific therapies.

Residual Urine As noted above, bladder percussion/palpation can be used to assess residual urine in slender patients. As ultrasound technology becomes less expensive, simple bladder scanners may become practical for primary care groups. Catheterized residual checks are highly accurate but much less acceptable in men than in women and should be avoided unless it is critical to obtain a sterile urine specimen.

14.2   Abnormal Bladders

Overactivity: The Overactive Bladder (OAB) OAB is a symptom syndrome (also urgency-frequency syndrome) defined as "urgency, with or without urge incontinence, usually with frequency and nocturia" occurring in the absence of infection or other proven pathology [2]. The cardinal symptom is urgency, "the complaint of a sudden, compelling desire to pass urine, which is difficult to defer" [2]. The primary point of the syndrome name is to include patients who suffer from urinary urgency but do not have incontinence. It is a syndrome, likely composed of several different subgroups which are yet to be defined. The definition implies an underlying pathophysiology of involuntary bladder contractions, but these are seen in only about 50 % of OAB patients during urodynamic testing. Of course, it is composed of a broad spectrum, but it is emphasized that the condition should be bothersome and that frequent urination alone (without urinary urgency) is not enough to assign this diagnosis.

Epidemiology No urologic diagnosis (with the possible exception of erectile dysfunction) has entered the public eye to the degree of OAB. The vast majority of the research and patient education efforts have been directed toward women; this likely makes men less aware of the abnormality and less likely to seek treatment. Nevertheless, epidemiologic studies make it clear that OAB is common in men.

OAB is typically divided into "wet" (with urgency incontinence) and "dry" (without urgency incontinence). While OAB is very common in men, OAB wet is relatively uncommon. For both men and women, OAB is common in all ethnic groups studied and is the prevalence correlates with age.

In a US population-based telephone survey, the prevalence of OAB in women was approximately 30 % for all racial groups, whereas the prevalence in men ranged from 15 % in US whites to 18 % in Hispanics and 20 % for African-Americans [2]. The same study found the prevalence of urgency incontinence to be 6–10 % among men but 15–19 % among women. If a stricter definition is used for OAB (symptoms occurring a few times a month as opposed to "sometimes"), the prevalence falls to 10–15 % in women and 4–6 % in men, still very significant numbers. The symptom burden falls heavily on older men. The prevalence increased steadily by decade of life but accelerates markedly after age 50. The specific problem of OAB in elderly men has been nicely reviewed by Griebling [3].

A study designed to model the worldwide prevalence of lower urinary tract disease from existing data estimates an increase in males with OAB from 205 million in 2008 to 247 million in 2018; similar estimates for women were 250 million and 299 million, respectively. While more common in women, it is clear that OAB is not simply a female disorder.

Etiology: Obstruction vs. Idiopathic? As noted in the introduction, all LUTS in men have traditionally been assumed to be due to benign prostatic obstruction (BPO). There is, of course, an underlying rationale for this—animal models of partial bladder outlet obstruction are among the most commonly used to study OAB, isolated storage symptoms are much less common in men than in women, and OAB symptoms are observed to resolve in the majority of men who undergo surgical relief of obstruction. However, OAB without obstruction also occurs in men—both as a primary problem and as persistence of storage symptoms after relief of obstruction.

The etiology of idiopathic OAB is still unknown and most probably will ultimately be determined to be due to different causes in different patient populations. Postulated causes include urothelial dysfunction, myogenic dysfunction, and occult neurologic (central or peripheral) dysfunction. There is some theoretical and basic science evidence to support each of these, but at this time, there is no agreed-upon means to stratify OAB patients into these criteria, and we are not currently able to determine how our treatments might be optimized by identifying specific phenotypes [4].

Diagnosis The basic approach to diagnosis has been stated—history, physical examination, frequency-volume chart, urinalysis, and post-void residual. In male OAB patients, the primary distinction that needs to be made initially is whether the OAB symptoms occur in the context of significant emptying symptoms (or elevated residual urine) or if the storage symptoms occur in isolation.

Additional testing that may be considered:

- Urinary flow rate/PVR: A normal urinary flow rate and low residual are highly predictive of normal voiding dynamics; BOO is largely excluded. However, a low urinary flow rate argues against pure OAB but does not provide a clear diagnosis; it could be due to either BOO or detrusor underactivity.
- Pressure-flow urodynamics: Pressure-flow urodynamics are the "gold standard" in understanding lower urinary tract dysfunction. Bladder outlet obstruction can be definitively diagnosed as can normal voiding. While data remain inadequate, it appears that patients with documented bladder outlet obstruction have a better outcome with surgical therapy and are less likely to respond to treatment for OAB than those who are not obstructed. When BOO is excluded, treatment options aimed at the bladder are more attractive. However, many patients fall into an equivocal or indeterminate classification where optimal management is uncertain.
- Cystoscopy: Cystoscopy is useful for patients who are considering surgical therapy as the size and configuration of the prostate influences surgical decision making. There is, however, no utility for cystoscopy in diagnosing BOO or OAB.
- Imaging: Upper tract imaging is not indicated in the evaluation of lower urinary tract symptoms (but may be indicated for specific findings such as hematuria or a markedly elevated PVR). Prostate sizing by ultrasound may be useful if surgery is contemplated, and the digital rectal exam is felt to be inadequate to estimate size.

For those interested in more detailed information, the updated American Urologic Association OAB Guidelines and the European Association of Urology 2015 Guidelines are recommended [5, 6].

Treatment Treatment of OAB in men remains controversial. If there are any emptying symptoms whatsoever, the treatment algorithm will follow that outlined in the BPH chapter (INSERT REFERENCE)—even when the storage symptoms clearly predominate. Sequential therapy (α-blocker first, followed by specific OAB therapy) is advocated in guidelines [7]. This discussion will focus on treatment of men with persistent OAB after treatment of BOO and those with monosymptomatic OAB. The AUA OAB Guidelines and Algorithm do not specify different therapies for male patients.

- Behavioral therapy: Substantial improvement in OAB can be obtained with simple means. Demonstrably effective, non-pharmacologic therapy includes:
  - Education. Changing behaviors begins with education about normal lower urinary tract function and about the condition; overactive bladder can be explained as an imbalance between bladder and sphincter activities. The bladder is overactive and this can be treated directly as explained below. However, improved urinary control can also come from improving sphincter function. In particular, learning to perform rapid contractions of the pelvic muscles or "quick flicks" when faced with urgency can abort the episode by activating a sacral inhibitory reflex.

- Pelvic floor muscle training. Improving the strength and responsiveness of the pelvic floor is effective for all types of urinary incontinence.
- Frequency-volume chart. A great deal of insight is also obtained by completing the FVC. Many patients identify problems—excessive fluid intake, urgency stimulated by caffeinated beverages, long delays between voids that lead to urgency episodes, etc. and begin to change behaviors without specific coaching.
- Bladder training. A short voiding interval is selected based on the FVC, and patients are instructed to void at that time, regardless of the sense of urge. The goal is to dissociate normal voiding and urgency. The interval is gradually increased as continence and control are achieved.
- Urge inhibition. Although less well studied, urge inhibition techniques are combined with quick flicks to allow the sense of urgency to pass, again dissociating normal voiding from urgency [8]. A study using cognitive behavioral therapy in children with refractory OAB showed very promising results. Superior results in older children suggest that such a program could be adapted to adult outpatient therapy.

- Pharmacotherapy: Anticholinergic (ACh) medications remain the first-line therapy for such men with OAB. Several clinical trials have examined ACh meds in OAB, either with or without α-blockers. It has long been recognized that studies of ACh monotherapy (against placebo) have shown good safety (no increase in acute urinary retention) even in the presence of documented bladder outlet obstruction [9]. It is less clear which men will benefit equally from monotherapy as compared to combination therapy with an α-blocker. One large RCT examining tamsulosin vs. solifenacin vs. combination therapy demonstrated improvement in all treatment arms against placebo with superiority of the combination arm in relief of urgency [10]. Then newest treatment for OAB, the β-3 agonist mirabegron, has also been demonstrated to be safe in the treatment of men with LUTS and BOO; clinical efficacy and optimal utilization are yet to be determined [11].
- Neuromodulation: Neuromodulation is an attractive option for men with refractory OAB when BOO has been ruled out. There is no risk of urinary retention with neuromodulation, and urethral instrumentation is avoided. There are two FDA-approved modalities for neuromodulation—percutaneous tibial nerve stimulation (PTNS) and InterStim sacral neuromodulation.
  - PTNS is delivered in an office setting with stimulation of the nerve through an acupuncture-type needle for 30 min, weekly × 12 weeks. It has been proven to be superior to sham therapy [12], to have equal efficacy and better tolerability than ACh (tolterodine) [13], and to have reasonably sustained long-term effect with maintenance therapy. Fifty patients who initially responded in randomized trials have been followed for 3 years [14]. Twenty-eight of 29 patients completing the follow-up maintained improvement for an overall response rate of 77 % while receiving an average of 1.1 treatments per month. The optimal utilization has yet to be determined. There is inadequate experience with male patients to know if there is any gender response bias.

Ideal candidates would seem to be patients who seek a non-pharmacologic solution and those who improve on ACh but are intolerant of the side effects.

- InterStim: Approved by the FDA for the treatment of urinary urgency incontinence in 1997 and subsequently for urgency-frequency without incontinence in 1999, InterStim has been the mainstay of treatment for OAB patients who are refractory to pharmacologic therapy. It can be effective for even severe and complex cases. This device is permanently implanted, essentially a "bladder pacemaker." There is a test phase which can be performed in the office with a temporary external wire or in the operating room with an implanted electrode. In either case, the patient has an opportunity to evaluate the response before going on to the permanent generator implant. Surgery is generally performed under light sedation.

- Approximately 2/3 of patients with refractory OAB respond to InterStim. Intermediate term results are good with one study showing mean 4-year responses of 70 % for urgency incontinence and 68 % for urgency-frequency [15]. Less than 20 % of the patients were male; this is similar to other published literature. Surgical reintervention remains common with an average of 1.7 procedures/patient in the 41 % who required additional surgery. The most common reasons for intervention were treatment failure (explantation) and lead repositioning. Infection, pain, need for MRI, and battery depletion are also reasons for reoperation. InterStim should be considered for patients with refractory OAB and reasonable life expectancy who are healthy enough to tolerate a surgical procedure.

- Botox injections: Botulinum toxin, officially named onabotulinumtoxinA to distinguish it from other botulinum toxin products, paralyzes muscle by blocking the release of acetylcholine at the neuromuscular junction. It cleaves SNAP-25, a protein receptor, so that the vesicles containing acetylcholine (and other neurotransmitters) cannot bind to the nerve terminal and release their contents. This is a reversible process with duration of effect lasting 2–6 months—seemingly longer in the bladder than in many other applications.

- InterStim presented a dramatic advance in treatment of refractory OAB, offering effective therapy to patients who previously only had the option of major surgery. Botox was approved by the FDA in 2013 and was even more of a game changer; patients could now be offered effective treatment in a 15-min office procedure under local anesthesia. However, Botox has some key differences that diminish its appeal—the procedure must be repeated over time, and the treatment can be "too effective" leading to urinary retention.

- It is not possible to define gender differences in response to Botox. The two multicenter registration trials leading to approval in the USA and Europe included over 1110 patients, only 135 of whom were men [16, 17]. As only half of these were actually randomized to receive Botox, the numbers are simply too small to draw conclusions. The overall data show marked improvement in incontinence and urinary urgency episodes with Botox. The global response rate (moderately or markedly improved) is 61 % with Botox compared to 29 % with placebo. Risks include urinary tract infection (difficult to analyze due to study definitions but potentially as high as 24 %) and urinary retention. In the two trials, the percentages of patients who developed an increase in post-void residuals of ≥ 200 cm³ were 8.7 and 8.8 % and 6.1–6.9 % initiated intermittent catheterization. Many studies have examined the long-term durability of injection therapy. It appears that it is uncommon to see loss of efficacy over time. The duration of response is typically 5–9 months, and the initial response predicts long-term results.

- While the bias is that men may be more likely to suffer urinary retention with Botox, the risk is probably very similar for well-selected patients with normal voiding dynamics. A more relevant issue for most men is the need for frequent instrumentation (typically every 6 months). Men are less accepting of this than women in an office setting, and a requirement for anesthetic makes the procedure extremely expensive over time.

Underactivity Detrusor underactivity (DUA) or hypocontractility is a poorly researched and poorly appreciated condition. There is not even a generally agreed definition. The International Continence Society proposed that detrusor underactivity was "a contraction of reduced strength and/or duration, resulting in prolonged bladder emptying and/or failure to achieve complete bladder emptying within a normal time span" [18]. This definition lacks the specificity needed for clinical or epidemiologic research. The patients complain of weak and interrupted urine flow, straining, hesitancy, and a sense of incomplete emptying. Patients with DUA can also experience storage symptoms such as urgency and urge incontinence; Neil Resnick named this condition detrusor hyperactivity with impaired contractility and suggested that it was a common and unrecognized cause of urinary incontinence in the elderly [19]. An excellent literature review on this topic was presented by Osman and colleagues for those who are interested in further study [20].

Epidemiology It is certain that many men and women, particularly the elderly, are affected by DUA. However, there are no useful epidemiologic studies to understand how prevalent this condition may be. The barrier to doing epidemiologic studies is considerable as this is a urodynamically defined condition; the clinical symptoms are nonspecific, overlapping considerably with bladder outlet obstruction.

Etiology In men, there is an underlying assumption that poor emptying is due to bladder outlet obstruction and that poor emptying may persist after relief of obstruction due to DUA. Yet it is well known that many men with high-grade bladder outlet obstruction have been followed for years without deterioration in bladder function. The mechanisms by which obstruction results in DUA, why it occurs in one patient and not another, and how to clinically identify patients at risk are entirely unknown. Furthermore, it is certain that there are other etiologies for DUA; many older women are diagnosed with DUA who have no reasonable cause of obstruction. It is highly likely that this occurs in aging men, also. Many neurologic diseases can produce DUA, but these are generally classified as neurogenic bladder disorders and are discussed below.

Diagnosis The diagnosis of DUA requires a pressure-flow urodynamic study to determine the quality of the detrusor contraction. There are not yet adequate data to create specific diagnostic criteria. In general, patients with DUA have low-pressure contractions ($\leq$20 cm H_2O), but in some cases, there is an initially adequate contraction that is poorly sustained. It has been suggested that a post-void residual of $\geq$ 40 % of the pre-void bladder volume could serve as a screen for potential DUA [6].

Treatment Treatment for DUA is rather unsatisfactory. Bethanechol is a cholinergic agonist that is approved for the treatment of acute postoperative and postpartum nonobstructive (functional) urinary retention and for neurogenic atony of the urinary bladder with retention. There is scant clinical evidence for its efficacy. In the author's experience, it may have some benefit for the patient with a large residual—perhaps emptying 50 % of bladder volume—but has no effect on patients in overt retention. Dosing is 25 to 50 mg TID to QID, and it is generally advisable to gradually titrate the dose upward as the expected cholinergic side effects (diarrhea, cramping, lacrimation, salivation, etc. are often problematic). A good outcome is tolerable side effects and enough improvement to obviate the need for catheterization.

Therefore, most treatment of DUA is focused on improving emptying. Alpha-blockers are accepted as first-line therapy for men with difficulty emptying—most studies of these drugs obviously include men with DUA as pressure-flow urodynamics are rarely used in clinical trials and symptoms cannot differentiate DUA from true bladder outlet obstruction. DUA is perhaps more easily recognized/accepted in women; one study from Taiwan of women with "chronic, bothersome voiding symptoms" treated all patients with 0.2 mg tamsulosin (half of the FDA-approved dose for men in the USA). They found that the response rate (defined as moderate to marked improvement in symptoms) was 66.6 % for those diagnosed with BOO compared to 50 % for those with DUA. Similar nonstatistically significant trends toward a better response in BOO were seen for objective measures, but it certainly seems that DUA patients can respond to α-blockers. There is no indication that any one of the approved drugs is superior in this patient population.

Only one study investigated combination therapy for DUA. Yamanishi and colleagues randomized 119 patients with DUA to treatment an α-blocker, a cholinergic agent, or both [21]. Various outcome measures clearly favored combination therapy. For the subgroup of men, there was statistically and clinically significant improvement in total symptom score (measured by IPSS) with combination and with α-blocker alone but not with the cholinergic.

The diagnosis of DUA is particularly important and controversial when symptoms are refractory or post-void residual becomes worrisomely high (particularly if $\geq$ the voided volume). There is no doubt that some of these patients will respond to surgical intervention and sometimes even a second operation. However, there have been a great many men over the years that have been subjected to multiple prostate operations with diminishing results and ultimately end up on intermittent catheterization because the underlying problem was DUA not BOO. There is at least general agreement that pressure-flow urodynamic studies are appropriate for:

- Men with chronic or large-volume urinary retention
- Men with LUTS who are still voiding but have very large residual urine (usually considered > 250 cm^3)
- Men with persistent LUTS after surgical intervention

If preoperative studies indicate DUA, this does not mean that surgery is inappropriate; rather, the patient should be counseled about a lower likelihood of successful outcome and offered the option of intermittent catheterization.

Of course, the ultimate intervention for DUA is intermittent self-catheterization (ISC). While many men are unable to accept this, it can dramatically improve quality of life. New hydrophilic catheters significantly diminish discomfort. Catheter supplies fit easily into a "belly bag" or briefcase and can be used in almost any public restroom. The difference between taking 2 min to catheterize 3–5×/day and straining to empty a failing bladder 15–20 times/day can be dramatic. The primary complications are transient discomfort, occasional mild hematuria, and urinary tract infections. Most men on ISC may have 1–2 episodes of simple cystitis per year which are easily treated. It is important to realize that these men will always have bacteriuria, and no effort should be made to treat this unless there are clear symptoms of infection (pain, frequency, etc.).

Bladder Pain If bladder problems are already decidedly "unmanly," there is little doubt that bladder pain is very difficult for men to acknowledge. Not surprisingly, there is essentially no research into this problem as it applies to men. Bladder pain conditions are currently grouped as bladder pain syndrome/interstitial cystitis (BPS/IC). These patients present with urinary frequency and urgency that is driven by increasing pain with bladder filling. However, interstitial cystitis (IC) is best considered as a distinct condition. It is characterized by discrete flat, erythematous lesions that are visualized at cystoscopy and demonstrate severe acute and chronic inflammation on biopsy. In contrast, bladder pain syndrome (BPS) is defined by the American Urologic Association and the Society for Urodynamics and Female Urology as "An unpleasant sensation (pain, pressure, discomfort) perceived to be related to the urinary bladder, associated with lower urinary tract symptoms of more than 6 weeks duration, in the absence of infection or other identifiable causes" [22]. While the symptoms are identical, these patients have normal appearing bladders at cystoscopy, and biopsies do not show inflammation [23].

Epidemiology It was commonly thought that only about 10 % of patients with BPS/IC were male. Only two published clinical studies specifically report on the occurrence of BPS/IC in men. Both are single-institution, retrospective chart reviews and tell us nothing about the overall epidemiology. Novicki and colleagues identified 29 men diagnosed at the Mayo Clinic over 8 years, 86 % of whom were previously diagnosed with prostatitis or BPH [24]. These were older patients (average 67.3 years) and 70 % had ulcers. Similarly, Forrest and Vo found that 83 % of their 52 male patients were referred with diagnoses of chronic prostatitis, BPH, or epididymitis [25]. On the other hand, their average age was only 44 years, and only 10 % of their patients had bladder ulcers. They also reported a female to male ratio in their practice was 7.6:1. There is nothing in either paper to suggest that male patients have a different clinical course or behave differently in response to treatment than do women.

The thinking that BPS/IC is uncommon in men has been recently challenged. The National Institutes of Diabetes, Digestive, and Kidney Diseases sponsored a nationwide, population-based survey on the prevalence of bladder pain symptoms. The Rand Interstitial Cystitis Epidemiology (RICE) developed case definitions of disease that could be ascertained by phone interview, validated them on a subset of responders who were willing to come in for an in-person evaluation, and then performed the nationwide survey. The results were surprising to many. In adult women, the prevalence estimates for BPS/IC range from a possible high of 6.53 % using a high-sensitivity definition to a low of 2.7 % using a high-specificity definition [26]. Only 10 % of those surveyed had actually been diagnosed with BPS/IC. When the same group performed a population-based screen in men, they found that the comparable prevalence estimates for BPS/IC were 4.2 % to 1.9 %—much closer to that of women than most expected [27]. In addition, they found that 1.8 % of men met a single high-sensitivity/high-specificity case definition for chronic pelvic pain syndrome (CPPS). The overlap between these two groups was only 17 %. It is clear from this study that

- BPS/IC is common in the male population; the female to male ratio is about 3:2.
- There may be as many (or more) men with BPS/IC as the more commonly diagnosed CPPS.
- Pelvic pain syndrome is an enormous problem for adult males.

Etiology Little is known about the etiology of BPS/IC. The most widely discussed theory, lower urinary dysfunctional epithelium (LUDE), is on the wane as there is no reliable test for this condition, and only a minority of patients respond to specific treatment with pentosanpolysulfate or heparin, and recent studies show no dose response to a nearly tenfold increase in pentosanpolysulfate dosage. Promising basic science work that detected a specific protein (antiproliferative factor) in BPS/IC patients urine that inhibits bladder epithelial growth has also disappointed. The protein has been fully identified, but the work has not been reproduced in other labs, and there is as yet no clinically useful test for the protein nor any treatment.

It is the feeling of the author (and many others) that while IC is a specific condition and may well ultimately be shown to have a clear etiology, BPS is really a syndrome that is best considered the common expression of different identifiable phenotypes [28]. It is likely that we will one day be able to identify a specific BPS bladder phenotype, and it may well be due to a urothelial abnormality. However, the most common phenotype may well be due to myofascial pain/pelvic floor dysfunction. Here, both the bladder pain and lower urinary tract symptoms are actually initiated by myofascial trigger points in the abdomen and pelvis in combination with poor relaxation/coordination of the pelvic floor muscles. Pudendal neuralgia can produce symptoms that mimic BPS/IC, and it is likely that other phenotypes can be described that respond to specific therapies. Finally, it is important to recognize that many patients with urologic chronic pelvic pain syndromes have significant comorbid systemic pain syndromes such as fibromyalgia [29]. This represents an important phenotype in which it is not always wise to focus on the pelvic pain.

Diagnosis Guidelines for the diagnosis of BPS/IC have been published by the American Urological Association, including an algorithm for evaluation and treatment [30]. The basic evaluation for all patients includes a history and physical examination, frequency-volume chart, determination of post-void residual, urinalysis, urine culture, and use of validated instruments to assess overall symptoms and pain. Urine cytology is recommended if there is a smoking history. The presence of hematuria or pyuria in the urinalysis should prompt a cystoscopic examination (as well as upper tract imaging). Other studies are usually not helpful. In men, an important consideration is bladder outlet obstruction due to prostatic enlargement or bladder neck dysfunction. Therefore, the post-void residual is an important screening test, and pressure-flow urodynamics should be considered if this is elevated or there are significant bladder emptying symptoms. In all cases, the need for additional diagnostic testing should be reassessed if the patient does not respond well to treatment.

Treatment The AUA Guidelines treatment algorithm describes six levels of treatment beginning with education and behavioral therapies and ending (in rare patients) with cystectomy and reconstruction or urinary diversion. There is also a detailed discussion of the principles of treatment; it is critical to properly evaluate each treatment modality, optimize successful treatments, and avoid polypharmacy. There is little if any evidence that men with BPS/IC respond differently to treatments than women, but some perspectives on the common treatment modalities are presented:

- Oral medications: Pentosanpolysulfate, amitriptyline, cimetidine, and hydroxyzine are all presented as acceptable second-line treatments. While amitriptyline is arguably the single most effective medication for bladder pain, the prominent anticholinergic side effects of this drug (and the anticholinergics indicated for overactive bladder which are also commonly used in this condition) can aggravate/expose any difficulty in emptying. The antihistaminic effects of hydroxyzine can do the same. This issue may be more of a problem for male patients.
- Intravesical therapies: A variety of intravesical "cocktails" using dimethyl sulfoxide or some combination of pentosanpolysulfate or heparin with local anesthetic agents have been employed in BPS/IC. Patients who respond can often be taught to perform home instillations as part of the chronic therapy. Men may be more reluctant to accept catheterization, but newer hydrophilic catheters ease this discomfort, and these therapies should not be discouraged.
- Hydrodistention under anesthesia: Some have argued that ulcerative IC is more common in men. While this cannot be demonstrated, an endoscopic examination to look for ulcers should certainly be performed whenever a patient is not responding to therapy.

The author has argued that we have typically been too passive in our approach to BPS/IC therapy, willing to settle for any improvement. In "An Oncologic Approach to UCPPS" [31], the idea of working to normalize bladder capacity and eliminate all symptoms when possible is proposed as a means of allowing the sensitized nervous system to revert back to normal achieving a sustainable complete remission. It is important to follow the patient's frequency-volume chart and symptom scores and understand to what degree symptoms are still present when the patient reports improvement.

14.2.1 Neurogenic Bladder

Overview Neurogenic bladder (NGB) is one of the least useful and most misused terms in urology. It can appropriately be defined as any lower urinary tract dysfunction that occurs in a patient with a neurologic disorder that could reasonably be attributed to that disorder. In truth, we are rarely able to prove that a neurologic disease is the proximate cause of LUTS; we can simply note that the time courses of the two conditions are parallel and that the neurologic condition is the most likely source of the symptoms.

Common neurogenic disorders and lower urinary tract outcome:

- Stoke: The cerebral edema of acute stroke often produces detrusor areflexia and urinary retention. This almost always resolves as the patient recovers unless there is massive injury. Stoke patients always have coordinated voiding and typically empty well so men with persistent retention after stroke should be investigated for bladder outlet obstruction. The most common long-term problem in stroke patients is overactive bladder (properly referred to here as neurogenic detrusor overactivity) with urge incontinence. The likelihood of persistent OAB after stroke is related to the severity of the injury/greater cerebral damage. These patients are much more likely to have incontinence without sensation (in contrast to typical urgency incontinence) than neurologically intact individuals.
- Multiple sclerosis: The unfortunate fact about multiple sclerosis (MS) is that lower urinary tract manifestations are as varied as the disease itself. The most common manifestation of MS is overactive bladder, but it is very common that these patients suffer from combined storage and emptying problems. Although upper urinary tract complications are uncommon with MS, they are more likely to occur in men; male patients deserve closer monitoring.
- Parkinson's disease: It is widely recognized that LUTS are common in patients with PD. Parkinson's disease (PD) has been an area of considerable controversy in urology; the most common manifestation is detrusor overactivity, but there may also be emptying dysfunction due to poor relaxation of the urinary sphincter. It has long been argued that men with LUTS and PD were poor candidates for surgical therapy because of the high prevalence of DO that would persist after surgery. However, current thinking is simply that it is important to make an

accurate diagnosis. A small study of men and women presenting for treatment of PD who were willing to undergo pressure-flow urodynamic testing found that 75 % had detrusor overactivity and only 14 % had bladder outlet obstruction (enlarged prostate was an exclusion criteria). Not surprisingly, men were more likely to be obstructed. If clear prostatic obstruction is present (and particularly if there is also increased post-void residual urine), surgery should not be denied.

- Spinal cord injury: The most serious NGB disorder is spinal cord injury (SCI) and the related myelomeningocele. These disorders are much more likely to lead to upper tract complications including renal failure. As with stroke, there is a period of spinal shock in the acute injury phase. As this resolves, the ultimate pattern takes shape. The type of LUTD in complete injury is largely predictable by the level of injury, but this is not true with incomplete injuries. Sacral injuries destroy both the sacral micturition center and the connection to the cortical micturition center leading to urinary retention. Suprasacral lesions allow the sacral micturition center to function without cortical inhibition and produce detrusor overactivity and incontinence. Lesions above T6 are the most serious as the coordination of urination is also affected. There is detrusor overactivity with external sphincter dyssynergia; these patients are at a particularly high risk for upper tract complications and deserve the closest monitoring.
- Radical pelvic surgery: Surgery for pelvic cancers, particularly radical hysterectomy and colectomy, presents a risk for bladder denervation and urinary retention. In male patients, this may lead to a prostatectomy with disastrous results. The bladder may actually be areflexic but noncompliant leading to severe urinary incontinence after TURP. Thoughtful evaluation and high-quality pressure-flow urodynamic evaluation are mandatory for these patients.

Management Principles In the same way that "neurogenic bladder" is a very nonspecific term, the management of patients with NGB must be individualized. Important considerations include:

- The natural history of the neurologic disease. Is progression likely? Will it impact the LUTD? Will it impact the patient's ability to manage the LUTD (make it to the toilet when faced with urgency, perform self-catheterization).
- The risk of upper urinary tract complications. When urodynamic studies show high pressures during storage (common in spinal cord injury and sometimes seen in MS), there is a clear risk of upper urinary tract damage over time. Monitoring is mandatory, and intervention may be required even when symptoms are not severe.
- The overall condition of the patient. It is common that NGB patients may have multiple disabilities and some of these (cognitive impairment, limited mobility, limited hand function) may impact management.

Each patient deserves careful evaluation and an individualized plan for both monitoring and treatment.

Nocturia Nocturia is the most bothersome lower urinary tract symptom and often the reason that men seek treatment. It is, unfortunately, the least likely to respond to standard therapy. Despite this, little research had been done on this problem until recent years. Our knowledge of nocturia is substantially improved by new knowledge. We understand that nocturia is most commonly not due to the bladder and that the lack of treatment response is indicative of not identifying the underlying cause. Nocturia is easy to evaluate, many effective interventions exist once properly classified, and it is best managed by the primary care physician.

Epidemiology The ICS defines nocturia as "the complaint that the individual has to wake at night one or more times to void" [2]. The individual must wake from sleep and return to sleep after voiding. Nocturia increases steadily with age and the point at which nocturia becomes abnormal and/or bothersome is not totally clear; most clinical research includes only subjects with a minimum of two episodes of nocturia.

Nocturia is clearly age related. An excellent literature review (recommended reading for those interested in the subject) by Bosch and Weiss found that "men in their 20s and 30s, 11 % to 35.2 % reported at least 1 void per night while 2 % to 16.6 % reported 2 or more voids nightly. Of men in their 70s and 80s, 68.9 % to 93 % reported at least 1 void per night while 29 % to 59.3 % reported at least 2 voids per night" [32]. The authors note that nocturia is much more common in younger women (perhaps due to sleep issues, responsibilities with children, etc.), but in older individuals, the gender difference disappears. There is no indication at this time that race or ethnicity contributes to nocturia.

Differential Diagnosis and Evaluation Strategy The basic diagnostic tools for all bladder conditions—history, physical examination, frequency-volume chart (FVC), urinalysis, and post-void residual determination—suffice in nearly all cases where nocturia is the chief complaint. It is important to know the medical history since so many conditions can cause nocturia. The history generally allows for classification of nocturia as an isolated condition (no daytime complaints) or as part of a global LUTS. The presence of snoring or other related nighttime issues can suggest sleep apnea or other sleep disturbances. On the physical exam, it is critical to look for peripheral edema, one of the most common and treatable causes of nocturia. The FVC is, however, indispensable as the cornerstone of effective diagnosis and management of nocturia.

The FVC must record the volume of all voids for at least 24 h (preferably 2–3 days) and the hours of sleep. While "normal" is necessarily a range, the FVC allows the clinician to analyze urine production and bladder function together. Some basic calculations are used to classify nocturia:

- 24-h urine production. This enables the diagnosis of global polyuria which is suspected with urine outputs >2500 cm^3 or 40 cm^3/kg.
- The percentage of urine produced during sleep. Nocturnal urine output includes the first morning void. This enables the diagnosis of nocturnal polyuria—generally defined as >33 % of urine made during sleep hours—a lower percentage for younger patients. 90 cm^3/h of sleep has also been suggested [33].

Table 14.2 Classification of lower urinary tract dysfunction

Classification of nocturia by frequency-volume chart	
Findings on FVC	Suggested etiologies
Low bladder volumes day and night	Lower urinary tract dysfunction—OAB, BPO, BPS/IC
Low bladder volumes night only	Sleep disorder
Nocturnal polyuria	Peripheral edema, CHF, behavioral issues
Global polyuria	Behavioral issues/polydipsia, uncontrolled diabetes, etc.

- Daytime/nighttime average and maximum void volumes. Lower volumes (average voids <200 cm^3, maximum voids <300 cm^3) identify patients who may have underlying lower urinary tract dysfunction).

This classification provides the insights needed to look for correctable/treatable causes of nocturia (Table 14.2). Proper treatment depends on proper classification. Nocturia is often multifactorial, and the initial management is typically focused on optimizing medical conditions such as CHF and peripheral edema. Diuretics can be used at in the late afternoon when compression stockings and elevation of the feet are insufficient to manage the edema. Treatments aimed at the bladder are usually only successful when nocturia is part of a day and night symptom complex; these should be reserved for those who have such a diagnosis. Sleep disorders can be identified and treated.

Desmopressin is a medication which is specifically approved for nocturnal enuresis in children. It is a synthetic analog of vasopressin that temporarily decreases urine production. It has been shown to be effective in adults [34] although it has not yet gained FDA approval for this indication. A common starting dose is 50 mcg and the drug can be titrated to 400 mcg. Patients should be monitored for hyponatremia, particularly the elderly. There is some evidence that men are less sensitive to the effects of desmopressin and may require higher doses.

14.3 Summary

Bladder problems are common in men, in many cases with similar frequency to that found in women. In most cases, men respond well to the same treatments that are effective for women so the primary challenge is in identifying and diagnosing these conditions. The primary care physician can do this effectively in the majority of cases and call for urologic consultation whenever the diagnosis is in doubt or the patient fails to respond to appropriate therapy.

References

1. Wein AJ. Pathophysiology and classification of lower urinary tract dysfunction: overview. In: Wein AJ, Kavoussi RL, Novick AC, Partin AW, Peters CA, editors. Campbell's urology). 10th ed. Philadelphia, PA: Elsevier-Saunders; 2012. p. 1834–46.

2. Coyne KS, Sexton CC, Bell JA, et al. The prevalence of lower urinary tract symptoms (LUTS) and overactive bladder (OAB) by racial/ethnic group and age: results from OAB-POLL. Neurourol Urodyn. 2013;32(3):230–7. doi:10.1002/nau.22295. Epub 2012 Jul 27.

3. Griebling TL. Overactive bladder in elderly men: epidemiology, evaluation, clinical effects, and management. Curr Urol Rep. 2013;14(5):418–25. doi:10.1007/s11934-013-0367-0.

4. Hanna-Mitchell AT, Kashyap M, Chan WV, et al. Pathophysiology of idiopathic overactive bladder and the success of treatment: a systematic review from ICI-RS 2013. Neurourol Urodyn. 2014;33(5):611–7. doi:10.1002/nau.22582. Epub 2014 May 20.

5. Gormley EA, Lightner DJ, Faraday M, et al. Diagnosis and treatment of overactive bladder (non-neurogenic) in adults: AUA/SUFU guideline amendment. J Urol. 2015;193(5):1572–80. doi:10.1016/j.juro.2015.01.087. Epub 2015 Jan 23. http://www.auanet.org/content/media/OAB_guideline.pdf.

6. Gratzke C, Bachmann A, Descazeaud A, et al. EAU Guidelines on the assessment of non-neurogenic male lower urinary tract symptoms including benign prostatic obstruction. Eur Urol. 2015;67(6):1099–109. doi:10.1016/j.eururo.2014.12.038. pii: S0302-2838(14)01394-3.

7. Oelke M, Bachmann A, Descazeaud A, et al. Guidelines on the management of male lower urinary tract symptoms including benign prostatic obstruction. Eur Urol. 2015. doi:10.1016/j.eururo.2014.12.038. pii: S0302-2838(14)01394-3.

8. Meijer EF, Nieuwhof-Leppink AJ, Dekker-Vasse E, et al. Central inhibition of refractory overactive bladder complaints, results of an inpatient training program. J Pediatr Urol. 2015;11(1):21.e1–5. doi:10.1016/j.jpurol.2014.06.024. Epub 2014 Aug 11.

9. Abrams P, Kaplan S, De Koning Gans HJ, et al. Safety and tolerability of tolterodine for the treatment of overactive bladder in men with bladder outlet obstruction. J Urol. 2006;175: 999–1004.

10. van Kerrebroeck P, Chapple C, Drogendijk T, et. al for NEPTUNE Study Group. Combination therapy with solifenacin and tamsulosin oral controlled absorption system in a single tablet for lower urinary tract symptoms in men: efficacy and safety results from the randomised controlled NEPTUNE trial. Eur Urol. 2013;64(6):1003–12. doi:10.1016/j.eururo.2013.07.034. Epub 2013 Aug 3.

11. Nitti VW, Rosenberg S, Mitcheson DH. Urodynamics and safety of the β_3-adrenoceptor agonist mirabegron in males with lower urinary tract symptoms and bladder outlet obstruction. J Urol. 2013;190(4):1320–7. doi:10.1016/j.juro.2013.05.062.

12. Peters KM, Carrico DJ, Perez-Marrero RA, et al. Randomized trial of percutaneous tibial nerve stimulation versus Sham efficacy in the treatment of overactive bladder syndrome: results from the SUmiT trial. J Urol. 2010;183(4):1438–43. doi:10.1016/j.juro.2009.12.036. Epub 2010 Feb 20.

13. Peters KM, MacDiarmid SA, Wooldridge LS, et al. Randomized trial of percutaneous tibial nerve stimulation versus extended-release tolterodine: results from the overactive bladder innovative therapy trial. J Urol. 2009;182(3):1055–61. doi:10.1016/j.juro.2009.05.045. Epub 2009 Jul 18.

14. Peters KM, Carrico DJ, Wooldridge LS, et al. Percutaneous tibial nerve stimulation for the long-term treatment of overactive bladder: 3-year results of the STEP study. J Urol. 2013;189(6):2194–201. doi:10.1016/j.juro.2012.11.175. Epub 2012 Dec 3.

15. Peeters K, Sahai A, De Ridder D, Van Der Aa F. Long-term follow-up of sacral neuromodulation for lower urinary tract dysfunction. BJU Int. 2014;113(5):789–94. doi:10.1111/bju.12571.

16. Nitti VW, Dmochowski R, Herschorn S, et al; EMBARK Study Group. OnabotulinumtoxinA for the treatment of patients with overactive bladder and urinary incontinence: results of a phase 3, randomized, placebo controlled trial. J Urol. 2013;189(6):2186–93. doi:10.1016/j.juro.2012.12.022. Epub 2012 Dec 14.

17. Chapple C, Sievert KD, MacDiarmid S, et al. OnabotulinumtoxinA 100 U significantly improves all idiopathic overactive bladder symptoms and quality of life in patients with overactive bladder and urinary incontinence: a randomised, double-blind, placebo-controlled trial. Eur Urol. 2013;64(2):249–56. doi:10.1016/j.eururo.2013.04.001. Epub 2013 Apr 10.

18. Abrams P, Cardozo L, Fall M, et al. The standardisation of terminology of lower urinary tract function: report from the Standardisation Sub-committee of the International Continence Society. Neurourol Urodyn. 2002;21:167–78.
19. Resnick NM, Yalla SV. Detrusor hyperactivity with impaired contractile function. An unrecognized but common cause of incontinence in elderly patients. JAMA. 1987;257:3076–81.
20. Osman NI. 2014.
21. Yamanishi T, Yasuda K, Kamai T, et al. Combination of a cholinergic drug and an alpha-blocker is more effective than monotherapy for the treatment of voiding difficulty in patients with underactive detrusor. Int J Urol. 2004;11(2):88–96.
22. Hanno P, Dmochowski R. Status of international consensus on interstitial cystitis/bladder pain syndrome/painful bladder syndrome: 2008 snapshot. Neurourol Urodyn. 2009;28:274.
23. Leiby B, Landis J, Propert K, Tomaszewski J, Group ICDBS. Discovery of morphological subgroups that correlate with severity of symptoms in interstitial cystitis: a proposed biopsy classification system. J Urol. 2007;177(1):142–8.
24. Novicki DE, Larson TR, Swanson SK. Interstitial cystitis in men. Urology. 1998;52(4):621–4.
25. Forrest J, Vo Q. Observations on the management of interstitial cystitis in men. Urology. 2001;57(6 Suppl 1):107.
26. Berry SH, Elliott MN, Suttorp M, et al. Prevalence of symptoms of bladder pain syndrome/interstitial cystitis among adult females in the United States. J Urol. 2011;186(2):540–4. doi:10.1016/j.juro.2011.03.132. Epub 2011 Jun 16.
27. Suskind AM, Berry SH, Ewing BA, et al. The prevalence and overlap of interstitial cystitis/bladder pain syndrome and chronic prostatitis/chronic pelvic pain syndrome in men: results of the RAND Interstitial Cystitis Epidemiology male study. J Urol. 2013;189(1):141–5. doi:10.1016/j.juro.2012.08.088. Epub 2012 Nov 16.
28. Payne CK. A new approach to urologic chronic pelvic pain syndromes: applying oncologic principles to "benign" conditions. Curr Bladder Dysfunct Rep. 2015;10(1):81–6.
29. Payne CK, Potts JM.
30. Hanno PM, Burks DA, Clemens JQ, et al., Interstitial Cystitis Guidelines Panel of the American Urological Association Education and Research, Inc.: AUA guideline for the diagnosis and treatment of interstitial cystitis/bladder pain syndrome. J Urol. 2011;185(6):2162–70. doi:10.1016/j.juro.2011.03.064. Epub 2011 Apr 16.
31. Payne CK.
32. Bosch JL, Weiss JP. The prevalence and causes of nocturia. J Urol. 2013;189(1 Suppl):S86–92. doi:10.1016/j.juro.2012.11.033.
33. Nocturia Think Tank: focus on nocturnal polyuria: ICI-RS 2011.
34. Weiss JP, Bosch JL, Drake M, Dmochowski RR, Hashim H, Hijaz A, Johnson TM, Juul KV, Nørgaard JP, Norton P, Robinson D, Tikkinen KA, Van Kerrebroeck PE, Wein AJ. Nocturia Think Tank: focus on nocturnal polyuria: ICI-RS 2011. Neurourol Urodyn. 2012;31(3):330–9. doi:10.1002/nau.22219. Epub 2012 Mar 13.
35. Ebell MH, Radke T, Gardner J. A systematic review of the efficacy and safety of desmopressin for nocturia in adults. J Urol. 2014;192(3):829–35. doi:10.1016/j.juro.2014.03.095. Epub 2014 Apr 1.

Chronic Pelvic Pain in Men Is NOT Prostatitis!

15

Jeannette M. Potts

15.1   Introduction

Male pelvic pain continues to be misunderstood as a urological condition and erroneously approached as an infection or disorder of the prostate gland.

Although growing numbers of studies demonstrate a changing focus away from the prostate, research and treatment remain in the realm of urologists, who perpetuate the prostatocentricism through their persistent reference to the prostatitis classification system and the categorization of male pelvic pain within the designation of Category 3 prostatitis: chronic (nonbacterial) prostatitis/chronic pelvic pain syndrome (Table 15.1) As recently as 2015, published research continues to use the National Institutes of Health-**Chronic Prostatitis** Symptom Index (NIH-CPSI) as the research tool for inclusion criteria and instrument for assessing progress. Even more confusing is the application of NIH-CPSI for studies testing the efficacy of therapies which neither address infection nor prostate disease, e.g., physical therapy, stress management, and biofeedback.

Imagine a similarly flawed NIH classification system for something like encephalitis, and Category 3 includes the broad category of HEADACHE! Imagine that every headache is evaluated and empirically treated as an infection. While this seems so outrageous, it is precisely what has been going on for decades in both primary care and urological practice.

The broad differential diagnosis of male pelvic pain requires a comprehensive approach. After excluding serious or acute pathological conditions of the colon, rectum, neurological system, or urinary tract, the physician should consider dynamic or functional conditions such as pelvic muscle dysfunction, myofascial trigger points, pudendal neuralgia, and functional somatic syndromes, also described as

J.M. Potts, M.D. (✉)
Vista Urology & Pelvic Pain Partners, 2998 South Bascom Avenue, Suite 100,
San Jose, CA 95124, USA
e-mail: DrPotts@VistaUrology.com

© Springer Science+Business Media New York 2016
J.M. Potts (ed.), *Men's Health*, DOI 10.1007/978-1-4939-3237-5_15

Table 15.1 NIH-NIDDK prostatitis classification system

Category 1	Acute bacterial prostatitis
Category 2	Chronic bacterial prostatitis
Category 3	A. Chronic [abacterial] prostatitis/chronic pelvic pain; with inflammation
	B. Chronic [abacterial] prostatitis/chronic pelvic pain; without inflammation (historically termed prostadynia)
Category 4	Asymptomatic inflammation Identified as leukocytospermia or histological evidence of inflammation

central sensitization syndromes. Patients may have one or more of these conditions, and often, I have found that patients do indeed have overlapping syndromes. Anxiety and stress play a predisposing and/or perpetuating role in pelvic pain as well.

Either because of biopsychosocial predispositions or because of secondary depression and hopelessness due to the burden of pain, patients find themselves no longer in the "driver's seat" and may assume a role of victimization. This response to a painful or chronic condition must be identified and addressed, as it greatly influences a patient's confidence in the diagnostic process and impacts compliance with therapy, most of which involves self-care.

15.2 CPPS Is NOT Prostatitis

As early as **1963**, an investigator observed that antibiotics afforded no better response than placebo among men with symptoms of prostatitis [1]. This has been corroborated by many investigators since then.

In a randomized, placebo-controlled trial, 6 weeks of levofloxacin therapy for chronic prostatitis yielded no advantage over placebo [2], and a subsequent trial found that neither ciprofloxacin, the alpha-blocker tamsulosin, nor their combination reduced symptoms of chronic prostatitis compared with placebo [3].

There has been no correlation between symptom severity and the results of localization cultures, when using the Meares–Stamey technique, otherwise known as the four-glass test [4]. (The four-glass test involves collection of sequential urine specimens before and after prostate massage and of prostatic fluid during prostate massage [5].)

Localization cultures can be even more misleading in the CPPS population as demonstrated in yet another, relatively large study in which normal controls were just as likely as men with chronic prostatitis/CPPS to have positive localization cultures (about 8 % in both groups) [6]. Even earlier, the Giessen Consensus Group recommended antibiotics were to be withheld until a second localization culture corroborated the same organism [7].

Localization testing to identify inflammation in either the expressed prostatic secretions (EPS) or in semen is similarly nonspecific. Patient symptom severity is not correlated to the presence or degree of inflammation detected in these specimens [4]. Indeed, abnormally high white blood cell counts have been identified among asymptomatic men. For example, many asymptomatic men seeking care for infertility have leukocytospermia. While infection is one potential cause of leukocytospermia, it can also occur in the setting of neurological trauma or in the setting of varicoceles [8]. In another example, among asymptomatic men with elevated PSA, 42 % were found to have abnormally high white blood cell counts in their EPS, and subsequent prostate biopsies in this cohort showed a 50 % incidence of histologically proven inflammation [9].

In 2013, researchers concluded there was no microbiological contribution to UCPPS. They demonstrated no differences in bacterial cultures when comparing symptomatic patients with controls. Using state-of-the-art microbial detection methods, 257 patients with either presumed Category 3 prostatitis or interstitial cystitis/bladder pain syndrome and 261 asymptomatic controls were tested for uropathogens and compared. (Sixty percent of the subjects were males.) This provides the latest and best evidence regarding the absence of a microbiological contribution to urologic pelvic pain syndromes [10].

Chronic orchialgia, defined as either constant or intermittent scrotal or testicular pain, is a common component or frequently diagnosed manifestation of chronic pelvic pain in men. Unfortunately, it too is approached as an infectious disorder and too commonly treated "empirically" with long repeated courses of antibiotics. In a related study, 55 men diagnosed with chronic scrotal pain syndrome (CSPS) were thoroughly evaluated by means of history, physical examination, scrotal ultrasound, and methodical microbiological investigation. This consisted of urine localization study (four-glass test), semen cultures, and PCR tests for chlamydia trachomatis, ureaplasma urealyticum, mycoplasma hominis, and gonorrhea. Only 22 % of the men had positive cultures of clinical significance, leading the investigators to conclude that there is no evidence for the widely held belief that CSPS is the result of a chronic bacterial infection; therefore, "widespread use of antibiotics for this condition is unjustified" [11].

This author notes that investigations conducted by the NIH-NIDDK over the past 15 years have not included urine culture as entrance criteria for patients with presumed NIH Category 3 prostatitis. A single negative urinalysis sufficed as adequate screening prior to informed consent in pregabalin trial [12], alfuzosin trial [13], and physical therapy trial [14]. Study designs were formulated by a consensus of prostatitis experts, and no patients developed a urinary tract infection during these trials.

Besides antibiotics, other prostatocentric therapies are prescribed to men with CPPS. Investigators followed 100 patients with chronic prostatitis over 1 year, during which time they received sequential monotherapies that included antibiotics, alpha-blockers, and antiandrogen therapies [15]. One third of patients showed only modest symptom improvement, while only 19 % experienced significant improvement. (Placebo responses are often similar.)

15.2.1 What About LUTS?

In a study of men 50 years of age or younger with voiding dysfunction, urodynamic testing revealed bladder neck obstruction (54 %), pseudo-dyssynergia (contraction of the external sphincter during voiding) (DSD) (24 %), impaired bladder contractility (17 %), and acontractile bladder (5 %) [16]. These are often the findings among men previously diagnosed with "prostatitis." In a subsequent study, men with urodynamic evidence of pseudo-DSD, 83 % were successfully treated with biofeedback alone [17]. The investigators also noted that >90 % of the patients were first born males, which may indicate a possible biopsychosocial predisposition for this condition.

These findings were more recently reproduced in a Chinese study. Of 113 CPP patients between ages of 18 and 48, nearly 20 % were found to have urodynamic evidence of [non-neurogenic] DSD or pseudo-DSD. This was characterized as low Q max, high detrusor pressure, and high urethral pressures [18]. These patients, too, responded well to biofeedback.

Some men have bladder neck hyperplasia, which requires alpha-blockade or transurethral incision of the bladder neck. This condition needs to be proven urodynamically. While surgical intervention is highly effective, patients must be cautioned about subsequent retrograde ejaculation and secondary fertility challenges.

15.3   Dysorgasmia and Post-ejaculatory Pain

While many continue to diagnose dysorgasmia (pain with orgasm) and pain following ejaculation as "prostatitis" [19], this symptom is more commonly a component of CPP particularly in the setting of pelvic floor muscle dysfunction or pudendal neuralgia.

Approximately 50 % of men with CPP also suffer from orgasmic or post-ejaculatory pain. A Turkish study published in 2011 found that 37 % of men with CPP had painful ejaculations as compared to zero in controls [20]. A review of the literature demonstrates a range cited between 40 and 70 % [21]. In our small series of 36 consecutive patients with CPP, 25 had dysorgasmia, post-ejaculatory pain, and/or other sexual dysfunction. Forty-five percent of the patients improved with physical therapy focusing on manual release of myofascial trigger points and pelvic floor relaxation [22]. Anderson et al. studied 133 men, among whom 92 % had sexual dysfunction (including 56 % who had ejaculatory pain). Greater than 77 % improved with specialized physical therapy [23].

In my experience, many men who suffer from this condition are similarly troubled by the decrease or absence in semen volume. Their anxiety is exacerbated by their wondering if there is a blockage or a backup of semen. Anecdotally speaking, many patients who recovered from CPP by employing the approach of pelvic floor physical therapy reported improved sexual functioning, disappearance of pain, and a return of normal ejaculatory volume and force.

By coincidence, I have also had several patients who practice martial arts or Eastern religions. These ASYMPTOMATIC men described the practice of preserving Chi [Energy], by preventing ejaculation during climax. What they describe, essentially, is a form of volitional retrograde ejaculation, whereby the pelvic floor muscles are tightly contracted during orgasm, causing semen to flow into the bladder rather than forward out through the urethra, instead of through the bladder neck, leading to retrograde ejaculation. Further research revealed that learning this practice can be painful. Listening carefully to men with CPP and learning more about my other patients' practices allowed me to make the connection between these phenomena and to formulate my theory of **ejaculatory dyssynergia** (http://www.pelvicpainrehab. com/male-pelvic-pain/1994/shedding-light-on-male-pelvic-pain-and-sexual-dysfunction/). This would explain the pain and decrease in ejaculated volume during flares and the coincidence of pain relief with normal ejaculation, with enhanced pleasure, improved force, and increased volume of semen.

15.4 Pelvic Floor Muscle Dysfunction and Myofascial Trigger Points

When patients present with pain that can be associated with urinary symptoms, defecatory dysfunction, and sexual symptoms, it should be no surprise that for most patients, the pelvic floor support structures and musculature are promoting the symptomology. I ask students and patients alike to imagine this extraordinary hammock, carrying the urinary and anal sphincters within a beautifully choreographed weaving of muscles, and then to imagine when one or more of those fibers are tense, nonelastic, knotted, or broken. Without proper attention, more and more of those fibers overcompensate and eventually malfunction, hence the recruitment of larger and larger areas of pain or dysfunction. This is why we sometimes see patients with recent urinary symptoms and painful ejaculation who began their odyssey years ago in the department of colorectal surgery with a nonhealing anal fissure, for example.

We must learn from other specialties as various forms of physical therapy have been employed with success for the treatment of analogous pain syndromes diagnosed by gynecologists and colorectal surgeons. Several urologists have applied these principles in the assessment and treatment of men with symptoms of prostatitis or CPP (see Table 15.2).

In 2004, Clemens and colleagues employed biofeedback and pelvic floor reeducation/bladder training for men with chronic pelvic pain syndrome. Fourteen of the 19 men enrolled in the study underwent pretreatment urodynamics. The various urodynamic findings (detrusor instability, hypersensitivity to filling, pseudo-dyssynergia), however, did not predict treatment results [24]. Overall, there were statistically significant improvements in all symptom parameters measured by AUA symptom score, ten-point visual analog pain and urgency scores, and voiding logs. Interestingly, only half of the patients completed the full treatment course prescribed as six sessions.

Biofeedback was again the therapeutic modality in a series by Cornel and colleagues, in Holland [25]. Thirty-one of 33 men initially recruited completed the program, which included weekly and biweekly physical therapy up to six to eight treatment sessions. These patients responded quite favorably as demonstrated by the improvement in NIH-Chronic Prostatitis Symptom Index (pretreatment mean, 23.6; posttreatment mean, 11.4) and pelvic floor electromyogram measurements during

Table 15.2 Physical therapy and myofascial trigger point release definitions

Myofascial trigger point: taut bands or tender nodules that can be detected on examination which may cause painful contractions and/or referred pain when palpated or twitch responses. Areas in which trigger points are located exhibit weakness and limited range of motion
Myofascial trigger point release: a form of manual physical therapy, which addresses hyperirritable points on muscles or taut bands, which are responsible for pain or restricted movement. The release or treatment is done by compressing, strumming, or stripping muscle fibers manually or digitally
Biofeedback a technique used to control certain anxiety states or tension with the use of an external device, in this case surface EMG's which are used to train patients to relax their muscles
Skin rolling a simple technique to free subcutaneous fascia. The skin is gently picked up and pulled away from underlying structures. The skin is then released from the fingertips and adjacent skin is lifted. This is done repeatedly over afflicted body regions
Injection therapy a more immediate means of inactivating a trigger point. Helpful for patients who may not have access to further skilled manual therapy or for those with limited treatment times. Myotoxic substances should be avoided
Dry needling a form of "injection" therapy, without injectable substance. May be safer and less damaging to muscle fibers.
Effleurage: a massage technique which involves sliding or gliding over the body with continuous motion.
Theracane: a self-massage tool, which is the same size and shape of a walking cane, which can be used to more easily or comfortably reach trigger points in the back, flank, or buttocks.

rest which improved from mean 4.9 mV at initial visit to mean 1.7 mV (normal resting tone <2.0 mV).

Pelvic floor myofascial trigger point release of the pelvic floor was studied for the treatment of interstitial cystitis and [urinary] urgency-frequency syndrome. In this series by Weiss, 7 of the 52 patients were men. Of 42 patients with urgency-frequency syndrome, 83 % of patients experienced either complete resolution or moderate to marked relief of their symptoms. Of ten patients diagnosed with interstitial cystitis, 70 % reported moderate to marked improvement [26]. The author believes that pelvic floor physical therapy "arrests the neurogenic trigger leading to bladder changes, decreases central nervous system sensitivity and alleviates pain due to dysfunctional muscles."

More recently, Anderson and colleagues employed myofascial trigger point release and paradoxical (progressive relaxation in the setting of complete acceptance of the painful symptoms) relaxation for the treatment of 138 men diagnosed with CP/CPPS, refractory to "traditional" therapy [27]. Patients received a minimum of weekly treatments for 4 weeks, but some received biweekly treatments for 8 weeks thereafter. Approximately half of the patients treated had clinical improvements associated with a 25 % or greater decrease in all symptom scores, which included NIH-CPSI and PPSS. According to Global Response Assessment, 72 % of patients reported marked or moderate improvement. The authors proposed a new understanding of UCPPS, in which certain types of pelvic pain reflect a "self-feeding state of tension in the pelvic floor, perpetuated by cycles of tension, anxiety and pain."

In 2008, we completed an NIH-sponsored multicenter trial, testing the feasibility of "manual" PT for the treatment of UCPPS in men and women. This was a randomized single-blinded clinical trial evaluating myofascial physical therapy (MPT), targeted trigger point release and connective tissue manipulation (CTM) focusing on the muscles and connective tissues of the pelvic floor, hip girdle, and abdomen, **versus** global therapeutic massage (GTM), nonspecific somatic treatment with full-body Western massage. Patients received 10 weekly treatments and were evaluated within 2 weeks after the last treatment. Forty-seven patients were randomized, including 23 (49 %) men and 24 (51 %) women. Twenty-four (51 %) patients were randomized to GTM, 23 (49 %) to MPT; 44 (94 %) patients completed the study. The trial proved feasibility of manual treatments and excellent adherence to protocol. More importantly, the trial showed a statistically significant difference in the benefit of myofascial physical therapy over global therapeutic massage. The response rate of 57 % in the MPT group was significantly higher than the rate of 21 % in the GTM treatment group ($p = 0.03$). Even more striking was the significantly greater response of men to either modality when compared to women in this study [14]. Among men, 67 % responded favorably to MPT, while 44 % responded to GTM. Interestingly, only 7 % of women responded to GTM.

15.5 A Functional Somatic Syndrome or, More Accurately, Central Sensitivity Syndrome

In 2001, this author found a strong correlation between the diagnosis of nonbacterial prostatitis and functional somatic syndromes (FSS). A review of randomly selected cases demonstrated that 65 % of men seeking second opinion for CP/CPPS met the criteria for overlapping diagnoses considered to be FSS. These diagnoses included IBS (35 %), chronic headache (36 %), FM (5 %), nonspecific rheumatological symptoms (21 %), and psychological disturbances (48 %) [28].

These results are especially compelling when analyzed in the context of the general population, in which the lifetime prevalence of FSS is only 4 %.

The inspiration for this chart review had come from a paper published in the Lancet in 1999. It had been given to me by a good friend and colleague, Dr. Leonard Calabrese, at the Cleveland Clinic. As was intended, this article expanded my curiosity and broadened my view of CP/CPPS.

In this article, by Wessley and colleagues, FSS are defined as a constellation of symptoms, which are persistent and distressing and which, after appropriate medical assessment, cannot be explained in terms of a conventionally defined medical disease [29]. These conditions are estimated to represent 35 % of patients seeking outpatient consultation in every medical and surgical clinic (see Table 15.3). Wessley and colleagues state that there are FSS diagnoses in every organ system and in every medical specialty. They believe this is the by-product of medical subspecialization and that we may in fact be dealing with a single global syndrome. The review did acknowledge interstitial cystitis as urology's brand of FSS, but did not mention prostatitis. Like myself, however, others have begun to notice the association between FSS and CP/CPPS.

Table 15.3 Functional somatic syndromes by medical specialty

Psychology	Affective disorders
Rheumatology	Fibromyalgia
Neurology	Migraine and tension headache, cognitive difficulties
Infectious disease	Chronic fatigue syndrome, night sweats, sick building syndrome, gulf war illness
Gastroenterology	Irritable bowel syndrome, spastic colon, globus syndrome, non-ulcer dyspepsia
Cardiovascular	Noncardiac chest pain, mitral valve prolapse, neurally mediated hypotension
Respiratory	Hyperventilation syndrome
Ear, nose, and throat	Vestibular complaints, vasomotor rhinitis, globus syndrome, temporomandibular dysfunction
Dermatological	Non-dermatomal paresthesias
Allergy	Multiple chemical sensitivity
Gynecology	Premenstrual syndrome, vulvodynia
Colorectal	Proctalgia fugax, levator ani syndrome
Urology	Interstitial cystitis/painful bladder syndrome, female urethral syndrome, chronic [abacterial] prostatitis, prostatodynia, chronic pelvic pain syndrome

Modifications and additions from various sources [30, 31]

Self-reported medical problems were compared between 463 CP/CPPS patients and 121 controls. Domains queried included gastroenterology, cardiovascular, neurological, lymphatic, infectious, and psychological. The CP/CPPS group reported dramatically higher incidence of comorbidities (P values < 0.008) [32]. The significantly higher reported comorbidities in the CP/CPPS group are consistent with the patients' real or perceived tendency to suffer with overlapping diseases.

The first systematic exploration of the connection between UCPPS and other disorders (in women) was reported by Alagiri in 1997 [33]. They found, "Allergies, irritable bowel syndrome, and sensitive skin were the most common diseases in the interstitial cystitis population." They appropriately concluded that "Interstitial cystitis has, as yet, an unexplained association with certain other chronic disease and pain syndromes."

Clauw and colleagues examined cohorts of patients with FM, IC, and healthy controls [30]. They found that IC patients shared many characteristics of FM patients. They were much more likely than controls to have systemic tender points and to report fatigue, musculoskeletal, gastrointestinal, and cardiopulmonary symptoms. In yet another investigation, a twin control study demonstrated the aggregation of overlapping syndromes among the 127 co-twin individuals diagnosed with CFS. When compared to their non-fatigued co-twin, there was a significantly higher prevalence of FM, IBS, chronic bacterial prostatitis, pelvic pain, and interstitial cystitis in the CFS twin [34].

Central sensitization or a central sensitivity syndrome (CSS) is one of the best explanations for the phenomenon of FSS, which have both visceral and somatic manifestations. Sensitization is caused by chemical and anatomical changes leading to hyperexcitability in the dorsal horn cells from persistent afferent C fiber bombardment by painful stimuli. The presence of sensitization expands the pain field and creates a neuroanatomical basis for pain persistence and recurrence in the presence of minimal or no discernable pathology. This process will eventually cause a local upregulation and central "wind up" that creates a neuroanatomical basis for pain persistence in the presence of minimal disease or stimuli.

While recognition of FSS continues to lag, even more compelling mechanisms for CSS and its role in our daily clinical practices have become elucidated. In yet another milestone, Yunus advances the insights of Wessley to explain and justify the use of central sensitivity syndrome for conditions previously designated FSS [35]. (In terms of taxonomy and the implications of our medical terminology, Dr. Yunus is as passionate about the misuse of an FSS as this author is about the overuse of the term prostatitis!) Not only does he convincingly amalgamate strong evidence from various subspecialty studies but also unifies specific CPP conditions such as myofascial pain syndromes and psychological distress within the definition of CSS. This inspires improved ways to approach patient care and research. And like Wessley, he presents yet another compelling call to action, as all manifestations of CSS represent the majority of outpatient consultations, as listed in Table 15.3.

Yilmaz and colleagues were able to detect differences in autonomic nervous system functioning in men with CPPS. Comparing blood pressure and heart rate variability among CPP patients and controls during rest, supine positioning, or standing, revealed a significant decrease in the parasympathetic component of heart rate variability and an increase in the sympathetic component with postural change [36]. Interestingly, the sympathetic component in men with CPPS did not demonstrate the expected increase upon standing from the supine position. But this may have led to the compensatory increase in blood pressure seen in the CPPS patients. There was also higher mean BP in supine and standing positions in the CPPS group compared to controls, representing increased peripheral vascular sympathetic tone in the CPPS group. These findings suggest cardiovascular autonomic dysregulation in men with CPPS.

The concept of central sensitization is gaining recognition in the urological community; however, it is still detrimental to continue perpetuating a link between an infectious or inflammatory assault on the prostate as the trigger, when in fact, triggers for men with pelvic pain include many other urological as well as non-urological causes: passage of kidney stones, changes in sexual functioning, obsessive masturbation, vasectomy, cycling, running, anal fissure disease, hemorrhoidectomy, sports or other orthopedic trauma, etc.

Recognizing the broad spectrum of potential triggers helps to better elucidate potential pathophysiology and expand our treatment repertoire. For example, I had seen a man who had experienced scrotal pain for over 5 years. So terrific was his pain that he underwent an orchiectomy, which unfortunately afforded him no relief of symptoms. Upon further review of his history, I discovered that he had a skiing accident about 9 months prior to the onset of scrotal pain. Although his broken ankle had healed well, his gait was never completely corrected, causing asymmetrical stress to his knees, hips, and pelvis. He had developed trigger points with referred pain to the ipsilateral scrotum. His pain was resolved after physical therapy and aggressive home exercise, stretching, and orthotics.

For decades, CPP has been evaluated and managed as an end-organ diagnosis or urological condition, with little benefit to patients. We believe CPP should be approached more comprehensively as a more common and plausible FSS or central sensitivity syndrome [37].

The causes for and the perpetuation of CPP are multifactorial. Cognitive/behavioral and environmental variables can be significant predictors of patient adjustment in chronic pain. Men ($n = 253$) from a North American multi-institutional NIH-funded Chronic Prostatitis Cohort Study in six US (and one Canadian) centers participated in a survey examining pain and disability. Measures included demographics, urinary symptoms, depression, pain, disability, catastrophizing, control over pain, pain-contingent rest, social support, and solicitous responses from a significant other. Regressions showed that urinary symptoms, depression, and helplessness catastrophizing predicted overall pain. Cognitive/behavioral variables of catastrophizing and pain-contingent rest, respectively, predicted greater pain and disability. Catastrophic helplessness was a prominent pain predictor [31]. The patients' coping and adaptive skills may influence the predisposition or perpetuation of symptoms in CP/CPPS patients, as well as perceived quality of life.

These observations, for example, could provide insights for cognitive therapy and patient self-care regimens.

Other investigators examined whether perceived stress was associated (longitudinally) with pain intensity and pain-related disability. A cohort of 224 men with CP/CPPS were followed for 1 year. Perceived stress and pain intensity measures were done at 1, 3, 6, and 12 months after diagnosis. Greater perceived stress during the 6 months after the health-care visit was associated with greater pain intensity ($p = .03$) and disability ($p = .003$) at 12 months, even after controlling for age, symptom duration, and pain and disability during the first 6 months [38].

Chronic stress may have a role in initiating or exacerbating pain syndromes including CP/CPPS. To that end, Anderson and colleagues demonstrated potential disturbances in psychosocial profiles and hypothalamic-pituitary-adrenal (HPA) function among patients with CP/CPPS. Forty-five men with CP/CPPS and 20 age-matched controls completed the Type A Personality Test, Perceived Stress Scale, Beck Anxiety Inventory, and the Brief Symptom Inventory for distress and physical symptoms. Saliva samples were collected at specific times over a 2-day period in order to measure free cortisol, reflecting secretory activity of the hypothalamic-pituitary-adrenal axis. Perceived stress and anxiety were significantly higher among men with CP/CPPS than controls, as were all other psychosocial variables. Men with chronic pelvic pain syndrome had significantly increased awakening cortisol responses, mean slope of 0.85 vs. 0.59 for controls ($p < 0.05$) [39].

As also reviewed and summarized by Yunus [35], CSS are highly correlated to HPA axis dysfunction and hyperexcitability of the central neurons. We would expect, therefore, neuroendocrine dysfunction in this cohort of patients, which explains both the precipitating and perpetuating influences of stress and the bidirectional cascade of this vicious cycle.

Table 15.4 Differential diagnosis of male chronic pelvic pain

Infection: Sexually transmitted diseases, chronic bacterial prostatitis, fungal infection
Gastrointestinal: Appendicitis, diverticulitis, constipation, anal fissures, hemorrhoids
Abdominal wall defects: Inguinal or ventral wall hernias, myofascial trigger points
Musculoskeletal: Neoplasm (primary or metastatic), degenerative joint disease of the hips, sacroiliitis, leg length disparity, athletic or orthopedic issues, pelvic floor dysfunction, myofascial pelvic pain syndrome
Neurologic: Low thoracic or lumbar herniated nucleus pulposus, lumbar stenosis, Parkinson disease, diabetic cystopathy, demyelinating disease, pudendal neuralgia
Central sensitivity syndromes: See functional somatic syndrome in Table 15.2
Urologic: Renal calculi, varicocele, epididymitis, testicular neoplasm, interstitial cystitis

15.5.1 Evaluation and Management

The differential diagnosis should be reviewed in advance to better query the patient during his interview and guide the physical examination (see Table 15.4).

The UPOINT classification system has been proposed as a first step toward a more ideal approach to men with pelvic pain. It does, however, have several deficiencies. The nomogram represents U for urinary, P for psychological, O for organ (prostate), I for infection, N for neurological, and T for tenderness [of muscles]. The authors of this construct point out the benefits of treating patients according to the subclassifications to better tailor therapy [40].

While the authors should be applauded for widening the scope of our approach to these patients, they still cannot seem to extricate themselves from "O" (the prostate organ) nor the "I" for infection. By definition, Category 3 prostatitis is nonbacterial and, as mentioned before, not proven to be caused by any malady of the prostate gland. Additionally, the N for neurological is poorly defined, as it is meant to somehow encompass the role of functional somatic syndromes and perhaps other neuralgias or nerve entrapment syndromes such as pudendal neuralgia. And finally, T for tenderness does not do justice to the very broad and specialized field of physical medicine and the detection of myofascial trigger points, which are clearly different from "tender" points. The UPOINT system does not address or explain the treatment or release of the trigger points. There is no acknowledgment of "T" or the clusion of myofascial pain syndromes as a single domain, which can be causing symptoms in the other domains. Moreover, rather than treating each component of the patients' symptomatology via the nomogram, it may be of greater benefit to treat myofascial trigger points in order to relieve urinary symptoms (U), perceive pain in the bladder or prostate (O), and relieve pelvic muscle tension, which can exacerbate nerve entrapment (N). Likewise, exercises and stretching to enhance the treatment and durability of manual trigger point release can be empowering and therefore improve patients' psychological well-being (P) as well.

After excluding acute conditions, such as prostatitis (fever, abnormal urinalysis, positive urine cultures) or other urological conditions such as kidney stone or general surgical issues such as hernias, colorectal pathology (fissures, hemorrhoids, abscess, neoplasm), or spinal column diseases, I approach the patient from a broader vantage point.

The history should include queries about occupational risk factors, repetitive motions, prolonged sitting, and recreational activities and sports. There should also be query into sexual activities, family and work relationships, and stressful life events. I usually compose a genogram for each patient, which not only provides family medical history but also illustrates important family dynamics which are often implicated as unhealthy patterns which predispose or impact patient's ability to achieve self-care and resolution of his condition (see Fig. 15.1).

The history should also explore the potential for underlying FSS or CSS, which is quite common in this patient population.

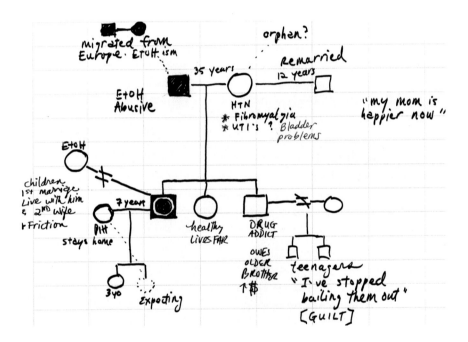

◉	=	patient
□	=	living family member
■	=	deceased family member
—	=	marriage
≠	=	divorce or separation

Appreciate the more comprehensive picture of this man with CPP as compared to that seen in a standard Past Medical and Family History. Note his need to take care of others parallels his Mom's enabling behavior and the predispositions to central sensitivity syndromes (as highlighted by *).

Fig. 15.1 A sample genogram

Table 15.5 Some common referred patterns of musculoskeletal sources of pain and symptoms	Psoas	Bladder or suprapubic pain; urgency
	Rectus abdominis	Penile pain
	External oblique	Suprapubic, bladder pressure, sometimes scrotal ache
	Quadratus lumborum	Scrotal/inguinal pain
	Obturator internus	Scrotum, perineum, urinary pressure
	Puborectalis	Tip of penis
	Bulbospongiosus	Perineum and penis
	Adductors	Groin, perineum, or base of penis

Based on the observations of others and my own experience [44, 45]

The examiner should be aware of characteristic referral patterns caused by myofascial trigger points, though variability exists between patients. These patterns can be confirmed during physical examination. Patients are often helpful by offering feedback during the exam, with respect to location of trigger points and character of referred pain [41]. In addition to complete physical and genitourinary examination, careful palpation of abdominal wall, pelvic floor, and thigh muscles may reveal taut bands characteristic of trigger points with associated twitch response and/or pain [42]. Many of the referred patterns illustrated by Travell and Simon were later corroborated by Anderson and colleagues [43] (see Table 15.5).

I believe this part of the evaluation is best performed with the patient in a supine lithotomy position, allowing for thorough examination of the external and internal muscles of the pelvic floor [46]. I carefully examine the coccyx for range of motion and pain as well as corresponding tension or knots in the levator ani muscle groups. The obturator internus is palpated and provocative testing can be applied by having the patient externally rotate against the resistance of the examiner's other hand. Alcock's canal should be gently explored to test for Tinel sign, indicating pudendal nerve hypersensitivity. Further testing may reveal nerve irritability with referred pain patterns in the distribution of the pudendal nerve branches. Obviously, the prostate is also examined for nodules and texture changes. But I reserve the exam of the prostate until the very end of the internal pelvic exam, so as to better educate the patient about his anatomy and the genuine sources of his discomfort.

I reposition the patient to assess posture, pelvic obliquity, and leg length symmetry along with strength, flexibility, and range of motion.

Urinalysis is performed to exclude bacteriuria, funguria, pyuria, or hematuria. Localization cultures should be considered in patients who have had previously documented positive bacterial urine cultures or past episodes associated with fever. Localization cultures should be performed to guide future evaluation and treatment and more importantly avoid or discontinue unnecessary antibiotics. Prescribing antibiotics empirically is very rarely appropriate and inexcusable without first performing localization cultures. History will also guide the appropriateness of STI testing. In addition to testing for chlamydia and gonorrhea, microscopic exam of the

VB1 may reveal trichomoniasis, and one may consider testing for ureaplasma urealyticum and Mycoplasma hominis [44]. I have found this useful in men with history of chlamydia infection in the past, who have recurrence of their symptoms without evidence of chlamydia after PCR testing.

As observed by Wessley and later by Yunus, regardless of the type of CSS diagnosed, patients respond favorably to similar factors. These include empathy, engagement of caregiver, explanation of the physiological nature of symptoms, limitation of investigations, emphasis on management rather than cure, antidepressants, cognitive behavioral therapy, and exercise. These qualities and interventions should be similarly considered for the man suffering from CPP.

Patient empowerment is paramount to management of symptoms of CPP. For men who are diagnosed with pelvic floor muscle dysfunction and/or myofascial trigger points, empowerment begins with muscle and postural reeducation to prevent further tissue compromise and to increase patient awareness and enhance balance and muscle tone [45].

Physical therapy for men with CPP involves connective tissue manipulation (CTM) and trigger point release to all body wall tissues of abdomen, back, buttocks, and thighs that are found to contain myofascial trigger points or other connective tissue abnormalities. In the prone position, CMT can be applied posteriorly, from inferior thoracic level 10 to the popliteal creases. These techniques are applied until the therapist notices a favorable texture change within the affected tissue.

In the supine position, CTM can be applied to anterior tissues. This allows the inclusion of the thighs, laterally, anteriorly, and medially from the knee up to and including the thigh crease. CTM can be performed on the abdominal wall from the suprapubic rim to the anterior costal cartilages, with a concentration of manual interventions to focus on the periumbilical tissues. This usually involves a skin rolling technique, which should be taught to patients as part of their self-care regimen. Manual trigger point release techniques are utilized to treat any noted trigger points or scars in the anterior or posterior lower quadrants. Options for the treatment of trigger points include manual release, manual stretching with and without cold spray, myofascial release, muscle play, dry needling, or injection therapy. Therapy for dysfunctional muscles includes stripping, strumming, skin rolling, and effleurage [47]. Sometimes, myofascial trigger point release requires adjuvant therapies, which include dry needling or injection therapies. Self-care of the external trigger points can be performed using a tennis ball against the wall or against the floor. A theracane can also be employed by the patient to reach his own trigger points comfortably and apply pressure according to his own leverage and tolerance. Tennis balls are also helpful, targeting external trigger points by leaning against them either on the wall or on the floor for increased pressure.

Transrectal treatment of the soft tissues of the pelvic floor with CTM can be done with the patient in supine lithotomy, lateral sims, or prone positions depending on the patient's trigger point locations, comfort of the patient, and ergonomics of the therapist. Regions evaluated and treated include periurethral tissues, white line, muscle origins, and insertions. Myofascial manipulation to each muscle group is performed with the focus on restrictive bands and trigger points. Self-care for internal trigger points has been both challenging and controversial. In 2011, investigators did prove feasibility and safety of an internal wand which comes equipped with a pressure gauge, allowing patients to measure the amount of pressure applied and to gradually titrate gentle force against the trigger points [48]. Of course, this requires special individualized instruction, as yet not available to the public.

Providing a form of biofeedback to patients by observing their progress in recruiting muscles and relaxing the pelvic floor helps patients to learn valuable pelvic floor "drop" techniques [47] which has been shown to help diminish pain as well as extinguish urinary urgency.

Severe discomfort may prohibit or limit transrectal therapy, but can be employed as treatments progress. However, I have also found that some patients improve without internal therapy, as the external therapies along with patient exercise and stretching at home can lead to what I call a beneficial cascading effect on the pelvic floor muscles.

Encouraging patients to resume some form of physical activity cannot be overemphasized. (Some patients are so frightened by the pain that they require medical permission to engage in any form of exercise.) Walking, for example, can lead to a positive feedback, whereby the stride increases, gait normalizes, and the patient in essence is providing his own pelvic floor muscle strengthening and lengthening.

Home exercise programs are tailored according to the patient's condition, his lifestyle, and abilities. These are prescribed to promote further muscle lengthening and pelvic floor reeducation as well as enhance durability of PT.

In the book, *A Headache in the Pelvis*, Anderson and Wise provide patients with much needed validation. Their valuable insights educate patients about the pathophysiology of most pelvic pain syndromes along with specific anatomical information which empowers patients to seek a non-urological approach to their diagnosis and to accept subsequent responsibility for the regimen involving physical therapy, self-care, and specialized relaxation techniques mentioned earlier in the chapter.

Ending Male Pelvic Pain, by Isa Herrera, includes many photographs to help guide patients through various exercises and stretches targeting muscle groups usually implicated in CPP [49]. The author provides a urological and pelvic floor overview along with detailed instructions for exercise and self-care. Some exercises and poses are adopted from traditional yoga practices. In addition to *A Headache in the Pelvis*, I also recommend this book, which helps relieve the loneliness and catastrophizing experienced by so many men with CPP. Both books are very accessible and inspiring.

A variety of stress management and psychological counseling options should be made available to men with CPP. These psychologically based alternatives should be explained as a synergistic part of medical modalities and physical interventions. Over 20 years of practice, I have noted that some of my patients are comfortable with church-based counseling and support, while others have found solace in meditation and yoga. Still others have remedied their anxiety through a series of relaxation tapes, guided imagery, or the paradoxical relaxation techniques as described in *A Headache in the Pelvis*, by Wise and Anderson [27].

In the early twentieth century, Edmund Jacobson, "the father of relaxation therapy," developed progressive relaxation techniques. Based on his work and other more contemporary psychologists, Dr. Wise developed *Paradoxical Relaxation*. While employing some of the Jacobson's progressive relaxation methods, Dr. Wise incorporates forgiveness and acceptance into his practice. Simply summarized, the paradox in this version of relaxation is the acceptance and embracing of one's pelvic pain rather than fighting or resenting it. In his book entitled *Paradoxical Relaxation*, the development, rationale, and instruction for this form of self-care is beautifully detailed [50]. The author emphasizes the need to practice these techniques regularly so as to be prepared for the inevitable flare-ups, which occur during recovery. He uses the metaphor of trying to build a well while trying to put out a house fire. A well, of course, must be in place in order to be prepared for such events.

Some institutions provide psychological support to men through programs such as "Executive Coaching," which may afford patients a more comfortable avenue toward psychotherapy. Some relaxation techniques might also be incorporated with physiotherapy using biofeedback, creative visualization, deep breathing, and hand warming techniques.

It is not feasible for clinicians to conduct all of these types of treatments; however, clinicians must be familiar with and conversant about the options and resources available to each patient. Patients should be convinced and therefore confident about their management strategies. Because there is no "quick fix" for CPP, I believe the patient's investment must be derived, in part, from his physician's level of engagement.

15.6   A Brief Word about Prostatitis (Affecting only 5 % of Symptomatic Men)

Acute prostatitis (NIH Category 1) is the easiest of the prostatitis syndromes to recognize. Patients present with moderate to severe lower urinary tract symptoms (LUTS) characteristic of bladder infection, associated with fever, chills, malaise, perineal, rectal, lower back pain, and, sometimes, generalized arthralgias/myalgias. On physical exam, patients may have urinary retention, and the prostate gland is typically exquisitely tender. Urinalysis and cultures are usually positive; the most common organism cultured in this setting is *Escherichia coli* (80 %). Other pathogens include *Pseudomonas aeruginosa*, *Serratia*, *Klebsiella*, *Proteus*, and enterococci; however there are shifts in the bacterial spectrum due to regional uses or overuses of antibiotics and the emergence of more resistant strains.

Fluoroquinolones remain the mainstay of therapy. Initial therapy should be administered intravenously. Antibiotic alternatives for acute bacterial prostatitis are ampicillin/gentamicin combination, doxycycline, and trimethoprim-sulfamethoxazole. Treatment duration should total 4–6 weeks and can be completed using oral regimens after acute symptoms subside to prevent chronic bacterial prostatitis and/or prostatic abscess. In men with urinary retention, urethral catheterization may increase the likelihood of prostatic abscess formation; therefore, one should strongly consider suprapubic catheter placement.

Chronic bacterial prostatitis (NIH Category 2) is more commonly found in older men as a relapsing disease with occasional exacerbations. Patients typically have a history of recurring urinary tract infections, but asymptomatic bacteriuria may also be the presenting sign. In this form of prostatitis, the prostate serves as a reservoir for bacteria. Bacterial localization cultures using the Meares–Stamey 4-glass technique, described earlier in this chapter, are necessary to confirm the diagnosis and identify the culpable organism. A modification of this technique is the pre-post massage test [51], which may be more feasible in a busy clinic setting. Recurrent infection caused by the same organism is considered one of the hallmarks of this disease.

Despite therapy, cure rates for chronic bacterial prostates are less than optimal. Prescribing antibiotics that can achieve adequate concentrations in prostatic fluid is essential; fluoroquinolones have been shown to be most efficacious. Other antibiotic alternatives include carbenicillin, doxycycline, and cephalexin. Treatment duration may vary from a minimum of 4 weeks up to 4 months. Weidner and colleagues [52] demonstrated the eradication of pathogens from expressed prostatic secretions (EPS) in 92 % of patients 3 months after a 4-week course of ciprofloxacin. After 12–24 months, 70–80 % of patients remained "cured." The presence of prostatic calculi did not influence treatment outcome in this study. In patients with frequent or serious recurrences, suppressive antibiotic regimens should be prescribed using low doses of TMP-sulfa, nitrofurantoin, or tetracycline on a daily basis. I usually consider suppressive therapy sooner in patients who have no prodrome of infection and present with fulminant uroseptic events. I also consider suppressive therapy earlier among patients who are chronically anticoagulated, in order to avoid frequent fluctuations in therapeutic warfarin levels. Transurethral resection of the prostate may afford cure in some patients; however, this remains highly controversial and usually reserved only for those patients with strong BPH indication for surgery.

15.7 Conclusion

Men suffering from chronic pelvic pain deserve a more compassionate and comprehensive approach, incorporating the lessons learned from other subspecialties. We must also consistently apply the concepts of central sensitization as they apply directly to pain perception, neuroendocrine dysfunction and stress, and myofascial and pelvic floor muscle dysfunction which can affect defecation, voiding, and sexual activity. Management often requires a component of self-care, which can be very challenging for patients with chronic and debilitating conditions such as this. Antibiotics must be avoided in men who are afebrile and have normal urine sediment! Patient empowerment derived from a positive physician-patient relationship is essential to therapy.

References

1. Gonder MJ. Prostatitis. Lancet. 1963;83:305–6.
2. Nickel JC, Downey J, Clark J, et al. Levofloxacin for chronic prostatitis/chronic pelvic pain syndrome in men: a randomized placebo- controlled multicenter trial. Urology. 2003;62: 614–7.
3. Alexander RB, Propert KJ, Schaeffer AJ, et al. Ciprofloxacin or tamsulosin in men with chronic prostatitis/chronic pelvic pain syndrome: a randomized, double-blind trial. Ann Intern Med. 2004;141:581–9.
4. Schaeffer AJ, Knauss JS, Landis JR, et al. Leukocyte and bacterial counts do not correlate with severity of symptoms in men with chronic prostatitis: the National Institutes of Health Chronic Prostatitis Cohort Study. J Urol. 2002;168:1048–53.
5. Meares EM, Stamey TA. Bacteriologic localization patterns in bacterial prostatitis and urethritis. Invest Urol. 1968;5:492–518.
6. Nickel JC, Alexander RB, Schaeffer AJ, et al. Leukocytes and bacteria in men with chronic prostatitis/chronic pelvic pain syndrome compared to asymptomatic controls. J Urol. 2003;170:818–22.
7. Nickel JC. Recommendations for the evaluation of patients with prostatitis. World J Urol. 2003;21(2):75–81. From the Giessen Consensus Meeting, Giessen 2002.
8. Sharma RK, Pasqualotto FF, Nelson DR, et al. Role of leukocytospermia in oxidative stress. J Androl. 2001;22:575–83.
9. Potts JM. Prospective Identification of NIH-Category IV prostatitis in men with elevated PSA levels. J Urol. 2000;164:1550–3.
10. Nickel JC, Stephens A, Chen J, et al. Application of State-of-the-Art Methods to Search for Microbial Contributions to the Etiology of Urological Chronic Pelvic Pain Syndrome (UCPPS) Abstract 1147, presented at American Urologic Association Annual Meeting, 2013.
11. Strebel RT, Schmidt C, Beatrice J, Sulser T. Chronic scrotal pain syndrome (CSPS): the widespread use of antibiotics is not justified. Andrology. 2013;1(1):155–9.
12. Pontari MA, Krieger JN, Litwin MS, et al. Pregabalin for the treatment of men with chronic prostatitis/chronic pelvic pain syndrome: a randomized controlled trial. Arch Intern Med. 2010;170(17):1586–93.
13. Nickel JC, Krieger JN, McNaughton-Collins M, et al. Alfuzosin and symptoms of chronic prostatitis- chronic pelvic pain syndrome. NEJM. 2008;359:2663–73.
14. Fitzgerald M, Anderson R, Potts J, et al. UPPCRN: randomized multicenter feasibility trial of myofascial physical therapy for the treatment of urologic chronic pelvic pain syndromes. J Urol. 2009;182:570–80.
15. Nickel JC, Downey J, Ardern D, Clark J, Nickel K. Failure of a monotherapy strategy for difficult chronic prostatitis/chronic pelvic pain syndrome. J Urol. 2004;172:551–4.
16. Kaplan SA, Ikeguchi EF, Santarosa RP, et al. Etiology of voiding dysfunction in men less than 50 years of age. Urology. 1996;47:836–9.
17. Kaplan SA, Santarosa RP, D'Alisera PM, et al. Psuedodyssynergia (contraction of the external sphincter during voiding) misdiagnosed as chronic non-bacterial prostatitis and the role of biofeedback as a therapeutic option. J Urol. 1997;157:2234–7.
18. Zu XB, Ye ZQ, Zhou SW, Qi L, Yang ZQ. Chronic prostatitis with non-neurogenic detrusor sphincter dyssynergia: diagnosis and treatment. Zhonghua Nan Ke Xue. 2010;16(2): 146–9.
19. Nickel JC, Elhilali M, Emberton M, Vallancien G. The Alf-One Study Group. The beneficial effect of alfuzosin 10 mg once daily in real life practice on lower urinary tract symptoms, quality of life and sexual dysfunction in men with LUTS and painful ejaculation. BJU Int. 2006;97:1242–6.
20. Sönmez NC, Kiremit MC, Güney S, et al. Sexual dysfunction in type III chronic prostatitis (CP) and chronic pelvic pain syndrome (CPPS) observed in Turkish patients. Int Urol Nephrol. 2011;43(2):309–14.

21. Magri V, Wagenlehner F, Perletti G, Schneider S, Marras E, Naber KG, Weidner W. Use of the UPOINT chronic prostatitis/chronic pelvic pain syndrome classification in European patient cohorts: sexual function domain improves correlations. J Urol. 2010;184(6):2339–45.
22. Potts JM, Decker S. Specialized physiotherapy for sexual discomfort and dysorgasmia associated with UCPPS. Presented at the 6th Annual Meeting of the International Society for Men's Health, Nice, France, 2010.
23. Anderson RU, Wise D, Sawyer T, Chan CA. Sexual dysfunction in men with chronic prostatitis/chronic pelvic pain syndrome: improvement after trigger point release and paradoxical relaxation training. J Urol. 2006;176(4 Pt 1):1534–8.
24. Clemens JQ, Nadler RB, Schaeffer AJ, Belani J, Albaugh J, Bushman W. Biofeedback, pelvic floor re-education, and bladder training for male chronic pelvic pain syndrome. Urology. 2000; 56(6):951–5.
25. Cornel EB, van Haarst EP, Schaarsberg RW, Geels J. The effect of biofeedback physical therapy in men with chronic pelvic pain syndrome type III. Eur Urol. 2005;47:607–11.
26. Weiss JM. Pelvic floor myofascial trigger points: manual therapy for interstitial cystitis and the urgency-frequency syndrome. J Urol. 2001;166:2226–31.
27. Anderson RU, Wise D, Sawyer T, Chan C. Integration of myofascial trigger point release and paradoxical relation training treatment of chronic pelvic pain in men. J Urol. 2005;174: 155–60.
28. Potts JM, Moritz N, Everson D, et al. Chronic abacterial prostatitis: a functional somatic syndrome? [abstract]. Presented at: Annual Meeting of the American Urological Association; June 2, 2001; Anaheim, CA. Abstract 2005126.
29. Wessley S, Nimnuin C, Sharpe M. Functional somatic syndromes: one or many? Lancet. 1999;354:936–9.
30. Clauw DJ, Schmidt M, Radulovic D, et al. The relationship between fibromyalgia and interstitial cystitis. J Psychiatr Res. 1997;31(1):125–31.
31. Tripp DA, Nickel JC, Wang Y, Litwin MS, McNaughton-Collins M, Landis JR, Alexander RB, Schaeffer AJ, O'Leary MP, Pontari MA, Fowler Jr JE, Nyberg LM, Kusek JW, NIH-CPCRN Study Group. Catastrophizing and pain-contingent rest predict patient adjustment in men with chronic prostatitis/chronic pelvic pain syndrome. J Pain. 2006;7(10):697–708.
32. Pontari MA, McNaughton-Collins M, O'leary MP, et al. A case-control study of risk factors in men with chronic pelvic pain syndrome. BJU Int. 2005;96(4):559–65.
33. Alagiri M, Chottiner S, Ratner V, et al. Interstitial cystitis: unexplained associations with other chronic disease and pain syndromes. Urology. 1997;49(5A suppl):52–7.
34. Aaron LA, Herrell R, Ashton S, et al. Comorbid clinical conditions in chronic fatigue: a co- twin control study. J Gen Intern Med. 2001;16:24–31.
35. Yunus MB. Fibromyalgia and overlapping disorders: the unifying concept of central sensitivity syndromes. Semin Arthritis Rheum. 2007;36:339–56.
36. Yilmaz U, Liu YW, Berger RE, Yang CC. Autonomic nervous system changes in men with chronic pelvic pain syndrome. J Urol. 2007;177:2170–4.
37. Potts JM, Payne CK. Critical review: urologic chronic pelvic pain in men and women. Pain. 2012;153(4):755–8.
38. Ullrich PM, Turner JA, Ciol M, Berger R. Stress is associated with subsequent pain and disability among men with nonbacterial prostatitis/pelvic pain. Ann Behav Med. 2005;30(2): 112–8.
39. Anderson RU, Orenberg EK, Chan CA, Morey A, Flores V. Psychometric profiles and hypothalamic-pituitary-adrenal axis function in men with chronic prostatitis/chronic pelvic pain syndrome. J Urol. 2008;179(3):956–60.
40. Shoskes DA, Nickel JC, Dolinga R, et al. Clinical phenotyping of patients with chronic prostatitis/chronic pelvic pain syndrome and correlation with symptom severity. Urology. 2009;73:538.
41. Benjamin PJ, Tappan FM. Handbook of healing massage techniques – classic, holistic, and emerging methods. Upper Saddle River, NJ: Pearson Education; 2005.
42. Travell JG. Myofascial pain and dysfunction: the trigger point manual. Baltimore: Williams and Wilkins; 1983.

43. Anderson RU, Sawyer T, Wise D, et al. Painful myofascial trigger points and pain sites in men with chronic prostatitis/chronic pelvic pain syndrome. J Urol. 2009;182(6):2753–8.
44. Potts JM, Sharma R, Pasqualotto F, et al. Association of Ureaplasma urealyticum with abnormal reactive oxygen species levels and absence of leukocytospermia. J Urol. 2000;163: 1775–8.
45. Potts JM, O'Dougherty E. Pelvic floor physical therapy for patients with prostatitis. Curr Urol Rep. 2000;1:155–8.
46. Potts J. Physical therapy for CP/CPPS. In: Shoskes DA, editor. Prostatitis. Totowa, NJ: Humana Press; 2008.
47. Kotarinos RK. CP/CPPS pelvic floor dysfunction: evaluation and treatment. GU-IT IS Humana Press; 2007.
48. Anderson R, Wise D, Sawyer T, Nathanson BH. Safety and effectiveness of an internal pelvic myofascial trigger point wand for urologic chronic pelvic pain syndrome. Clin J Pain. 2011;27(9):764–8.
49. Herrera I. Ending male pelvic pain. New York: Duplex; 2013.
50. Wise D. Paradoxical relaxation: the theory and practice of dissolving anxiety by accepting it. Occidental, CA: National Center for Pelvic Pain Research; 2010.
51. Nickel JC. The Pre and Post Massage Test (PPMT): a simple screen for prostatitis. Tech Urol. 1997;3:38–43.
52. Weidner W, Ludwig M, Brahler E, Schiefer HG. Outcome of antibiotic therapy with ciprofloxacin in chronic bacterial prostatitis. Drugs. 1999;58 suppl 2:103–6.

Male Mental Health: A Peek Inside the Black Box

16

Dean A. Tripp and Hayley Yurgan

16.1 Introduction

Mental illness is a worldwide leading cause of poor health and disability, with approximately 450 million people currently suffering from mental illness [1]. The prevalence of mental health struggles in North America makes it an important topic of discussion. This chapter will examine the impact of mental health in adult males.

Approximately 10 % of Canadian and 16.8 % of American males suffer from mental illness [2, 3]. Men tend to be diagnosed with externalizing [e.g., schizophrenia, antisocial personality disorder, attention deficit hyperactivity disorder (ADHD), conduct disorder] and substance disorders more often than women [4]. In the United States, approximately 17 % of men and 8 % of women develop alcohol dependence during their lives [5].

Women are more often diagnosed with mood and anxiety disorders than men. The fairly stable 2:1 ratio seen across cultures might reason for a biological rationalization for depression, but research across countries suggests that social explanations are at play [6–8]. Interestingly, research suggests that this gender gap may even widen as we age [4]. A study on gender differences in mental disorders that included over 70,000 adults from 15 different countries and 4 different age groups showed that gender differences in major depressive disorder (MDD) and substance disorders were significantly smaller in younger cohorts [4]. The gender role hypothesis suggests that gender differences in mental health disturbances may become more prominent as the societal roles of males and females become more distinct. This is especially noted in more developed areas of the world such as North

D.A. Tripp, Ph.D. (✉)
Department of Psychology, Anesthesiology & Urology, Queen's University,
62 Arch Street, Kingston, ON K7L 3N6, Canada
e-mail: dean.tripp@queensu.ca

H. Yurgan, B.Sc.H.
Department of Psychology, Queen's University, Kingston, ON, Canada

© Springer Science+Business Media New York 2016
J.M. Potts (ed.), *Men's Health*, DOI 10.1007/978-1-4939-3237-5_16

America, where gender roles of males and females are becoming more alike. Thus, recognizing the importance and role of gender norms and psychosocial factors in male mental health is crucial in improving their overall health and quality of life (QoL).

16.1.1 Screening Tools

Physicians play an essential role in identifying depression, which is considered a first step to improving mental health. Valid and reliable screening instruments are imperative. Accurate yet easy-to-administer depression screens can make it more convenient for physicians to incorporate psychological screening into clinical routines. Ideally, a diagnostic test should meet three criteria: provide accurate diagnostic information, support the need for therapy, and provide an index for improved patient outcomes [9].

Although there are many mental health and depression screening tools (for a review, see Anderson et al. [9]), two valid and reliable screening tools used in our clinic and research lab are the general health questionnaire twelve (GHQ-12; to assess general mental health) and the primary care evaluation of mental disorders (PRIME-MD; to assess depression) (see Table 16.1) [9]. The GHQ-12 is a self-administered screen used to identify current mental disturbances and disorders [10]. With only 12 items, the GHQ-12 is convenient for clinicians to use as an initial screening tool. It assesses a wide variety of mental disorders defined by the DSM-IV

Table 16.1 Mental health screening tools

Name	Abbreviation	Authors	Number of items	Administration	Description
General health questionnaire twelve	GHQ-12	Goldberg and Hillier	12	Self-administered	Measures the risk of developing psychological disorders
Patient health questionnaire nine	PRIME-MD/ PHQ-9	Kroenke, Spitzer, and Williams	9	Self-administered	Screens for depression
Patient health questionnaire two	PRIME-MD/ PHQ-2	Kroenke, Spitzer, and Williams	2–6	Clinician administered	Screens for depression. If answers to the first two questions are positive, four more specific questions are asked

including substance abuse, psychiatric disorders, mood disorders, and anxiety disorders.

To screen for depression, a self-report version of the PRIME-MD known as the patient health questionnaire nine (PHQ-9) can be easily completed in approximately 3 min by the patient [11]. The PHQ-9 provides a potential diagnosis and a depression severity score, making it a convenient tool to follow outcomes of therapeutic intervention [9]. The PHQ-9 is also a valid and reliable tool, making it applicable to both clinical and research purposes. To quickly screen for depression, a brief version of the PRIME-MD, the patient health questionnaire two (PHQ-2), requires the patient to answer 2 questions: (1) Have you been bothered by little interest or pleasure in doing things? (2) Have you been feeling down, depressed, or hopeless in the last month? If the patient responds yes to these questions, the healthcare provider should inquire further with questions related to sleep disturbance, appetite change, low self-esteem, and anhedonia (i.e., inability to experience pleasure). If the patient reports two or more of these additional disturbances, the provider should consider more comprehensive questioning of current stressors, supports, and physical comorbidities alongside immediate and longer-term treatment options [12].

16.2 Depression in Men

The incidence of depression is on the rise, with approximately 5 % suffering from the condition [13]. As many as 6 % of Canadians and 8 % of Americans are currently suffering from depression [14, 15]. Depression is the leading cause of disability for Americans between the ages of 15 and 44 years [16]. More specifically, within the United States, approximately six million men report depression each year [17]. A person diagnosed with a depressive disorder is experiencing a sad, empty, or irritable mood, accompanied by somatic and cognitive changes that greatly affect their ability to function [18]. Depressive disorders can range in severity and symptoms depending on the individual case. Therefore, targeting therapy to fit the individual is an important consideration.

Fewer men than women are diagnosed with depression in developed countries with a ratio of 2:1 [6, 7], but the underreporting of mental illness in men may account for this discrepancy. In addition, men may not exhibit the conventionally viewed symptoms of depression [19]. Men's depression symptoms may be expressed in terms of increases in fatigue, irritability and anger (sometimes abusive in nature), loss of interest in work or hobbies, and sleep disturbances rather than the traditional depressive sad affect [20]. It has also been suggested that men use more drugs and alcohol than women, perhaps to self-medicate their depression, which can hide symptoms of depression, making diagnosis and treatment more difficult. Therefore, a lower prevalence in men may be part underreporting, misdiagnosis due to nontraditional symptoms, and avoidance of services.

Although reported rates of depression in men are lower, suicide death rates are four times higher in men than women [21]. Suicide in men has been described as a "silent epidemic" due to its high prevalence and a lack of public awareness [22].

The incidence of male suicide increases with age, peaking in the late 40s [22]. Men's traditionally low levels of help-seeking behaviors may contribute to discrepancies in suicide rates. Indeed, in the year before suicide, an average of 58 % of women visited a mental health professional, while only 35 % of men sought out mental healthcare in the year before suicide [23]. Importantly, 78 % of men who died by suicide were in contact with their primary care provider (e.g., physician) within the year of their suicide. Receiving medical and/or psychological assistance from a healthcare professional can help counteract suicidal thinking, further supporting the role of primary care providers in mental health. Some men may even feel more comfortable going to see their physician than a psychologist. If the physician is able to screen for depression and suicidal tendencies, they will be in a much better position to encourage men to seek further help from a mental health professional.

16.3   What Promotes Mental Health Struggles in Males?

Understanding is a key start in any treatment approach. The dominant narrative about men is that men are more reluctant to seek help than women, regardless of the health concern. Likewise, according to the mental health literature, men are more likely to be resistant to seeking help for distress [24, 25]. However, research shows the links between gender and mental health struggles are more complex than once believed. In particular, the following areas have been promoted as key factors in male mental health:

16.3.1 Stigma

Stigma is the most prominent obstacle to seeking out and accessing mental health services for men [26]. Stigma refers to a set of negative beliefs, attitudes, and behaviors that labels individuals and disseminates stereotypes. Reducing stigma is necessary to increase the use of mental health services, in turn, enhancing mental health in general. When it comes to mental health, there are three main stereotypical elements involved in public stigma: dangerousness, avoidance, and character weakness [27]. A person with a mental illness is often believed to be violent or unpredictable [28, 29], leading others to avoid contact. These beliefs are unfortunately embedded in North American culture and may lead to reluctance in reporting poor mental health.

Men tend to have higher stigmatizing attitudes than women when it comes to mental health. In studies of depression stigmatization, men report higher proportions of stigmatizing attitudes than women. More specifically, men believed that depressed individuals could "snap out of it," should be avoided, and are unpredictable [26]. Previous research has indicated that education programs that raise awareness and increase mental health knowledge can help to reduce stigma [27]. By reducing stigmatizing beliefs in men, their own mental health may be improved, especially if this leads to greater engagement in available mental health resources.

16.3.2 Help-Seeking Behaviors

There are several important factors that inhibit help-seeking behaviors in men: treatment fears (i.e., social stigma), fear of emotional display or experiences, anticipated risks, and self-disclosure [30]. Treatment fears refer to hesitation to seek assistance due to negative expectations, which is in part stigma, regarding mental health services. Help-seeking behaviors may also be impeded if the person is afraid to discuss painful emotions. The risk of opening up to another person and being misunderstood can lead to avoidance of mental health services. Finally, many men may not feel initial comfort in disclosing personal information with a healthcare provider or mental health professional.

Men's reluctance to seek help leads to underreported suffering in men [24, 31, 32]. Men are also more likely to deny the presence of a mental illness and engage in traditional positive self-management practices (e.g., talking therapy). Indeed, men are more likely to self-medicate with drugs and alcohol and engage in excessive working and infidelity than to communicate their distress [25].

Health-promoting behaviors seem to be associated with femininity, whereas risk-taking behaviors are interconnected with masculinity [33]. Illness is associated with weakness and vulnerability, contradicting the stoicism associated with masculinity [33]. This stereotypical thinking is thought to contribute to health differences between men and women. Therefore, this perception of "weakness" may contribute to men's hesitancy toward seeking treatment. Identifying and overcoming these traditional masculine stereotypes may play an important role in enhancing help-seeking behaviors.

16.3.3 Coping/Self-Regulation

Understanding how men manage stressful situations increases understanding of how to improve their mental health. Coping refers to a person's fluctuating cognitive and behavioral attempts to manage an internal or external demand [34]. The primary stressors men report are often related to work/finances and relationships with friends and lovers [35]. Men often use emotional suppression (e.g., ignoring or pretending that the stressor is not there) and problem-focused coping methods when they encounter a stressor [35]. Problem-focused coping involves active attempts to deal with stress, whereas emotion-focused coping involves ruminative and emotional responses, and for men problem-focused coping has better mental health outcomes [36, 37]. Emotional suppression in men is related to negative mood, decreased interpersonal functioning, and higher levels of psychopathology [38–40]. Therefore, coping strategies, especially a reduction in the use of emotional suppression, can be an important area of development for men in psychotherapy.

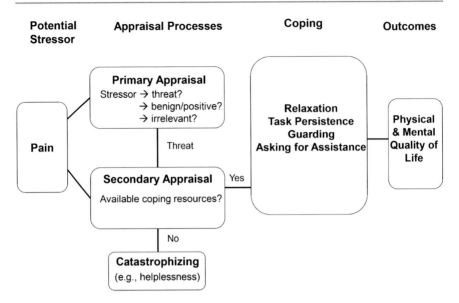

Fig. 16.1 Transactional model of stress applied to pain

Self-regulation theory describes an individual's ability to control or cope with their thoughts, feelings, and behaviors [41]. Self-regulation theory suggests that coping is influenced by appraisals of the stressor and expectancies for effective coping [42]. Lazarus and Folkman's transactional stress model suggests that the chosen coping strategy is a result of a series of appraisals (Fig. 16.1) [34]. For example, a chronic pain patient perceives their pain as a stressor. In their primary appraisal of the pain, they may interpret it as threatening, benign positive, or irrelevant [43]. If the pain is considered a threat, then the individual engages in secondary appraisal. At this stage, the individual contemplates their available coping resources in order to manage the situation. If the individual perceives that their coping resources are inadequate, negative appraisals can manifest such as feelings of helplessness.

16.4   Case in Point: Importance of Mental Health in Males with Urological Conditions

Mental health, including depression, has been a long-standing concern in urological health for decades. There are several urological conditions affecting men [e.g., benign prosthetic hypoplasia (BPH; enlargement of the prostate gland), prostate cancer, lower urinary tract symptoms (LUTS), erectile dysfunction (ED), interstitial cystitis (IC), chronic prostatitis/chronic pelvic pain syndrome (CP/CPPS)]. Urological disturbances can lead to pain and a reduced QoL, especially when the condition is unmanaged. Men with urological diseases experience elevated levels of anxiety and depression [44, 45]. For instance, the risk of suicide in men with prostate cancer is over four times greater than men without it [46], and men with LUTS experience higher levels of psychological distress including anxiety and depression [47]. Approximately 10 % of men with ED experience depression [19, 48]. Further, depression is significantly comorbid in CP/CPPS [49]. Therefore, psychological factors related to the distress experienced by men with urological conditions are an important area of research. Considering that urological conditions are common in aging men, it is important to examine the psychosocial impact these disorders can have.

Our research group has examined the implications of urological health for over 20 years. Recently, our research with men has focused on chronic prostatitis/chronic pelvic pain syndrome (CP/CPPS), a disease characterized by a painful, persistent, nonbacterial inflammation of the prostate. Symptoms include urinary urgency and frequency and chronic pelvic pain. Prevalence rates are surprisingly high for CP/CPPS symptoms, between 2 and 16 % in North America [50, 51]. Unfortunately, symptoms experienced by these men may not subside, with 66 % of patients in a community-based sample continuing to experience symptoms 1 year after diagnosis [52]. The etiology of CP/CPPS is poorly understood, stressing symptom management and mental health.

Research suggests that 80 % of patients with CP/CPPS report some form of depression [49] and that 5 % of these men report suicidal thinking. Pain and urinary symptoms are exacerbated with depression [53], which can contribute to a diminished QoL. Depression has been described as a psychosomatic factor in CP/CPPS symptoms [54] and depression, urinary scores, and pain are predictors of poorer physical QoL [55, 56].

We know that how a patient copes with their symptoms can contribute to poorer QoL. There are two main behavioral coping strategies now considered in the urologic research: "wellness-focused" or active coping (WFC) and "illness-focused" or passive coping (IFC). WFC, such as relaxation and a person's persistence to stay on attempts to complete a chore or task, allows the individual to function despite pain [57]. IFC, which involves behaviors such as adopting a sedentary lifestyle (pain-contingent resting) and guarding (taking comforting physical positions when in pain), may lead the individual to surrender control to symptoms like pain. Indeed, pain-contingent resting is a predictor of poorer physical QoL in patients with CP/CPPS [56] and IFC has also been shown to be a mechanism that promotes higher pain and thus poorer mental and physical QoL in CP/CPPS [58]. Therefore, behavioral coping strategies play an important role in the management of CP/CPPS QoL and depression.

How CP/CPPS patients appraise symptoms is important to understand when considering disease management. Catastrophizing, a negative cognitive appraisal process for pain (see Sullivan, Bishop, and Pivik 1995 for the scale) [59], plays a critical role in mental QoL [58, 60]. Catastrophizing includes three components: rumination (inability to redirect thoughts away from the pain), magnification (expectancies for negative outcomes), and helplessness. Catastrophizing in men with CP/CPPS is associated with greater disability, depression, urinary symptoms, and pain [61]. More specifically, it has been shown that the helplessness component of catastrophizing predicts diminished mental QoL in men with CP/CPPS [56]. It is suggested that experiencing chronic symptoms (e.g., pain) alongside no effective standard medical therapy may generate a sense of helplessness in patients over time [62].

Social support plays an important role in patient management. Patients who report lower support also report diminished QoL, greater depression, disability, and pain severity [63]. There are three primary categories of social support from a significant other: (1) solicitous (e.g., "tries to get me to rest," "does some of my chores"), (2) distracting (e.g., "tries to get me involved in some activity"), and (3) negative or punishing (e.g., "gets angry with me"). In chronic pain conditions, these spousal responses to a partner's pain are associated with depression, disability, pain catastrophizing, and greater pain [64–67]. In men with CP/CPPS, highly solicitous responses to pain increase the negative impact of pain on disability [68]. Solicitous responses may encourage pain behaviors such as pain-contingent resting, as discussed earlier. In contrast, distracting responses to pain decrease the negative impact of pain on disability. Therefore, encouraging men to stay active in their lives and providing distraction techniques (e.g., puzzles, watching media programs, calling friends) may be an important component in preventing disability in CP/CPPS [62].

16.4.1 A Biopsychosocial Approach to Treating CP/CPPS?

The biomedical model is limited in scope, but a biopsychosocial model accounts for demographic, physical function, cognitive/ behavioral, and environmental patient domains. The biomedical CP/CPPS model has been criticized for its ineffectiveness in symptom management [69]. The integration of psychosocial interventions can contribute to better patient outcomes. For example, an eight-week psychosocial management program for CP/CPPS that was designed to teach patients to identify/

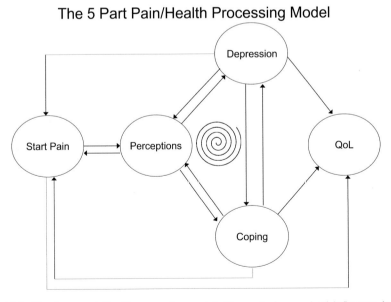

Fig. 16.2 The 5-part pain/health processing model. How pain is perceived influences how a patient copes. Perceptions of unmanageability can lead a patient to experience depressive symptoms. Depressive symptoms and poor coping strategies can exacerbate pain and decrease quality of life

dispute catastrophic thinking and to encourage health-focused behaviors has achieved reductions in patient pain, disability, and catastrophizing [70] (see Fig. 16.2). The authors suggest that by targeting both physical and psychosocial contributions to the patient experience, overall patient outcomes can be improved.

16.5 Psychological Support in Males

The data is clear; men suffering from CP/CPPS or male mental health in general are an underserviced group in need of psychological supports. Cognitive behavioral therapy (CBT) is a form of psychological treatment that focuses on the relationship between thoughts, feelings, and actions (e.g., Tripp et al. [70]). CBT practitioners often use an ABCDE model [71] to explain how positive self-regulation can go awry and be mended. As shown in Fig. 16.3, the event that creates upset or difficulty or triggers stress or worry for the patient is identified as an activating event (A). The patient may have rational (adaptive) or irrational (maladaptive) beliefs (B) regarding the cause or course of the activating event (e.g., "I created this pain," "It will never get any better," "My doctor cannot help me at all"). Positive beliefs about one's ability to manage or see hope in the future are likely to lead to more positive emotional, cognitive, and behavioral consequences, whereas negative beliefs, as suggested above, are likely to lead to anxiety, fear, and/or sadness (C). Operating with a therapist, patients work to identify irrational beliefs and then dispute them (D). Patients are encouraged to challenge their irrational beliefs by replacing negative/irrational thinking with a more adaptive evaluation of the situation (e.g.,

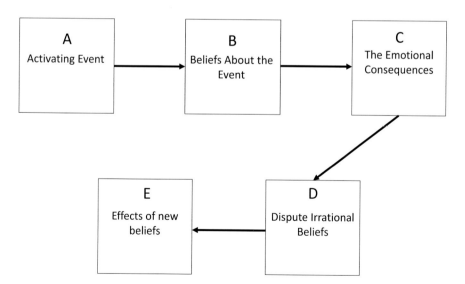

Fig. 16.3 ABCDE model of cognitive behavioral therapy [71]

consider alternate ways to cope versus sticking to one style that has not produced any improvements in the past—drinking alcohol, suppressing emotions, etc.). The last step is to employ the alternate beliefs or behaviors and to analyze the effects of such a change (E). With repeated attempts to work through this ABCDE cycle across a range of upsetting life events, patients in successful therapy will move toward having more self-enhancing responses (appraisals) to the situation and be more likely to cope in a manner that will promote more positive emotional, cognitive, and behavioral reactions.

Men are almost three times less likely to seek mental health services [72, 73], have negative attitudes toward therapy [74], and drop treatment prematurely compared to women [75]. Men's reluctance to be part of therapy can be manifest from their beliefs on how a "man" should feel and behave [74]. The commonly held belief for therapy in the popular media is that emotionally difficult self-disclosure is paramount to treatment. Unfortunately, many men would see this process in stark contrast to the traditional social norms they have been raised under. If emotional disclosure in therapy is suggested as an important component of patient success [76] and many men will rigidly view this as contrary or unacceptable with how they "see" their place in the world, we will need to adjust therapy or at least the male perception of therapy. This is ironic because CBT therapies are well suited to identify and dispute rigid/irrational thinking. For example, male gender role norms may manifest emotional suppression, superiority, and self-sufficiency, making many men more likely to respond to techniques that focus on beliefs and their behaviors, rather than on how they feel about an event. Indeed, in our therapy [70], men were provided with a focused behavioral approach to help manage stressful life events and told that the therapy was designed to help them "beat" pain and symptoms and "live" in spite of these factors. This sense of opposition and confrontation of their physical situation was well received, at least anecdotally. Clinicians focused on the treatment of men can also add subtle changes to connect with and accommodate men. For example, office space that has a traditional male-based theme, such as sports-themed art or memorabilia, or using male-friendly terms like "meetings" rather than "therapy sessions" may provide a more comfortable environment for men.

16.6   Conclusions

This chapter reports on data stressing that men's mental health is a warranted healthcare issue and an often-misinterpreted issue when it comes to quality of life. From mental health screening to treatment, male patient care maps must be considered and individualized as required. Depression is a salient aspect of male mental health and this chapter provides some insight into factors that may contribute (e.g., stigma, masculine gender norms, low help-seeking behaviors, and coping). A biopsychosocial model with concern for the gender-based norms of men is suggested as a preferred approach in understanding men's health. Such a tactic will allow the consideration of physical, psychological, and environmental factors as key to enhancing patient well-being. Improved psychological support is necessary and psychological interventions such as cognitive behavioral therapy can benefit men, especially if they are tailored to approach men from a gender-based norm perspective.

References

1. The World Health Organization. The world health report 2001 – Health: New Understanding, New Hope Geneva; 2001 [cited 2015]. Available from: http://www.who.int/whr/2001/media_centre/press_release/en/
2. Association CMH. Men and Mental Illness Ottawa, Canada; 2007 [cited 2015 Jan. 12, 2015]. Available from: http://www.cmha.ca/get-involved/find-your-cmha/
3. Substance Abuse and Mental Health Services Administration. Results from the 2010 National Survey on Drug Use and Health: Mental Health Findings Rockville, MD; 2012 [cited 2015]. Available from: http://archive.samhsa.gov/data/NSDUH/2k10MH_Findings/2k10MHResults.htm – High.
4. Seedat S, Scott KM, Angermeyer MC, Berglund P, Bromet EJ, Brugha TS, et al. Cross-national associations between gender and mental disorders in the World Health Organization World Mental Health Surveys. Arch Gen Psychiatry. 2009;66(7):786–95.
5. Hasin DS, Stinson FS, Ogburn E, Grant BF. Prevalence, correlates, disability, and comorbidity of DSM-IV alcohol abuse and dependence in the United States: results from the National Epidemiologic Survey on Alcohol and Related Conditions. Arch Gen Psychiatry. 2007;64(7): 830–42.
6. Kessler RC. Epidemiology of women and depression. J Affect Disord. 2003;74(1):5–13.
7. Oliffe JL, Phillips MJ. Men, depression and masculinities: a review and recommendations. J Mens Health. 2008;5(3):194–202.
8. Van de Velde S, Bracke P, Levecque K. Gender differences in depression in 23 European countries. Cross-national variation in the gender gap in depression. Soc Sci Med. 2010;71(2): 305–13.
9. Anderson JE, Michalak EE, Lam RW. Depression in primary care: tools for screening, diagnosis, and measuring response to treatment. B C Med J. 2002;44(8):415–9.
10. Goldberg DP, Hillier VF. A scaled version of the General Health Questionnaire. Psychol Med. 1979;9(1):139–45.
11. Kroenke K, Spitzer RL, Williams JBW. The PHQ-9: validity of a brief depression severity measure. J Gen Intern Med. 2001;16(9):606–13.
12. Kroenke K, Spitzer RL, Williams JBW. The Patient Health Questionnaire-2: validity of a two-item depression screener. Med Care. 2003;41(11):1284–92.
13. The World Health Organization. Depression Fact Sheet. 2012 [cited 2015]. Available from: http://www.who.int/mediacentre/factsheets/fs369/en/
14. Public Health Agency of Canada. What is depression? 2012 [cited 2015]. Available from: http://www.phac-aspc.gc.ca/cd-mc/mi-mm/depression-eng.php
15. Center for Disease Control. QuickStats: Prevalence of Current Depression* Among Persons Aged ≥12 Years, by Age Group and Sex – United States, National Health and Nutrition Examination Survey, 2007–2010; 2012 [cited 2015]. Available from: http://www.cdc.gov/mmwr/preview/mmwrhtml/mm6051a7.htm?s_cid=mm6051a7_w-x2013; %20United%20States,%20National%20Health%20and%20Nutrition%20Examination%20 Survey,%202007-2010</a>

16. Center for Disease Control. National Depression Screening Day; 2010 [cited 2015]. Available from: http://www.state.ky.us/agencies/behave/misc/DBWHandouts/BI12/CDC%20Ho%20on%20Depression%20-%20Diana%20Session%204%20Thurs%201pm.pdf
17. National Alliance on Mental Illness. Men and Depression Fact Sheet; 2009 [cited 2015]. Available from: http://www.nami.org/Content/NavigationMenu/Mental_Illnesses/Depression/Depression_and_Men_Fact_Sheet.htm
18. Diagnostic and statistical manual of mental disorders: DSM-5 (5th ed.). Arlington, VA: American Psychiatric Publishing; 2013.
19. Matthew A, Elterman D. Men's mental health: Connection to urologic health. Can Urol Assoc J. 2014;8(7–8 Suppl 5):S153–5.
20. Brownhill S, Wilhelm K, Barclay L, Schmied V. 'Big build': hidden depression in men. Aust N Z J Psychiatry. 2005;39(10):921–31.
21. Moscicki EK. Identification of suicide risk factors using epidemiologic studies. Psychiatr Clin N Am. 1997;20(3):499–517.
22. Bilsker D, White J. The silent epidemic of male suicide. B C Med J. 2011;53(10):529–34.
23. Luoma JB, Martin CE, Pearson JL. Contact with mental health and primary care providers before suicide: a review of the evidence. Am J Psychiatry. 2002;159(6):909–16.
24. Harding C, Fox C. It's not about "Freudian couches and personality changing drugs": An investigation Into men's mental health help-seeking enablers. Am J Mens Health. 2014:1–13.
25. Moller-Leimkuhler AM. Barriers to help-seeking by men: a review of sociocultural and clinical literature with particular reference to depression. J Affect Disord. 2002;71(1–3):1–9.
26. Cook TM, Wang J. Descriptive epidemiology of stigma against depression in a general population sample in Alberta. BMC Psychiatry. 2010;10:29.
27. Rusch N, Angermeyer MC, Corrigan PW. Mental illness stigma: concepts, consequences, and initiatives to reduce stigma. Eur Psychiatry. 2005;20(8):529–39.
28. Link BG, Phelan JC, Bresnahan M, Stueve A, Pescosolido BA. Public conceptions of mental illness: labels, causes, dangerousness, and social distance. Am J Public Health. 1999;89(9):1328–33.
29. Wang J, Lai D. The relationship between mental health literacy, personal contacts and personal stigma against depression. J Affect Disord. 2008;110(1-2):191–6.
30. Vogel DL, Wade NG, Wester SR, Larson L, Hackler AH. Seeking help from a mental health professional: the influence of one's social network. J Clin Psychol. 2007;63(3):233–45.
31. McKelley RA. Men's resistance to seeking help: Using individual psychology to understand counseling-reluctant men. J Individ Psychol. 2007;63(1):48.
32. Peate I. The mental health of men and boys: an overview. Br J Nurs. 2010;19(19):1231–5.
33. Evans J, Frank B, Oliffe JL, Gregory D. Health, illness, men and masculinities (HIMM): a theoretical framework for understanding men and their health. J Mens Health. 2011;8(1):7–15.
34. Lazarus RS, Folkman S. Stress, appraisal, and coping. New York: Springer; 1984.
35. Matud MP. Gender differences in stress and coping styles. Personal Individ Differ. 2004;37(7):1401–15.
36. Beasley M, Thompson T, Davidson J. Resilience in responses to life stress: the effects of coping style and cognitive hardiness. Personal Individ Differ. 2003;34(1):77–95.
37. Higgins JE, Endler NS. Coping, life stress, and psychological and somatic distress. Eur J Personal. 1995;9(4):253–70.
38. Dennis TA. Interactions between emotion regulation strategies and affective style: implications for trait anxiety versus depressed mood. Motiv Emot. 2007;31(3):200–7.
39. Gross JJ, John OP. Individual differences in two emotion regulation processes: implications for affect, relationships, and well-being. J Pers Soc Psychol. 2003;85(2):348–62.
40. Moore SA, Zoellner LA, Mollenholt N. Are expressive suppression and cognitive reappraisal associated with stress-related symptoms? Behav Res Ther. 2008;46(9):993–1000.
41. Carver CS, Scheier M. On the self-regulation of behaviour. New York: Cambridge University Press; 1998. 439 p.

42. Johnson JE. Self-regulation theory and coping with physical illness. Res Nurs Health. 1999;22(6):435–48.
43. Sullivan MJL, Rodgers WM, Kirsch I. Catastrophizing, depression and expectancies for pain and emotional distress. Pain. 2001;91(1-2):147–54.
44. Barczak P, Kane N, Andrews S, Congdon AM, Clay JC, Betts T. Patterns of psychiatric morbidity in a genito-urinary clinic: a validation of the Hospital Anxiety Depression scale (HAD). May 1988. Br J Psychiatry. 1988;152:698–700.
45. Seivewright H, Salkovskis P, Green J, Mullan N, Behr G, Carlin E, et al. Prevalence and service implications of health anxiety in genitourinary medicine clinics. Int J STD AIDS. 2004;15(8):519–22.
46. Llorente MD, Burke M, Gregory GR, Bosworth HB, Grambow SC, Homer RD, et al. Prostate cancer: a significant risk factor for late-life suicide. Am J Geriatr Psychiatry. 2005;13(3):195–201.
47. Pinto JDO, He H-G, Chan SWC, Toh PC, Esuvaranathan K, Wang W. Health-related quality of life and psychological well-being in patients with benign prostatic hyperplasia. J Clin Nurs. 2014;24(3–4):511–22.
48. Corretti G, Baldi I. The Relationship Between Anxiety Disorders and Sexual Dysfunction. Psychiatr Times. 2007;24:9.
49. Alexander RB, Trissel D. Chronic prostatitis: results of an Internet survey. Urology. 1996;48(4):568–74.
50. Nickel JC, Downey J, Hunter D, Clark J. Prevalence of prostatitis-like symptoms in a population based study using the National Institutes of Health chronic prostatitis symptom index. J Urol. 2001;165(3):842–5.
51. Nickel JC, Teichman JM, Gregoire M, Clark J, Downey J. Prevalence, diagnosis, characterization, and treatment of prostatitis, interstitial cystitis, and epididymitis in outpatient urological practice: the Canadian PIE Study. Urology. 2005;66(5):935–40.
52. Nickel JC, Downey JA, Nickel KR, Clark JM. Prostatitis-like symptoms: one year later. BJU Int. 2002;90(7):678–81.
53. Ku JH, Jeon YS, Kim ME, Lee NK, Park YH. Psychological problems in young men with chronic prostatitis-like symptoms. Scand J Urol Nephrol. 2002;36(4):296–301.
54. Ku JH, Kim SW, Paick JS. Quality of life and psychological factors in chronic prostatitis/chronic pelvic pain syndrome. Urology. 2005;66(4):693–701.
55. Tripp DA, Curtis Nickel J, Landis JR, Wang YL, Knauss JS, Group CS. Predictors of quality of life and pain in chronic prostatitis/chronic pelvic pain syndrome: findings from the National Institutes of Health Chronic Prostatitis Cohort Study. BJU Int. 2004;94(9):1279–82.
56. Nickel JC, Tripp DA, Chuai S, Litwin MS, McNaughton-Collins M, Landis JR, et al. Psychosocial variables affect the quality of life of men diagnosed with chronic prostatitis/chronic pelvic pain syndrome. BJU Int. 2008;101(1):59–64.
57. Brown GK, Nicassio PM. Development of a questionnaire for the assessment of active and passive coping strategies in chronic pain patients. Pain. 1987;31(1):53–64.
58. Krsmanovic A, Tripp DA, Nickel JC, Shoskes DA, Pontari M, Litwin MS, et al. Psychosocial mechanisms of the pain and quality of life relationship for chronic prostatitis/chronic pelvic pain syndrome (CP/CPPS). Can Urol Assoc J. 2014;8(11–12):403–8.
59. Sullivan MJL, Bishop SR, Pivik J. The pain catastrophizing scale: development and validation. Psychol Assess. 1995;7(4):524–32.
60. Sullivan MJL. The communal coping model of pain catastrophising: clinical and research implications. Can Psychol. 2012;53(1):32–41.
61. Tripp DA, Nickel JC, Wang Y, Litwin MS, McNaughton-Collins M, Landis JR, et al. Catastrophizing and pain-contingent rest predict patient adjustment in men with chronic prostatitis/chronic pelvic pain syndrome. J Pain. 2006;7(10):697–708.
62. Tripp DA, Nickel JC. The Psychology of Urological Chronic Pelvic Pain: A Primer for Urologists Who Want to Know How to Better Manage Chronic Prostatitis and Interstitial Cystitis. Am Urol Assoc. 2011;30:386–95.
63. Leonard MT, Cano A, Johansen AB. Chronic pain in a couples context: a review and integration of theoretical models and empirical evidence. J Pain. 2006;7(6):377–90.

64. Cano A, Gillis M, Heinz W, Geisser M, Foran H. Marital functioning, chronic pain, and psychological distress. Pain. 2004;107(1–2):99–106.
65. Cano A, Johansen AB, Franz A. Multilevel analysis of couple congruence on pain, interference, and disability. Pain. 2005;118(3):368–79.
66. Buenaver LF, Edwards RR, Haythornthwaite JA. Pain-related catastrophizing and perceived social responses: inter-relationships in the context of chronic pain. Pain. 2007;127(3): 234–42.
67. Cano A, Weisberg JN, Gallagher RM. Marital satisfaction and pain severity mediate the association between negative spouse responses to pain and depressive symptoms in a chronic pain patient sample. Pain Med. 2000;1(1):35–43.
68. Ginting JV, Tripp DA, Nickel JC. Self-reported spousal support modifies the negative impact of pain on disability in men with chronic prostatitis/chronic pelvic pain syndrome. Urology. 2011;78(5):1136–41.
69. Nickel JC, Downey J, Ardern D, Clark J, Nickel K. Failure of a monotherapy strategy for difficult chronic prostatitis/chronic pelvic pain syndrome. J Urol. 2004;172(2):551–4.
70. Tripp DA, Nickel JC, Katz L. A feasibility trial of a cognitive-behavioural symptom management program for chronic pelvic pain for men with refractory chronic prostatitis/chronic pelvic pain syndrome. Can Urol Assoc J. 2011;5(5):328–32.
71. Ellis A. Reason and emotion in psychotherapy. Oxford, England: Lyle Stuart; 1962. 442 pp.
72. Rhodes AE, Goering PN, To T, Williams JI. Gender and outpatient mental health service use. Soc Sci Med. 2002;54(1):1–10.
73. Smith LD, Peck PL, McGovern RJ. Factors contributing to the utilization of mental health services in a rural setting. Psychol Rep. 2004;95(2):435–42.
74. Addis ME, Mahalik JR. Men, masculinity, and the contexts of help seeking. Am Psychol. 2003;58(1):5–14.
75. Cottone JG, Drucker P, Javier RA. Gender differences in psychotherapy dyads: Changes in psychological symptoms and responsiveness to treatment during 3 months of therapy. Psychotherapy: Theory, Research, Practice, Training, 2002;39(4):297-308.
76. Kahn JH, Achter JA, Shambaugh EJ. Client distress disclosure, characteristics at intake, and outcome in brief counseling. J Couns Psychol. 2001;48(2):203–11.

Index

© Springer Science+Business Media New York 2016
J.M. Potts (ed.), *Men's Health,* DOI 10.1007/978-1-4939-3237-5

Printed in the United States
By Bookmasters